primer of biostatistics

SIXTH EDITION

primer of biostatistics

SIXTH EDITION

stanton a. glantz, PhD

Professor of Medicine
Director, Center for Tobacco Control Research and Education
Member, Cardiovascular Research Institute
Member, Institute for Health Policy Studies
Member, Cancer Center
University of California, San Francisco

McGRAW-HILL
Medical Publishing Division

New York Chicago San Francisco Lisbon London Madrid Mexico City
Milan New Delhi San Juan Seoul Singapore Sydney Toronto

The McGraw-Hill Companies

Primer of Biostatistics, Sixth Edition

1 2 3 4 5 6 7 8 9 0 DOC DOC 0 9 8 7 6 5

Set ISBN: 0-07-144781-4
Book ISBN: 0-07-143509-3
CD-ROM ISBN: 0-07-143822-X

Notice

Medicine is an ever-changing science. As new research and clinical experience broaden our knowledge, changes in treatment and drug therapy are required. The author and the publisher of this work have checked with sources believed to be reliable in their efforts to provide information that is complete and generally in accord with the standards accepted at the time of publication. However, in view of the possibility of human error or changes in medical sciences, neither the author nor the publisher nor any other party who has been involved in the preparation or publication of this work warrants that the information contained herein is in every respect accurate or complete, and they disclaim all responsibility for any errors or omissions or for the results obtained from use of the information contained in this work. Readers are encouraged to confirm the information contained herein with other sources. For example and in particular, readers are advised to check the product information sheet included in the package of each drug they plan to administer to be certain that the information contained in this work is accurate and that changes have not been made in the recommended dose or in the contraindications for administration. This recommendation is of particular importance in connection with new or infrequently used drugs.

This book was set in Times Roman by Progressive Information Technologies.
The editors were Jason Malley, Harriet Lebowitz, and Karen Davis.
The production supervisor was Richard Ruzycka.
The book cover was designed by Pehrsson Design.
The indexer was Frieda Glantz.
RR Donnelley was the printer and binder.

This book is printed on acid-free paper.

Library of Congress Cataloging-in-Publication Data

Glantz, Stanton A.
Primer of biostatistics / Stanton A. Glantz. —6th ed.
p. ; cm.
Includes bibliographical references and index.
ISBN 0-07-143509-3 (alk. paper)
1. Medical statistics. 2. Biometry.
[DNLM: 1. Biometry. WA 950 G545p 2005] I. Title.
RA409.G55 2005
610′.72′7—dc22

2005041630

To Marsha Kramar Glantz

Hunches and intuitive impressions are essential for getting the work started, but it is only through the quality of the numbers at the end that the truth can be told.*

Lewis Thomas
Memorial Sloan-Kettering Cancer Center

*L. Thomas, "Biostatistics in Medicine," *Science* **198:**675, 1977.

Contents

Location of Tables for Tests of Significance

Preface

I have always thought of myself as something of an outsider and troublemaker, so it is with some humility that I prepare the sixth edition of this book, 24 years after the first edition appeared. Then, as now, the book had an unusual perspective: that many papers in the medical literature contained avoidable errors. At the time, the publisher, McGraw-Hill, expressed concern that this "confrontational approach" would put off readers and hurt sales. They also worried that the book was not organized like a traditional statistics text.

Time has shown that the biomedical community was ready for such an approach, and the book has achieved remarkable success. Over time, it has evolved to include more topics, including power and sample size, more on multiple comparison procedures, relative risks and odds ratios, and survival analysis. Rather than adding more statistical tests in this edition, I have expanded the discussion of the qualitative issues in the use of statistics, such as what a random sample is, why it is important, the differences between experimental and observational studies, and bias and how to avoid it. I also completely rewrote the presentation of power in a continuing effort to make this daunting subject intuitive. This edition also continues the process of updating the examples and problems to use more contemporary material. At the same time, many of the original examples from the first edition remain;

they have worked well over time and nothing seemed to be gained in messing with success just to change things.

By far, the biggest change in this sixth edition is a complete redesign of the illustrations in the book to use color. I wanted to use color in this book from the beginning because I thought that color would make it easier to communicate the important intuitive ideas of populations, sampling, randomness, and sampling distributions that underlie applied biostatistics. The addition of color is more than cosmetic; it substantially improves the presentation of ideas in the book.

This book has its origins in 1973, when I was a postdoctoral fellow. Many friends and colleagues came to me for advice and explanations about biostatistics. Since most of them had less knowledge of statistics than I did, I tried to learn what I needed to help them. The need to develop quick and intuitive, yet correct, explanations of the various tests and procedures slowly evolved into a set of stock explanations and a 2-hour (color) slide show on common statistical errors in the biomedical literature and how to cope with them. The success of this slide show led many people to suggest that I expand it into an introductory book on biostatistics, which led to the first edition of *Primer of Biostatistics* in 1981.

As a result, this book is oriented as much to the individual reader—be he or she student, postdoctoral research fellow, professor, or practitioner—as to the student attending formal lectures.

This book can be used as a text at many levels. It has been the required text for the biostatistics portion of the epidemiology and biostatistics course required of medical students, covering the material in the first eight chapters in eight 1-hour lectures. The book has also been used for a more abbreviated set of lectures on biostatistics (covering the first three chapters) given to our dental students. In addition, it has served me (and others) well in a one quarter four unit course in which we cover the entire book in depth. This course meets for 4 lecture hours and has a 1-hour problem session. It is attended by a wide variety of students, from undergraduates through graduate students and postdoctoral fellows, as well as an occasional faculty member.

Since this book includes the technical material covered in any introductory statistics course, it is suitable as either the primary or supplementary text for a general undergraduate introductory statistics course (which is essentially the level at which this material is taught in medical schools), especially for a teacher seeking a way to make statistics relevant to students majoring in the life sciences.

This book differs from other introductory texts on biostatistics in several ways, and it is these differences which seem to account for the book's popularity.

First, it is based on the premise that much of what is published in the biomedical literature uses dubious statistical practices, so that a reader who takes what he reads at face value may often be absorbing erroneous information. Most of the errors (at least as they relate to statistical inference) center on misuse of the *t* test, probably because the people doing the research were unfamiliar with anything else. The *t* test is usually the first procedure presented in a statistics book that will yield the highly prized *P* value. Analysis of variance, if presented at all, is deferred to the end of the book to be ignored or rushed through at the end of the term. Since so much is published that should probably be analyzed with analysis of variance, and since analysis of variance is really the paradigm of all parametric statistical tests, I present it first, then discuss the *t* test as a special case.

Second, in keeping with the problems I see in the literature, there is a discussion of multiple comparison testing.

Third, the book is organized around hypothesis testing and estimation of the size of treatment effects, as opposed to the more traditional (and logical from a theory of statistics perspective) organization that goes from one-sample to two-sample to general *k*-sample estimation and hypotheses testing procedures. I believe my approach goes directly to the kinds of problems one most commonly encounters when reading about or doing biomedical research.

The examples are mostly based on interesting studies from the literature and are reasonably true to the original data. I have, however, taken some liberty in recreating the raw data to simplify the statistical problems (for example, making the sample sizes equal) so that I could focus on the important intuitive ideas behind the statistical procedures rather than getting involved in the algebra and arithmetic. When the text only discusses the case of equal sample sizes, the formulas for the more general unequal sample size case are included in an appendix.

It is worth mentioning a few items I have not added. Some people suggested that I add an explicit discussion of probability calculus and expected values, rather than the implicit discussion of them in the existing text. Others suggested that I make the distinction between *P* and α more precise. (I purposefully blurred this distinction.) I also was tempted to use the platform this book has created within the research community to popularize multivariate statistical methods—in particular multiple regression—within the biomedical community. These methods have been applied widely with good results in the social sciences and I have found them very useful in my work on cardiac function and tobacco control. I decided against making these changes, however, because they would have fundamentally changed the scope and tone of the book, which are the keys to its success.*

*These suggestions did, however, lead to a new book on the subject of multiple regression and analysis of variance, written with the same approach in *Primer of Biostatistics*. It is: *Primer of Applied Regression and Analysis of Variance* (2nd ed.), S. A. Glantz and B. K. Slinker, New York:McGraw-Hill, 2001.

As with all books, there are many people who deserve thanks. Julien Hoffman gave me the first really clear and practically oriented course in biostatistics that allowed me to stay one step ahead of the people who came to me for expert help. His continuing interest and discussion of statistical issues has helped me learn enough to even think of writing this book. Philip Wilkinson and Marion Nestle suggested some of the best examples in the original edition and many of them remain. They also offered very useful criticisms of the manuscript. Mary Giammona, Bryan Slinker, Jim Lightwood, Kristina Thayer, Joaquin Barnoya, and Jennifer Ibrahim helped develop problems. Virginia Ernster and Susan Sacks not only offered many helpful suggestions, but also unleashed their 300 first- and second-year medical students on the manuscript for the first edition when they graciously offered to use it as the required text for their course.

Since the first edition of this book in 1981, many things have changed. There is a much wider appreciation for the need to use appropriate statistical methods in biomedical research than there was in 1981. While the problem persists, many journals have recognized the problems caused by ignorance of statistical issues among many scientists and have explicitly included biostatistical considerations in the review process for manuscripts. Indeed, in a classic example of the fact that the individual who complains the loudest gets put in charge, I was honored to serve as an Associate Editor of the *Journal of the American College of Cardiology* for 10 years (1991–2001) with special responsibility for reviewing tentatively accepted manuscripts for statistical problems prior to publication. About half the papers still had some sort of problem (of varying severity), but we caught most of them *before* publication.

Finally, I thank the many others who have used the book, both as students and as teachers of biostatistics, who took the time to write me questions, comments, and suggestions on how to improve it. I have done my best to heed their advice in preparing this sixth edition.

Many of the pictures in this book are direct descendants of my original slides. In fact, as you read this book, you would do best to think of it as a slide show that has been set to print. Most people who attend my slide show leave more critical of what they read in the biomedical literature. After I gave it to the MD-PhD candidates at the University of California, San Francisco, I heard that the candidates gave every subsequent speaker a hard time about misuse of the standard error of the mean as a summary statistic and abuse of t tests. This book has had a similar effect on many others. Nothing could be more flattering or satisfying to me. I hope that this book will continue to make more people more critical and help improve the quality of the biomedical literature and, ultimately, the care of people.

Stanton A. Glantz

primer of biostatistics

SIXTH EDITION

Chapter 1

Biostatistics and Clinical Practice

In an ideal world, editors of medical journals would do such an excellent job of ensuring the quality and accuracy of the statistical methods of the papers they publish that readers with no personal interest in this aspect of the research work could simply take it for granted that anything published was correct. If past history is any guide, however, we will probably never reach that ideal. In the meantime, consumers of the medical literature—practicing physicians and nurses, biomedical researchers, and health planners—must be able to assess statistical methods on their own in order to judge the strength of the arguments for or against the specific diagnostic test or therapy under study.

While this necessity may seem daunting for non-statisticians, it is not. The great bulk of errors in the biomedical literature involve basic errors of design, such as failing to conduct proper randomization or include a control group, or misuse of the basic statistical methods that are discussed in this book, particularly misuse of the *t* test for multiple comparisons. Moreover, once armed with an understanding of basic statistical concepts and methods, both producers and consumers of biomedical research are better positioned to understand (and challenge) the statistical designs and methods that are used in most research reports.

"SCIENTIFIC" MEDICINE

Until the second quarter of the last century, medical treatment had little positive effect on when, or even whether, sick people recovered. With the discovery of ways to reverse the biochemical deficiencies that caused some diseases and the development of antibacterial drugs, it became possible to cure sick people. These early successes and the therapeutic optimism they engendered stimulated the medical research community to develop a host of more powerful agents to treat heart disease, cancer, neurologic disorders, and other ailments. These successes led society to continue increasing the amount of resources devoted to the delivery of medical services. In 2004, the United States spent $1.8 trillion (over 14 percent of the gross domestic product) on medical services. In addition, both the absolute amount of money and the fraction of the gross domestic product devoted to the medical sector have grown rapidly (Fig. 1–1). Today, many government and business leaders view this continuing explosion with concern. Tens of millions of Americans have simply been priced out of medical care, joining the swelling ranks of the uninsured, and containing (or shifting) the costs of medical care has taken center stage in more and more labor-management disputes. These costs also threaten to undermine longstanding popular government programs such as Medicare, which finances medical care for the elderly, and Medicaid, which finances care for poor people.

Once there were ample resources to enable physicians and other health care providers to try tests, procedures, and therapies with little or no restriction on their use. As a result, much of what is considered good medical practice developed without firm evidence demonstrating that these practices actually helped the patient. Even for effective therapies, there has been relatively little systematic evaluation of precisely which patients these therapies help.* In addition to wasting money,

*A. L. Cochrane, *Effectiveness and Efficiency: Random Reflections on Health Services,* Nuffield Provincial Hospitals Trust, London, 1972.

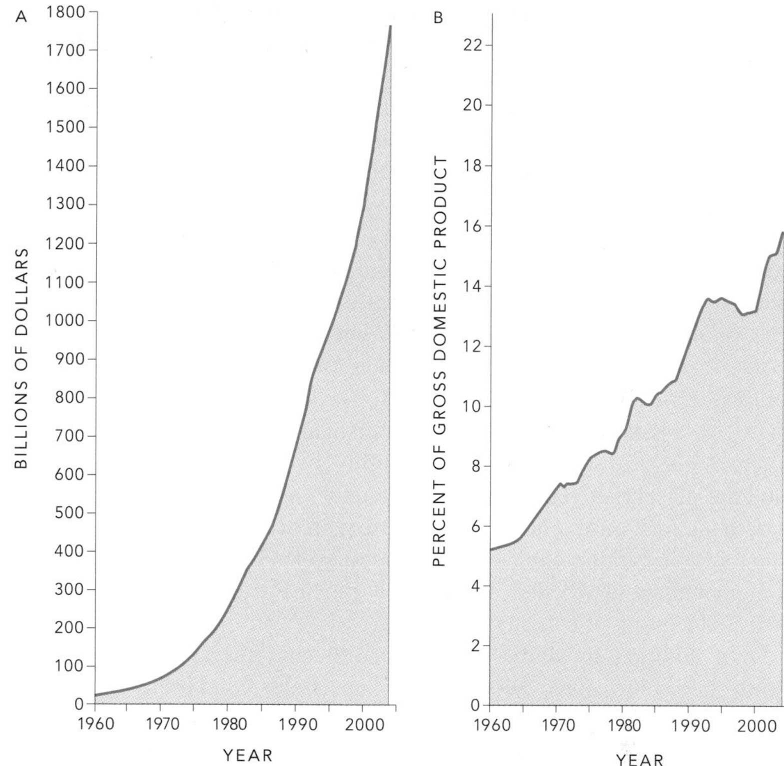

Figure 1–1 ***(A)*** Total annual expenditures for medical services in the United States between 1960 and 2004. ***(B)*** Expenditures for medical services as a percentage of the gross domestic product. (Source: *Statistical Abstract of the United States, 2003.* Washington DC: U.S. Department of Commerce, pp. 103.)

these practices regularly expose people to powerful drugs, surgery, or other interventions with potentially dangerous side effects in cases where such treatment does not do the patient any good.

What does this have to do with biostatistics?

In an effort to control costs and minimize unnecessary treatment, a consensus has been developed in support of *evidence-based medicine,* in which diagnostic tests and therapeutic interventions are limited to those modalities that have been shown to work. There is now substantial literature demonstrating that effective use of drugs and other therapies improve patient outcomes and reduce costs. In addition to assessing whether an intervention made a difference, it has become important to assess how great the difference is. The result has been a growth in formularies and other efforts to see that drugs and other therapies are used in accordance with the available evidence of efficacy. These ideals are often enforced through a system of prior approvals and clinical reviews, ideally to improve the quality of care and help contain costs. While reality often does not live up to this ideal, the simple fact is that this system is here to stay. Even if there is a major reorganization of the medical care system, such as replacing the dominant fee-for-service model with a single payer system or some form of national health insurance, the fundamental questions of clinical efficacy and resource allocation will remain.

These issues are, at their heart, statistical issues. Because of factors such as the natural biological variability between individual patients and the placebo effect,* one usually cannot conclude that some therapy was beneficial on the basis of simple experience. Biostatistics provides the tools for turning clinical and laboratory experience into quantitative statements about whether and by how much a treatment or procedure affected a group of patients.

In addition to studies of procedures and therapies, researchers study how physicians, nurses, and other health care professionals go about their work. For example, one study† demonstrated that patients with uncomplicated pyelonephritis, a common kidney infection, who were treated in accordance with the guidelines in the *Physicians' Desk Reference* remained in the hospital an average of 2 days less than those who were not treated appropriately. Since hospitalization costs constitute a sizable element of total medical care expenditures, it would seem desirable to minimize the length of stay when it does not affect the patient's recovery adversely.

*The placebo effect is a response attributable to therapy per se as opposed to the therapy's specific properties. For example, about one-third of people given placebos in place of pain killers experience relief. Examples of placebos are an injection of saline, sugar pill, and surgically opening and closing without performing any specific surgical procedure.

†D. E. Knapp, D. A. Knapp, M. K. Speedie, D. M. Yaeger, and C. L. Baker, "Relationship of Inappropriate Drug Prescribing to Increased Length of Hospital Stay," *Am. J. Hosp. Pharm.*, **36:**1334–1337, 1979. This study will be discussed in detail in Chaps. 3 to 5.

Hence, evidence collected and analyzed using biostatistical methods can potentially affect not only how clinicians choose to practice health professions but what choices are open to them. Intelligent participation in these decisions requires an understanding of biostatistical methods and models that will permit one to assess the quality of the evidence and the analysis of that evidence used to support one position or another.

Clinicians have not, by and large, participated in debates on these quantitative questions, probably because the issues appear too technical and seem to have little impact on their day-to-day activities. Clinicians need to be able to make more informed judgments about claims of medical efficacy so that they can participate more intelligently in the debate on how to allocate medical resources. These judgments will be based in large part on statistical reasoning.

WHAT DO STATISTICAL PROCEDURES TELL YOU?

Suppose researchers believe that administering some drug increases urine production in proportion to the dose and to study it they give different doses of the drug to five different people, plotting their urine production against the dose of drug. The resulting data, shown in Fig. 1–2*A*, reveal a strong relationship between the drug dose and daily urine production in the five people who were studied. This result would probably lead the investigators to publish a paper stating that the drug was an effective diuretic.

The only statement that can be made with absolute certainty is that as the drug dose increased, so did urine production *in the five people in the study.* The real question of interest, however, is: How is the drug likely to affect *all people who receive it?* The assertion that the drug is effective requires a leap of faith from the limited experience shown in Fig. 1–2*A* to all people. Of course, one cannot know in advance how all people will respond to the drug.

Now, pretend that we knew how every person who would ever receive the drug would respond. Figure 1–2*B* shows this information. There is no systematic relationship between the drug dose and urine production! The drug is not an effective diuretic.

How could we have been led so far astray? The shaded points in Fig. 1–2*B* represent the specific individuals who happened to be studied

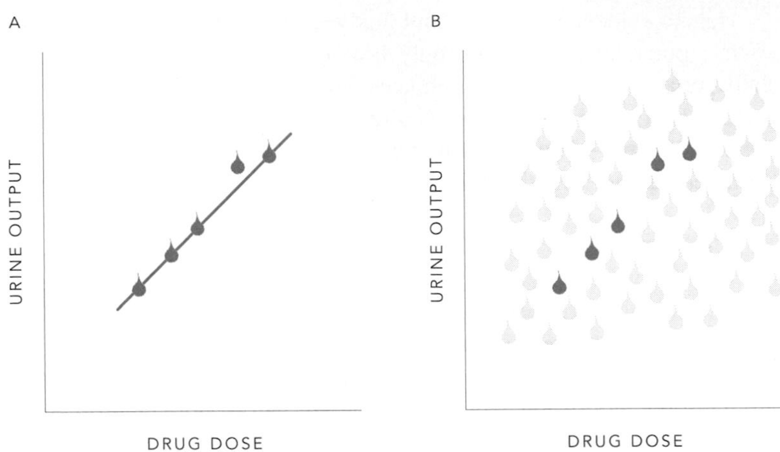

Figure 1–2 ***(A)*** Results of an experiment in which researchers administered five different doses of a drug to five different people and measured their daily urine production. Output increased as the dose of drug increased in these five people, suggesting that the drug is an effective diuretic in all people similar to those tested. ***(B)*** If the researchers had been able to administer the drug to all people and measure their daily urine output, it would have been clear that there is no relationship between the dose of drug and urine output. The five specific individuals who happened to be selected for the study in panel ***A*** are shown as shaded points. It is possible, but not likely, to obtain such an unrepresentative sample that leads one to believe that there is a relationship between the two variables when there is none. A set of statistical procedures called tests of hypotheses permits one to estimate the chance of getting such an unrepresentative sample.

to obtain the results shown in Fig. 1–2*A*. While they are all members of the population of people we are interested in studying, the five specific individuals we happened to study, taken as a group, were not really representative of how the entire population of people responds to the drug.

Looking at Fig. 1–2*B* should convince you that obtaining such an unrepresentative sample of people, though possible, is not very likely. One set of statistical procedures, called *tests of hypotheses,* permits you to estimate the likelihood of concluding that two things are related as Fig. 1–2*A* suggests when the relationship is really due to bad luck in selecting people for study and not a true effect of the drug investigated. In this example, we will be able to estimate that such a sample of people should turn up in a study of the drug only about 5 times in 1000 when the drug actually has no effect.

Of course it is important to realize that although biostatistics is a branch of mathematics, there can be honest differences of opinion about the best way to analyze a problem. This fact arises because all statistical methods are based on relatively simple mathematical models of reality, so the results of the statistical tests are accurate only to the extent that the reality and the mathematical model underlying the statistical test are in reasonable agreement.

WHY NOT DEPEND ON THE JOURNALS?

Aside from direct personal experience, most health care professionals rely on medical journals to keep them informed about the current concepts on how to diagnose and treat their patients. Since few members of the clinical or biomedical research community are conversant in the use and interpretation of biostatistics, most readers assume that when an article appears in a journal, the reviewers and editors have scrutinized every aspect of the manuscript, including the use of statistics. Unfortunately, this is often not so.

Beginning in the 1950s, several critical reviews* of the use of statistics in the general medical literature consistently found that about half the articles used incorrect statistical methods. This situation led many of the larger journals to incorporate formal statistical reviews (by a statistician) into the peer review process. More recent reviews of the use of statistical methods in the medical literature have concentrated on the efficacy of providing these secondary statistical reviews of tentatively accepted papers. These reviews have revealed that about half (or more) of the papers tentatively accepted for publication have statistical problems.† For the most part, these errors are resolved before

*O. B. Ross, Jr., "Use of Controls in Medical Research." *JAMA*, **145:**72–75, 1951; R. F. Badgley, "An Assessment of Research Methods Reported in 103 Scientific Articles from Two Canadian Medical Journals," *Can M.A.J.*, **85:**256–260, 1961; S. Schor and I. Karten, "Statistical Evaluation of Medical Journal Manuscripts," *JAMA*, **195:**1123–1128, 1966; S. Gore, I. G. Jones, and E. C. Rytter, "Misuses of Statistical Methods: Critical Assessment of Articles in B.M.J. from January to March, 1976," *Br. Med. J.* **1**(6053):85–87, 1977.

†For a discussion of the experiences of two journals, see M. J. Gardner and J. Bond, "An Exploratory Study of Statistical Assessment of Papers Published in the *British Medical Journal*," *JAMA* **263:**1355–1357, 1990 and S. A. Glantz, "It Is All in the Numbers," *J. Am. Coll. Cardiol.* **21:**835–837, 1993.

publication, together with substantive issues raised by the other (content) reviewers, and the rate of statistical problems in the final published papers is much lower.

By 1995, most (82 percent) of the large-circulation general medical journals had incorporated a formal statistical review into the peer review process. There was a 52 percent chance that a paper published in one of these journals would receive a statistical review before it was published.* This situation was not nearly as common among the smaller speciality and subspecialty journals. Only 31 percent of these journals had a statistical reviewer available and only 27 percent of published papers had been reviewed by a statistician. Indeed, reviews of specialty journals continue to show a high frequency of statistical problems in published papers.†

When confronted with this observation—or the confusion that arises when two seemingly comparable articles arrive at different

*S. N. Goodman, D. G. Altman, S. L. George, "Statistical Reviewing Policies of Medical Journals: Caveat Lector?" *J. Gen. Intern. Med.* **13:**753–756, 1998.

†More recent reviews, while dealing with a more limited selection of journals, have shown that this problem still persists. See S. J. White, "Statistical Errors in Papers in the *British Journal of Psychiatry*," *Br. J. Psychiatry,* **135:**336–342, 1979; M. J. Avram, C. A. Shanks, M. H. M. Dykes, A. K. Ronai, W. M. Stiers, "Statistical Methods in Anesthesia Articles: An Evaluation of Two American Journals during Two Six-Month Periods," *Anesth. Analg.* **64:**607–611, 1985; J. Davies, "A Critical Survey of Scientific Methods in Two Psychiatry Journals," *Aust. N.Z. J. Psych.,* **21:**367–373, 1987; D. F. Cruess, "Review of the Use of Statistics in *The American Journal of Tropical Medicine and Hygiene* for January–December 1988," *Am. J. Trop. Med. Hyg.,* **41:**619–626, 1990; C. A. Silagy, D. Jewell, D. Mant, "An Analysis of Randomized Controlled Trials Published in the US Family Medicine Literature, 1987–1991," *J. Fam. Pract.* **39:**236–242, 1994; M. H. Kanter and J. R. Taylor, "Accuracy of Statistical Methods in *Transfusion:* A Review of Articles from July/August 1992 through June 1993," *Transfusion* **34:**697–701, 1994; N. R. Powe, J. M. Tielsch, O. D. Schein, R. Luthra, E. P. Steinberg, "Rigor of Research Methods in Studies of the Effectiveness and Safety of Cataract Extraction with Intraocular Lens Implantation," *Arch. Ophthalmol.* **112:**228–238, 1994; A. M. W. Porter, "Misuse of Correlation and Regression in Three Medical Journals," *J. R. Soc. Med.* **92:**123–128, 1999; L. Rushton, "Reporting of Occupational and Environmental Research: Use and Misuse of Statistical and Epidemiological Methods," *Occup. Environ. Med.* **57:**1–9, 2000; J. B. Dimick, M. Diener-West, P. A. Lipsett, "Negative Results of Randomized Clinical Trials Published in the Surgical Literature," *Arch. Surg.* **136:**796–800, 2001; M. Dijkers, G. C. Kropp, R. M. Esper, G. Yavuzer, N. Cullen, Y. Bakdalieh, "Quality of Intervention Research Reporting in Medical Rehabilitation Journals," *Am. J. Physical Med. & Rehab.* **81:**21–33, 2002; G. E. Welch II, S.G. Gabbe, "Statistics Usage in the *American Journal of Obstetrics and Gynecology:* Has Anything Changed?" **186:**584–586, 2002; M. A. Maggard, J. B. O'Connell, J. H. Liu, D. A. Etzioni, C. Y. Ko, "Sample Size Calculations in Surgery: Are They Done Correctly" *Surgery.* **134:**275–279, 2003.

conclusions—people often conclude that statistical analyses are maneuverable to one's needs, or are meaningless, or are too difficult to understand.

Unfortunately, except when a statistical procedure merely confirms an obvious effect (or the paper includes the raw data), a reader cannot tell whether the data in fact support the author's conclusions or not. Ironically, the errors rarely involve sophisticated issues that provoke debate between professional statisticians but are simple mistakes, such as neglecting to include a control group, not allocating treatments to subjects at random, or misusing elementary tests of hypotheses. These errors generally bias the study on behalf of the treatments.

The existence of errors in experimental design and misuse of elementary statistical techniques in a substantial fraction of published papers is especially important in clinical studies. These errors may lead investigators to report a treatment or diagnostic test to be of statistically demonstrated value when, in fact, the available data fail to support this conclusion. Physicians who believe that a treatment has been proved effective on the basis of publication in a reputable journal may use it for their patients. Because all medical procedures involve some risk, discomfort, or cost, people treated on the basis of erroneous research reports gain no benefit and may be harmed. On the other hand, errors could produce unnecessary delay in the use of helpful treatments. Scientific studies which document the effectiveness of medical procedures will become even more important as efforts grow to control medical costs without sacrificing quality. Such studies must be designed and interpreted correctly.

In addition to indirect costs, there are significant direct costs associated with these errors: money is spent, animals may be sacrificed, and human subjects may be put at risk to collect data that are not interpreted correctly.

WHY HAS THE PROBLEM PERSISTED?

Because so many people are making these errors, there is little peer pressure on academic investigators to use statistical techniques carefully. In fact, one rarely hears a word of criticism. Quite the contrary, some investigators fear that their colleagues—and especially reviewers—will view a correct analysis as unnecessarily theoretical and complicated.

Most editors still assume that the reviewers will examine the statistical methodology in a paper with the same level of care that they examine the clinical protocol or experimental preparation. If this assumption were correct, one would expect all papers to describe, in detail as explicit as the description of the protocol or preparation, how the authors have analyzed their data. Yet, often the statistical procedures used to test hypotheses in medical journals are not even identified. It is hard to believe that the reviewers examined the methods of data analysis with the same diligence with which they evaluated the experiment used to collect the data.

In short, to read the medical literature intelligently, you will have to be able to understand and evaluate the use of the statistical methods used to analyze the experimental results as well as the laboratory methods used to collect the data. Fortunately, the basic ideas needed to be an intelligent reader—and, indeed, to be an intelligent investigator—are quite simple. The next chapter begins our discussion of these ideas and methods.

Chapter 2

How to Summarize Data

An investigator collecting data generally has two goals: to obtain descriptive information about the population from which the sample was drawn and to test hypotheses about that population. We focus here on the first goal: to summarize data collected on a single variable in a way that best describes the larger, unobserved population.

When the value of the variable associated with any given individual is more likely to fall near the mean (average) value for all individuals in the population under study than far from it and equally likely to be above the mean and below it, the *mean* and *standard deviation* for the sample observations describe the location and amount of variability among members of the population. When the value of the variable is more likely than not to fall below (or above) the mean, one should report the *median* and values of at least two other *percentiles.*

To understand these rules, assume that we observe *all* members of the population, not only a limited (ideally representative) sample as in an experiment.

For example, suppose we wish to study the height of Martians and to avoid any guesswork, we visit Mars and measure the entire population—all 200 of them. Figure 2–1 shows the resulting data with each Martian's height rounded to the nearest centimeter and represented by a circle. There is a *distribution* of heights of the Martian population. Most Martians are between about 35 and 45 cm tall, and only a few (10 out of 200) are 30 cm or shorter or 50 cm or taller.

Having successfully completed this project and demonstrated the methodology, we submit a proposal to measure the height of Venusians. Our record of good work assures funding, and we proceed to make the measurements. Following the same conservative approach, we measure the heights of *all* 150 Venusians. Figure 2–2 shows the measured heights for the entire population of Venus, using the same presentation as Fig. 2–1. As on Mars, there is a distribution of heights among members of the population, and all Venusians are around 15 cm tall, almost all of them being taller than 10 cm and shorter than 20 cm.

Comparing Figs. 2–1 and 2–2 demonstrates that Venusians are shorter than Martians and that the variability of heights within the Venusian population is smaller. Whereas almost all (194 of 200) the Martians' heights fell in a range 20 cm wide (30 to 50 cm), the analo-

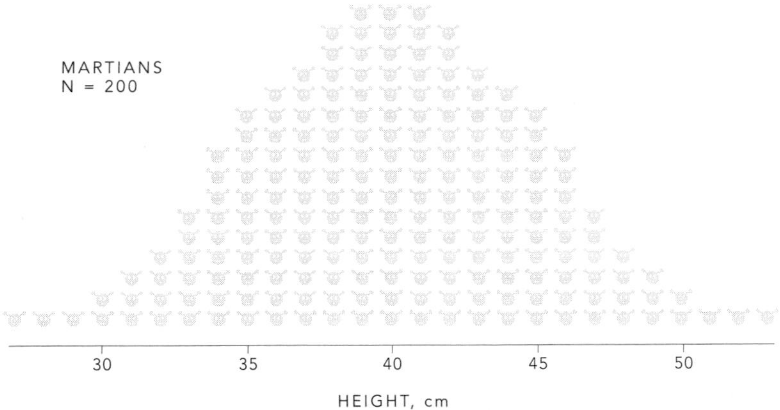

Figure 2–1 Distribution of heights of 200 Martians, with each Martian's height represented by a single point. Notice that any individual Martian is more likely to have a height near the mean height of the population (40 cm) than far from it and is equally likely to be shorter or taller than average.

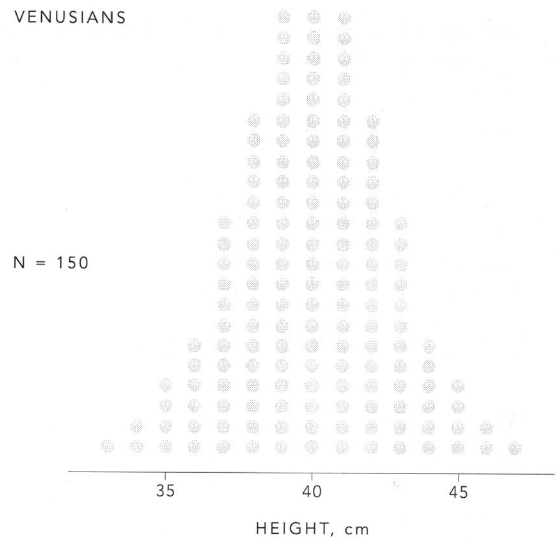

Figure 2–2 Distribution of heights of 150 Venusians. Notice that although the average height and dispersion of heights about the mean differ from those of Martians (Fig. 2–1), they both have a similar bell-shaped appearance.

gous range for Venusians (144 of 150) is only 10 cm (10 to 20 cm). Despite these differences, there are important similarities between these two populations. In both, any given member is more likely to be near the middle of the population than far from it and equally likely to be shorter or taller than average. In fact, despite the differences in population size, average height, and variability, the *shapes* of the distributions of heights of the inhabitants of both planets are almost identical. A most striking result!

We can now reduce all this information to a few numbers, called *parameters* of the distribution. Since the shapes of the two distributions are similar, we need only describe how they differ; we do this by computing the *mean* height and the *variability* of heights about the mean.

THE MEAN

To indicate the location along the height scale, define the *population mean* to be the average height of all members of the population.

Population means are often denoted by μ, the Greek letter mu. When the population is made up of discrete members,

$$\text{Population mean} = \frac{\text{sum of values, e.g., heights, for each member of population}}{\text{number of population members}}$$

The equivalent mathematical statement is

$$\mu = \frac{\Sigma X}{N}$$

in which Σ, Greek capital sigma, indicates the sum of the value of the variable X for all N members of the population. Applying this definition to the data in Figs. 2–1 and 2–2 yields the result that the mean height of Martians is 40 cm and the mean height of Venusians is 15 cm. These numbers summarize the qualitative conclusion that the distribution of heights of Martians is higher than the distribution of heights of Venusians.

MEASURES OF VARIABILITY

Next, we need a measure of dispersion about the mean. A value an equal distance above or below the mean should contribute the same amount to our index of variability, even though in one case the deviation from the mean is positive and in the other it is negative. Squaring a number makes it positive, so let us describe the variability of a population about the mean by computing the *average squared deviation from the mean.* The average squared deviation from the mean is larger when there is more variability among members of the population (compare the Martians and Venusians). It is called the *population variance* and is denoted by σ^2, the square of the lower case Greek sigma. Its precise definition for populations made up of discrete individuals is

$$\text{Population variance} = \frac{\text{sum of (value associated with member of population} - \text{population mean})^2}{\text{number of population members}}$$

The equivalent mathematical statement is

$$\sigma^2 = \frac{\Sigma(X - \mu)^2}{N}$$

Note that the units of variance are the square of the units of the variable of interest. In particular, the variance of Martian heights is 25 cm^2 and the variance of Venusian heights is 6.3 cm^2. These numbers summarize the qualitative conclusion that there is more variability in heights of Martians than in heights of Venusians.

Since variances are often hard to visualize, it is more common to present the square root of the variance, which we might call the *square root of the average squared deviation from the mean.* Since that is quite a mouthful, this quantity has been named the *standard deviation* σ. Therefore, by definition,

$$\text{Population standard deviation} = \sqrt{\text{population variance}} = \sqrt{\frac{\text{sum of (value associated with member of population} - \text{population mean})^2}{\text{number of population members}}}$$

or mathematically,

$$\sigma = \sqrt{\sigma^2} = \sqrt{\frac{\Sigma(X - \mu)^2}{N}}$$

where the symbols are defined as before. Note that the standard deviation has the same units as the original observations. For example, the standard deviation of Martian heights is 5 cm, and the standard deviation of Venusian heights is 2.5 cm.

THE NORMAL DISTRIBUTION

Table 2–1 summarizes what we found out about Martians and Venusians. The three numbers in the table tell a great deal: the population size, the

Table 2–1 Population Parameters for Heights of Martians and Venusians

	Size of population	Population mean, cm	Population standard deviation, cm
Martians	200	40	5.0
Venusians	150	15	2.5

mean height, and how much the heights vary about the mean. The distributions of heights on both planets have a similar shape, so that *roughly 68 percent of the heights fall within 1 standard deviation from the mean and roughly 95 percent within 2 standard deviations from the mean.* This pattern occurs so often that mathematicians have studied it and found that if the observed measurement is the sum of many independent small random factors, the resulting measurements will take on values that are distributed like the heights we observed on both Mars and Venus. This distribution is called the *normal (or gaussian) distribution.*

Its height at any given value of X is

$$\frac{1}{\sigma\sqrt{2\pi}}\exp\left[-\frac{1}{2}\left(\frac{X-\mu)}{\sigma}\right)^2\right]$$

Note that the distribution is completely defined by the population mean μ and population standard deviation σ. Therefore, the information given in Table 2–1 is not just a good abstract of the data, it is *all* the information one needs to describe the population fully *if the distribution of values follows a normal distribution.*

PERCENTILES

Armed with this theoretical breakthrough, we renew our grant by proposing not only to measure the heights of all Jupiter's inhabitants but also to compute the mean and standard deviation of the heights of all Jovians. The resulting data show the mean height to be 37.6 cm and the standard deviation of heights to be 4.5 cm. By comparison with Table 2–1, Jovians appear quite similar in height to Martians, since these two parameters completely specify a normal distribution.

The actual distribution of heights on Jupiter, however, tell a different story. Figure 2–3*A* shows that, unlike those living on the other two planets, a given Jovian is not equally likely to have a height above average as below average; the distribution of heights of all population members is no longer symmetric but *skewed.* The few individuals who are much taller than the rest increase the mean and standard deviation in a way that led us to think that most of the heights were higher than they actually are and that the variability of heights was greater than it actually is. Specifically, Fig. 2–3*B* shows a population of 100 individu-

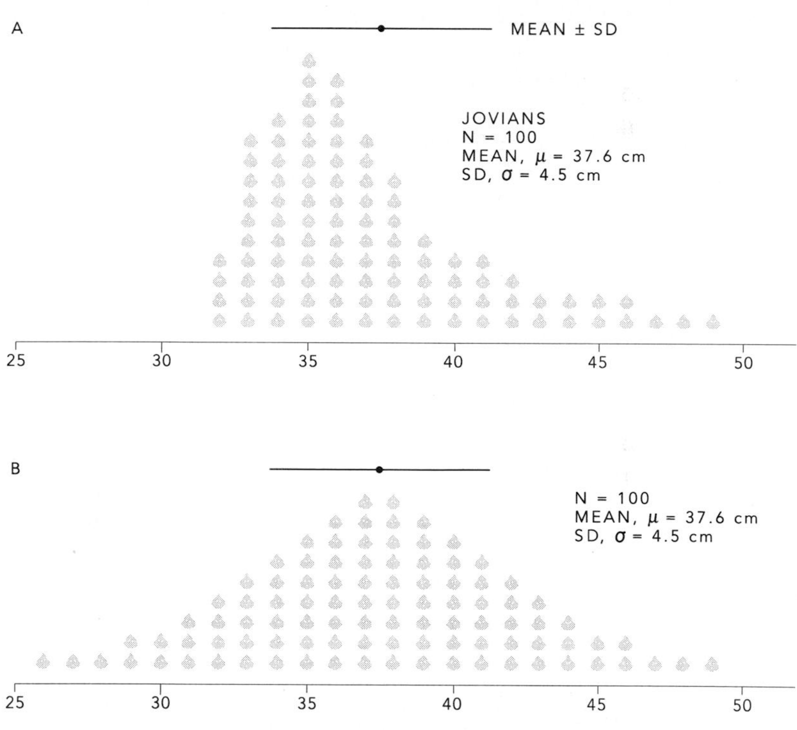

Figure 2–3 When the population values are not distributed symmetrically about the mean, reporting the mean and standard deviation can give the reader an inaccurate impression of the distribution of values in the population. Panel ***A*** shows the true distribution of the heights of the 100 Jovians (note that it is skewed toward taller heights). Panel ***B*** shows a normally distributed population with 100 members and the same mean and standard deviation as in panel ***A.*** Despite the fact that the means and standard deviations are the same, the distributions of heights in the two populations are quite different.

als whose heights are distributed according to a normal or gaussian distribution with the same mean and standard deviation as the 100 Jovians in Fig. 2–3*A*. It is quite different. So, although we can compute the mean and standard deviation of heights of Jupiter's—or, for that matter, any—population, these two numbers do not summarize the distribution of heights nearly so well as they did when the heights in the population followed a normal distribution.

An alternative approach that better describes such data is to report the *median.* The median is the value that half the members of the population fall below. Figure 2–4*A* shows that half the Jovians are shorter than 36 cm; 36 cm is the median. Since 50 percent of the population values fall below the median, it is also called the *50th percentile.*

Calculation of the *median* and other *percentiles* is simple. First, list the n observations in order. The median, the value that defines the lower half of the observations, is simply the $(n + 1)/2$ observation. When there are an odd number of observations, the median falls on one of the observations. For example, if there are 27 observations, the $(27 + 1)/2 = 14$th observation (listed from smallest to largest) is the median. When there is an even number of observations, the median falls between two observations. For example, if there are 40 observations, the median would be the $(40 + 1)/2 = 20.5$th observation. Since there is no 20.5th observation, we take the average of 20th and 21st observation.

Other percentile points are defined analogously. For example the 25th percentile point, the point that defines the lowest quarter of the observations, is just the $(n + 1)/4$ observation. Again, if the value falls between two observations, take the mean of the two surrounding observations. In general, the pth percentile point is the $(n + 1)/(100/p)$ observation.

To give some indication of the dispersion of heights in the population, report the value that separates the lowest (shortest) 25 percent of the population from the rest and the value that separates the shortest 75 percent of the population from the rest. These two points are called the *25th* and *75th percentile* points, respectively. For the Jovians, Fig. 2–4*B* shows that these percentiles are 34 and 40 cm. While these three numbers (the 25, 50, and 75 percentile points, 34, 36, and 40 cm) do not precisely describe the distribution of heights, they do indicate what the range of heights is and that there are a few very tall Jovians but not many very short ones.

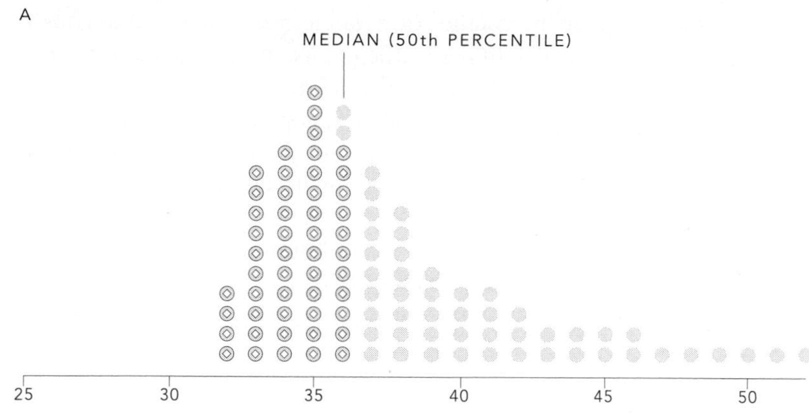

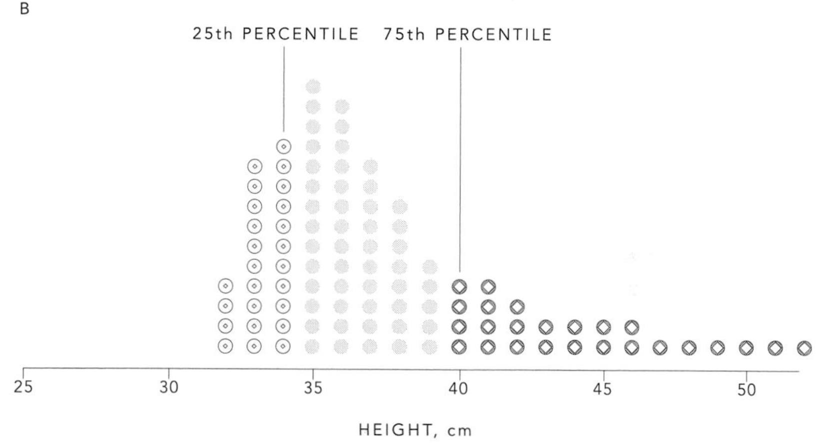

Figure 2–4 One way to describe a skewed distribution is with percentiles. The median is the point that divides the population in half. Panel ***A*** shows that 36 cm is the median height on Jupiter. Panel ***B*** shows the 25th and 75th percentiles, the points locating the lowest and highest quarter of the heights, respectively. The fact that the 25th percentile is closer to median than the 75th percentile indicates that the distribution is skewed toward higher values.

Although these percentiles are often used, one could equally well report the 5th and 95th percentile points, or, for that matter, report the 5-, 25-, 50-, 75-, and 95-percentile points.

Computing the percentile points of a population is a good way to see how close to a normal distribution it is. Recall that we said that in a population that exhibits a normal distribution of values, about 95 percent of the population members fall within 2 standard deviations of the mean and about 68 percent fall within 1 standard deviation of the mean. Figure 2–5 shows that, for a normal distribution, the values of the associated percentile points are:

2.5th percentile	mean − 2 standard deviation
16th percentile	mean − 1 standard deviation
25th percentile	mean − 0.67 standard deviation
50th percentile (median)	mean
75th percentile	mean + 0.67 standard deviation
84th percentile	mean + 1 standard deviation
97.5th percentile	mean + 2 standard deviation

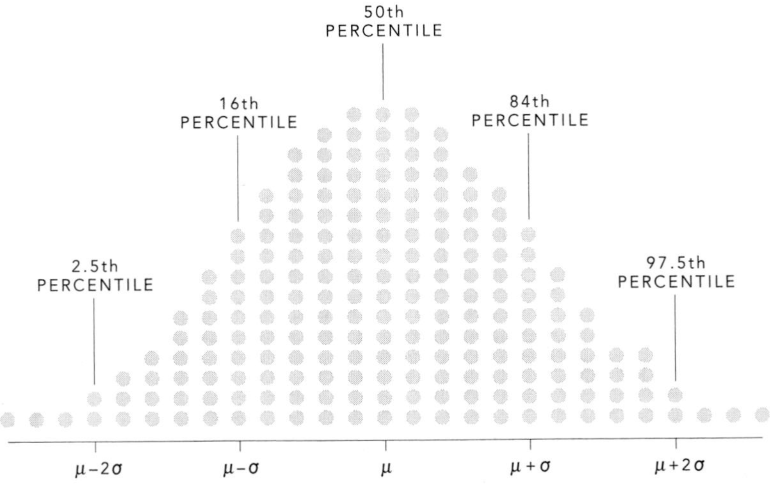

Figure 2–5 Percentile points of the normal distribution.

If the values associated with the percentiles are not too different from what one would expect on the basis of the mean and standard deviation, the normal distribution is a good approximation to the true population and then the mean and standard deviation describe the population adequately.

Why care whether or not the normal distribution is a good approximation? Because many of the statistical procedures used to test hypotheses—including the ones we will develop in Chaps. 3, 4, and 9—require that the population follow a normal distribution at least approximately for the tests to be reliable. (Chapters 10 and 11 present alternative tests that do not require this assumption.)

GETTING THE DATA

So far, everything we have done has been exact because we followed the conservative course of examining every single member of the population. Usually it is physically or fiscally impossible to do this, and we are limited to examining a *sample* of n individuals drawn from the population in the hope that it is representative of the complete population. Without knowledge of the entire population, we can no longer know the population mean μ and population standard deviation σ. Nevertheless, we can estimate them from the sample. To do so, however, the sample has to be "representative" of the population from which it is drawn.

Random Sampling

All statistical methods are built on the assumption that the individuals included in your sample represent a *random sample* from the underlying (and unobserved) population. In a random sample *every member of the population has an equal probability (chance) of being selected for the sample.* For the results of any of the methods developed in this book to be reliable, this assumption has to be met.

The most direct way to create a simple random sample would be to obtain a list of every member of the population of interest, number them from 1 to N (where N is the number of population members), then use a computerized *random number generator* to select the *n* individuals for the sample. Table 2–2 shows 100 random numbers between 1 and 150 created with a random number generator. Every number has the same chance of appearing and there is no relationship between adjacent numbers.

We could use this table to select a random sample of Venusians from the population shown in Fig. 2–2. To do this, we number the Venusians from 1 to 150, beginning with number 1 for the far left individual in Fig. 2–2, numbers 2 and 3 for the next two individuals in the second column in Fig. 2–2, numbers 4, 5, 6, and 7 for the individuals in the next column, until we reach the individual at the far right of the distribution, who is assigned the number 150. To obtain a simple random sample of 6 Venusians from this population, we take the first six numbers in the table—2, 101, 49, 54, 30, and 137—and select the corresponding individuals. Figure 2–6 shows the result of this process.

Table 2–2 One Hundred Random Numbers Between 1 and 150

2	135	4	138	57
101	26	116	131	77
49	99	146	137	129
54	83	4	121	129
30	102	7	128	15
137	85	71	114	7
40	67	109	34	123
6	23	120	6	72
112	7	131	58	38
74	30	126	47	79
108	82	96	57	123
55	32	16	114	41
7	81	81	37	21
4	52	131	62	7
7	38	55	102	5
37	61	142	42	8
116	5	41	111	109
76	83	51	37	40
100	82	49	11	93
83	146	42	50	35

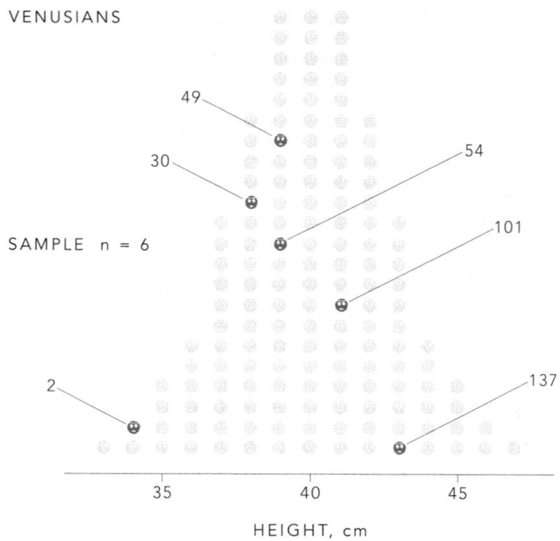

Figure 2–6 To select $n = 6$ Venusians at random, we number the entire population of $N = 150$ Venusians from 1 to 150, beginning with the first individual on the far left of the population as number 1. We then select six random numbers from Table 2–2 and select the corresponding individuals for the sample to be observed.

(When a number repeats, as with the two 7's in the first column of Table 2–2, simply skip the repeats because the corresponding individual has already been selected.)

We could create a second random sample by simply continuing in the table beginning with the seventh entry, 40, or starting in another column. The important point is not to reuse any sequence of random numbers already used to select a sample. (As a practical matter, one would probably use a computerized random number generator, which automatically makes each sequence of random numbers independent of the other sequences it generates.) In this way, we ensure that every member of the population is equally likely to be selected for observation in the sample.

The list of population members from which we drew the random sample is known as a *sampling frame.* Sometimes it is possible to obtain such a list (for example, a list of all people hospitalized in a given hospital on a given day), but often no such list exists. When there is no list, investigators use other techniques for creating a random sample, such as dialing telephone numbers at random for public opinion polling or selecting geographic locations at random from maps. The issue of how the sampling frame is constructed can be very important in terms of how well and to whom the results of a given study generalize to individuals beyond the specific individuals in the sample.*

The procedure we just discussed is known as a *simple random sample.* In more complex designs, particularly in large surveys or clinical trials, investigators sometimes use *stratified random samples* in which they first divide the population into different subgroups (perhaps based on gender, race, or geographic location), then construct simple random samples within each subgroup (strata). This procedure is used when there are widely varying numbers of people in the different subpopulations so that obtaining adequate sample sizes in the smaller subgroups would require collecting more data than necessary in the larger subpopulations if the sampling was done with a simple random sample. Stratification reduces data collection costs by reducing the total sample size necessary to obtain the desired precision in the results, but makes the data analysis more complicated. The basic need to create a random sample in which each member of each subpopulation (strata) has the same chance of being selected is the same as in a simple random sample.

Bias

The primary reason for random sampling—whether a simple random sample or a more complex stratified sample—is to avoid *bias* in selecting the individuals to be included in the sample. A bias is a systematic difference between the characteristics of the members of the sample and the population from which it is drawn.

Biases can be introduced purposefully or by accident. For example, suppose you are interested in describing the age distribution of the population. The easiest way to obtain a sample would be to simply select the people whose age is to be measured from the people in your biostatistics

*We will return to this issue in Chapter 12, with specific emphasis on doing clinical research on people being served at academic medical centers.

class. The problem with this *convenience sample* is that you will be leaving out everyone not old enough to be learning biostatistics or those who have outgrown the desire to do so. The results obtained from this convenience sample would probably underestimate both the mean age of people in the entire population as well as the amount of variation in the population. Biases can also be introduced by selectively placing people in one comparison group or another. For example, if one is conducting an experiment to compare a new drug with conventional therapy, it would be possible to bias the results by putting the sicker people in the conventional therapy group with the expectation that they would do worse than people who were not as sick and were receiving the new drug. Random sampling protects against both these kinds of biases.

Biases can also be introduced when there is a systematic error in the measuring device, such as when the zero on a bathroom scale is set too high or too low, so that all measurements are above or below the real weight.*

Another source of bias can come from the people making or reporting the measurements if they have hopes or beliefs that the treatment being tested is or is not superior to the control group or conventional therapy being studied. It is common, particularly in clinical research, for there to be some room for judgment in making and reporting measurements. If the investigator wants the study to come out one way or another, there is always the possibility for reading the measurements systematically low in one group and systematically high in the other.

The best way to avoid this measurement bias is to have the person making the measurements *blinded* to which treatment led to the data being measured. For example, suppose that one is doing a comparison of the efficacy of two different stents (small tubes inserted into arteries) to keep coronary arteries (arteries in the heart) open. To blind the measurements, the person reading the data on artery size would not know whether the data came from a person in the control group (who did not receive a stent) or which of the different stents was used in a given person.

Another kind of bias is due to the *placebo effect,* the tendency of people to report a change in condition simply because they received

*For purposes of this text, we assume that the measurements themselves are unbiased. Random errors associated with the measurement process are absorbed into the other random elements associated with the sampling process.

a treatment, even if the treatment had no biologic effect. For example, about one-third of people given an inert injection that they thought was an anesthetic reported a lessening of dental pain. To control for this effect in clinical experiments, it is common to give one group a placebo so that they think that they are receiving a treatment. Examples of placebos include an injection of saline, a sugar pill, or surgically opening and closing without performing any specific procedure on the target organ. Leaving out a placebo control can seriously bias the results of an experiment in favor of the treatment.* Ideally, the experimental subject would not know if they were receiving a placebo or an active treatment. When the subject does not know whether they received a placebo or not, the subject is *blinded.*

When neither the investigator nor the subject knows who received which treatment, the study is *double blinded.* For example, in double-blind drug studies, people are assigned treatments at random and neither the subject nor the person delivering the drug and measuring the outcome know whether the subject received an active drug or a placebo. The drugs are delivered with only a number code identifying them. The code is broken only after all the data have been collected.

Experiments and Observational Studies

There are two ways to obtain data: *experiments* and *observational studies.* Experiments permit drawing stronger conclusions than observational studies, but often it is only possible to do observational studies.

In an *experiment,* the investigator selects individuals from the population of interest (using an appropriate sampling frame), then assigns the selected individuals to different *treatment groups,* applies the treatments, and measures the variables of interest. Drug trials where people are randomly assigned to receive conventional therapy or a drug that is thought to improve their condition are common biomedical experiments. Since the only systematic difference between the different treatment groups is the treatment itself, one can be reasonably confident that the treatment *caused* the observed differences.

*We will discuss the placebo effect in detail in Chapter 12.

Selecting people and randomly assigning them to different experimental conditions is not always possible or ethical. In an *observational study,* the investigator selects individuals from the population of interest, measures the variables of interest, then assigns individuals in the sample to different groups based on some other characteristics of interest. For example, epidemiologists have compared the rates of lung cancer and heart disease in nonsmokers whose spouses or coworkers smoke with the rates observed in nonsmokers living in smokefree environments. These studies have shown higher rates of lung cancer and heart disease in the people exposed to secondhand smoke, leading to the conclusion that secondhand smoke increases the risk of disease (Fig. 2–7*A*).

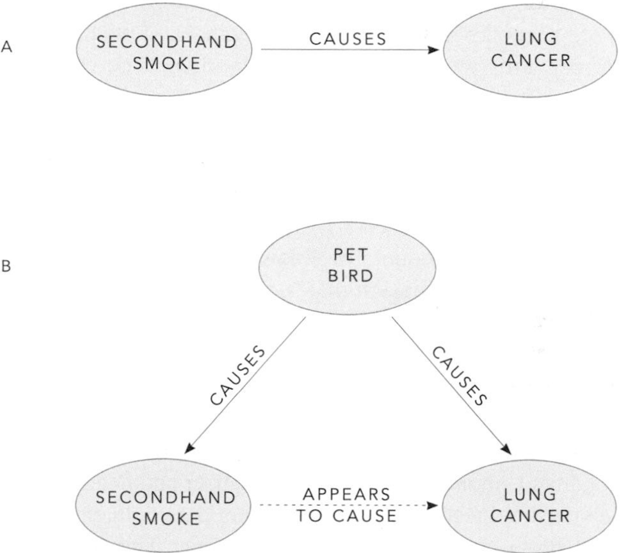

Figure 2–7 Panel ***A*** shows the situation that would exist if breathing secondhand smoke caused lung cancer. Panel ***B*** shows the situation that would exist if, as suggested by a tobacco industry consultant, people exposed to secondhand smoke were more likely to own pet birds and the birds carried diseases that caused lung cancer, while there was no connection between breathing secondhand smoke and lung cancer. Since owning a pet bird would be linked both to exposure to secondhand smoke and lung cancer this (unobserved) *confounding variable* could make it appear that secondhand smoke caused lung cancer when, in fact, there was no link.

When doing an observational study, however, one always has to worry that the association observed in the data is not due to a cause-and-effect link between the two variables (in this case, secondhand smoke causing lung cancer), but rather the presence of some unobserved *confounding variable* that was related causally to the other two variables and so makes it appear that the two observed variables were causally linked when they were not (Fig. 2–7*B*). For example, a tobacco industry consultant has claimed that nonsmokers married to smokers are more likely to own pet birds and that the birds spread diseases that increase the risk of lung cancer.*

The only way to completely exclude the possibility of confounding variables would be to conduct a randomized trial in which nonsmokers were randomly selected from the population, randomly allocated to marry other nonsmokers or smokers, then monitored for many years to see who developed heart disease or lung cancer. (Presumably the ownership of pet birds would be randomly distributed between the people assigned to marry nonsmokers and assigned to marry smokers.) Such an experiment could never be done.

It is, however, still possible to conclude that there are causal links between exposure to some agent (such as secondhand smoke) and an outcome (such as lung cancer) from observational studies. Doing so requires studies that account for known confounding variables either through an experimental design that separates people based on the effect of the confounding variable (by stratifying the confounding variable) or by controlling for their effects using more advanced statistical procedures,† and considering other related experimental evidence that helps explain the biologic mechanisms that cause the disease. These considerations have led reputable scientists and health authorities to conclude that secondhand smoke causes both lung cancer and heart disease.

The statistical techniques for analyzing data collected from experiments and observational studies are the same. The differences lie in how you interpret the results, particularly how confident you can be in using the word "cause."

*A. Gardiner and P. Lee, "Pet birds and lung cancer," *BMJ.* **306(6869):**60, 1993.

†For a discussion of the statistical approaches to control for confounding variables, see S. A. Glantz and B. K. Slinker, *Primer of Applied Regression and Analysis of Variance,* 2nd ed., New York: McGraw Hill, 2001, Chapter 12: Regression with a Qualitative Dependent Variable.

Randomized Clinical Trials

One procedure, called a *randomized clinical trial,* is the method of choice for evaluating therapies because it avoids the selection biases that can creep into observational studies. The randomized clinical trial is an example of what statisticians call an *experimental study* because the investigator actively manipulates the treatment under study, making it possible to draw much stronger conclusions than are possible from observational studies about whether or not a treatment produced an effect. Experimental studies are the rule in the physical sciences and animal studies in the life sciences but are less common in studies involving human subjects.

Randomization reduces biases that can appear in observational studies and, since all clinical trials are *prospective,* no one knows how things will turn out at the beginning. This fact also reduces the opportunity for bias. Perhaps for these reasons, randomized clinical trials often show therapies to be of little or no value, even when observational studies have suggested that they were efficacious.*

Why, then, are not all therapies subjected to randomized clinical trials? Once something has become part of generally accepted medical practice—even if it did so without any objective demonstration of its value—it is extremely difficult to convince patients and their physicians to participate in a study that requires withholding it from some of the patients. Second, randomized clinical trials are always prospective; a person recruited into the study must be monitored for some time, often many years. People move, lose interest, or die for reasons unrelated to the study. Simply keeping track of people in a randomized clinical trial is often a major task.

To collect enough patients to have a meaningful sample, it is often necessary to have many groups at different institutions participating. While it is great fun for the people running the study, it is often just one more task for the people at the collaborating institutions. All these factors often combine to make randomized clinical trials expensive and difficult to execute. Nevertheless, when done, they provide the most definitive answers to questions regarding the relative efficacy of different treatments.

*For a readable and classic discussion of the place of randomized clinical trials in providing useful clinical knowledge, together with a sobering discussion of how little of commonly accepted medical practice has ever been actually shown to do any good, see A. K. Cochran, *Effectiveness and Efficiency: Random Reflections on Health Services,* Nuffield Provincial Hospitals Trust, London, 1972.

HOW TO ESTIMATE THE MEAN AND STANDARD DEVIATION FROM A SAMPLE

Having obtained a random sample from a population of interest, we are ready to use information from that sample to estimate the characteristics of the underlying population. The estimate of the population mean is called the *sample mean* and is defined analogously to the population mean:

$$\text{Sample mean} = \frac{\text{sum of values, e.g., heights, of each observation in sample}}{\text{number of observations in sample}}$$

The equivalent mathematical statement is

$$\overline{X} = \frac{\Sigma X}{n}$$

in which the bar over the X denotes that it is the mean of the n observations of X.

The estimate of the population standard deviation is called the *sample standard deviation s* and is defined by

$$\text{Sample standard deviation} = \sqrt{\frac{\text{sum of (value of observation in the sample} - \text{sample mean)}^2}{\text{number of observations in sample} - 1}}$$

or, mathematically,*

$$s = \sqrt{\frac{\Sigma(X - \overline{X})^2}{n - 1}}$$

(The standard deviation is also often denoted SD.) The definition of the sample standard deviation, s, differs from the definition of the

*All equations in the text will be presented in the form most conducive to understanding statistical concepts. Often there is another, mathematically equivalent, form of the equation which is more suitable for computation. These forms are tabulated in Appendix A.

population standard deviation σ in two ways: (1) the population mean μ has been replaced by our estimate of it, the sample mean $\overline{X}$, and (2) we compute the "average" squared deviation of a sample by dividing by $n - 1$ rather than n. The precise reason for dividing by $n - 1$ rather than n requires substantial mathematical arguments, but we can present the following intuitive justification: The sample will never show as much variability as the entire population and dividing by $n - 1$ instead of n compensates for the resultant tendency of the sample standard deviation to underestimate the population standard deviation.

In conclusion, if you are willing to assume that the sample was drawn from a normal distribution, summarize data with the sample mean and sample standard deviation, the best estimates of the population mean and population standard deviation, because these two parameters completely define the normal distribution. When there is evidence that the population under study does not follow a normal distribution, summarize data with the median and upper and lower percentiles.

HOW GOOD ARE THESE ESTIMATES?

The mean and standard deviation computed from a random sample are estimates of the mean and standard deviation of the entire population from which the sample was drawn. There is nothing special about the specific random sample used to compute these statistics, and different random samples will yield slightly different estimates of the true population mean and standard deviation. To quantitate how accurate these estimates are likely to be, we can compute their *standard errors.* It is possible to compute a standard error for any statistic, but here we shall focus on the *standard error of the mean.* This statistic quantifies the certainty with which the mean computed from a random sample estimates the true mean of the population from which the sample was drawn.

What is the standard error of the mean?

Figure 2–8*A* shows the same population of Martian heights we considered before. Since we have complete knowledge of every Martian's height, we will use this example to explore how accurately statistics computed from a random sample describe the entire population. Suppose that we draw a random sample of 10 Martians from the entire population of 200, then compute the sample mean and sample

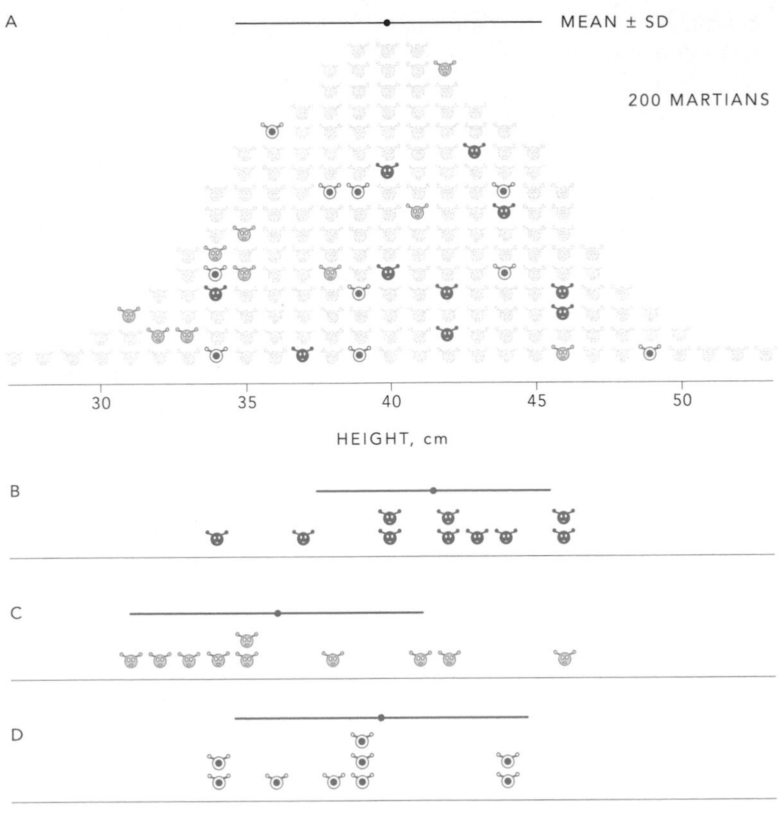

Figure 2–8 If one draws three different samples of 10 members each from a single population, one will obtain three different estimates of the mean and standard deviation.

standard deviation. The 10 Martians in the sample are indicated by solid points in Fig. 2–8*A*. Figure 2–8*B* shows the results of this random sample as it might be reported in a journal article, together with the sample mean ($\overline{X} = 41.5$ cm) and sample standard deviation ($s = 3.8$ cm). The values are close, but not equal, to the population mean ($\mu = 40$ cm) and standard deviation ($\sigma = 5$ cm).

There is nothing special about this sample—after all, it was drawn at random—so let us consider a second random sample of 10 Martians from the same population of 200. Figure 2–8*C* shows the results of this sample, with the corresponding Martians that comprise the sample identified in Fig. 2–8*A*. While the mean and standard deviation, 36 and 5 cm, of this second random sample are also similar to the mean and standard deviation of the whole population, they are not the same. Likewise, they are also similar, but not identical, to those from the first sample.

Figure 2–8*D* shows a third random sample of 10 Martians, identified in Fig. 2–8*A* with circles containing dots. This sample leads to estimates of 40 and 5 cm for the mean and standard deviation.

Now, we make an important change in emphasis. Instead of concentrating on the population of all 200 Martians, let us examine the *means of all possible random samples of 10 Martians.* We have already found three possible values for this mean, 41.5, 36, and 40 cm, and there are many more possibilities. Figure 2–9 shows these three means, using the same symbols as Fig. 2–8. To better understand the amount of variability in the means of samples of 10 Martians, let us draw another 22 random samples of 10 Martians each and compute the mean of each sample. These additional means are plotted in Fig. 2–9 as open points.

Now that we have drawn 25 random samples of 10 Martians each, have we exhausted the entire population of 200 Martians? No. There

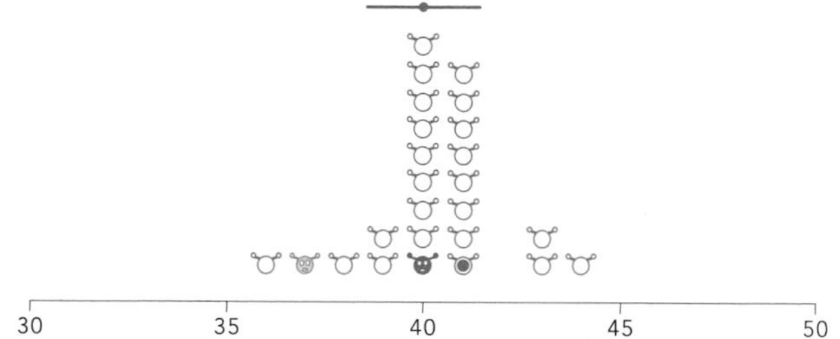

Figure 2–9 If one draws more and more samples—each with 10 members—from a single population, one eventually obtains the population of all possible sample means. This figure illustrates the means of 25 samples of 10 Martians each drawn from the population of 200 Martians shown in Figs. 2–1 and 2–8*A*. The means of the three specific samples shown in Fig. 2–8 are shown using corresponding symbols. This new population of all possible sample means will be normally distributed regardless of the nature of the original population; its mean will equal the mean of the original population; its standard deviation is called the standard error of the mean.

are more than 10^{16} different ways to select 10 Martians at random from the population of 200 Martians.

Look at Fig. 2–9. The collection of the means of 25 random samples, each of 10 Martians, has a roughly bell-shaped distribution, which is similar to the normal distribution. When the variable of interest is the sum of many other independent random variables, its distribution will tend to be normal, regardless of the distributions of the variables used to form the sum. Since the sample mean is just such a sum, its distribution will tend to be normal, with the approximation improving as the sample size increases. (If the sample were drawn from a normally distributed population, the distribution of the sample means would have a normal distribution regardless of the sample size.) Therefore, it makes sense to describe the data in Fig. 2–9 by computing their mean and standard deviation. Since the mean value of the 25 points in Fig. 2–9 is the mean of the means of 25 samples, we will denote it $\overline{X}_{\overline{X}}$. The standard deviation is the *standard deviation of the means* of 25 independent random samples of 10 Martians each, and so we will denote it $\sigma_{\overline{X}}$. Using the formulas for mean and standard deviation presented earlier, we compute $\overline{X}_{\overline{X}} = 40$ cm and $\sigma_{\overline{X}} = 1.6$ cm.

The mean of the sample means $\overline{X}_{\overline{X}}$ is (within measurement and rounding error) equal to the mean height μ of the entire population of 200 Martians from which we drew the random samples. This is quite a remarkable result, since $\overline{X}_{\overline{X}}$ is *not* the mean of a sample drawn directly from the original population of 200 Martians; $\overline{X}_{\overline{X}}$ is the mean of 25 random samples of size 10 drawn from the *population consisting of all 10^{16} possible values of the mean of random samples of size 10 drawn from the original population of 200 Martians.*

Is $\sigma_{\overline{X}}$ equal to the standard deviation σ of the population of 200 Martians? No. In fact, it is quite a bit smaller; the standard deviation of the collection of sample means $\sigma_{\overline{X}}$ is 1.6 cm while the standard deviation for the whole population is 5 cm. Just as the standard deviation of the original sample of 10 Martians s is an estimate of the variability of Martians' heights, $\sigma_{\overline{X}}$ is an estimate of the *variability of possible values of means of samples of 10 Martians.* Since when one computes the mean, extreme values tend to balance each other, there will be less variability in the values of the sample means than in the original population. $\sigma_{\overline{X}}$ is a measure of the precision with which a sample mean $\overline{X}$ estimates the population mean μ. We might name $\sigma_{\overline{X}}$ "standard deviation of means of random samples of size 10 drawn from the original population." To be brief, statisticians have coined a shorter name, the *standard error of the mean* (SEM).

Since the precision with which we can estimate the mean increases as the sample size increases, the standard error of the mean decreases as the sample size increases. Conversely, the more variability in the original population, the more variability will appear in possible mean values of samples; therefore, the standard error of the mean increases as the population standard deviation increases. The true standard error of the mean of samples of size n drawn from a population with standard deviation σ is*

$$\sigma_{\overline{X}} = \frac{\sigma}{\sqrt{n}}$$

The best estimate of $\sigma_{\overline{X}}$ from a single sample is

$$s_{\overline{X}} = \frac{s}{\sqrt{n}}$$

Since the possible values of the sample mean tend to follow a normal distribution, the true (and unobserved) mean of the original population will lie within 2 standard errors of the sample mean about 95 percent of the time.

As already noted, mathematicians have shown that the distribution of mean values will always approximately follow a normal distribution *regardless* of how the population from which the original samples were drawn is distributed. We have developed what statisticians call the *Central-Limit Theorem.* It says:

- *The distribution of sample means will be approximately normal regardless of the distribution of values in the original population from which the samples were drawn.*
- *The mean value of the collection of all possible sample means will equal the mean of the original population.*
- *The standard deviation of the collection of all possible means of samples of a given size, called the standard error of the mean, depends on both the standard deviation of the original population and the size of the sample.*

*This equation is derived in Chapter 4.

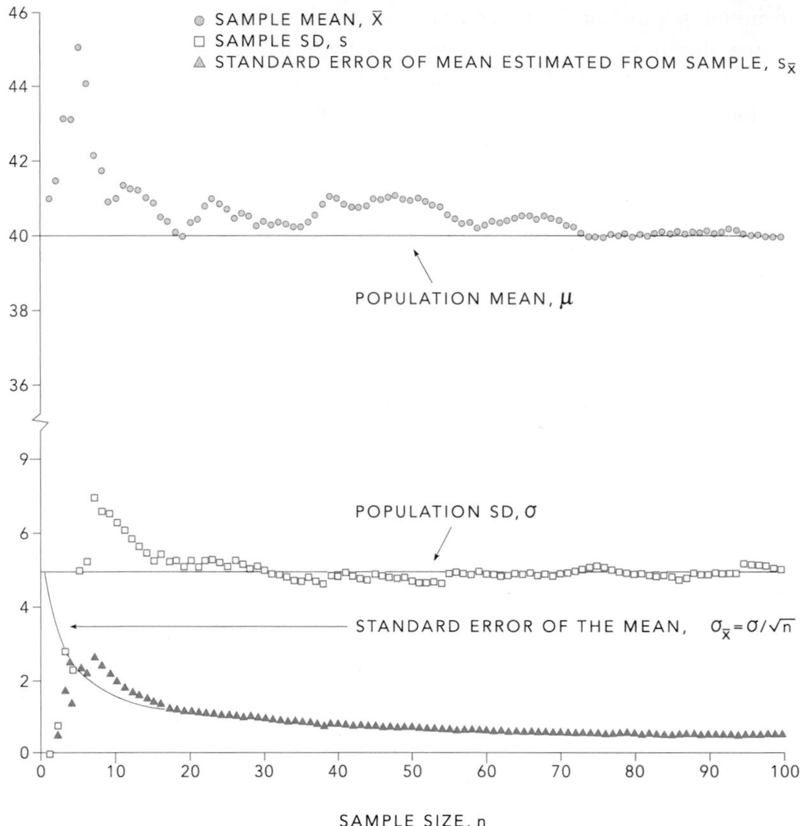

Figure 2–10 As the size of a random sample of Martians drawn from the population depicted in Fig. 2–1 grows, the precision with which the sample mean and sample standard deviation, $\overline{X}$ and *s*, estimate the true population mean and standard deviation, μ and σ, increases. This increasing precision appears in two ways: (1) the difference between the statistics computed from the sample (the points) moves closer to the true population values (the lines), and (2) the size of the standard error of the mean decreases.

Figure 2–10 illustrates the relationship between the sample mean, the sample standard deviation, and the standard error of the mean and how they vary with sample size as we measure more and more

Martians.* As we add more Martians to our sample, the sample mean $\overline{X}$ and standard deviation s estimate the population mean μ and standard deviation σ with increasing precision. This increase in the precision with which the sample mean estimates the population mean is reflected by the smaller standard error of the mean with larger sample sizes. Therefore, the standard error of the mean tells not about variability in the original population, as the standard deviation does, but about the certainty with which a sample mean estimates the true population mean.

The *standard deviation* and *standard error of the mean* measure two very different things and are often confused. Most medical investigators summarize their data with the standard error of the mean because it is always smaller than the standard deviation. It makes their data look better. However, unlike the standard deviation, which quantifies the *variability in the population,* the standard error of the mean quantifies *uncertainty in the estimate of the mean.* Since readers are generally interested in knowing about the population, data should generally not be summarized with the standard error of the mean.

To understand the difference between the standard deviation and standard error of the mean and why one ought to summarize data using the standard deviation, suppose that in a sample of 20 patients an investigator reports that the mean cardiac output was 5.0 L/min with a standard deviation of 1 L/min. Since about 95 percent of all population members fall within about 2 standard deviations of the mean, this report would tell you that, assuming that the population of interest followed a normal distribution, it would be unusual to observe a cardiac output below about 3 or above about 7 L/min. Thus, you have a quick summary of the population described in the paper and a range against which to compare specific patients you examine. Unfortunately, it is unlikely that these numbers would be reported, the investigator being more likely to say that the cardiac output was 5.0 ± 0.22 (SEM) L/min. If you confuse the standard error of the mean with the standard deviation, you would believe that the range of most of the population

*Figure 2–10 was obtained by selecting two Martians from Fig. 2–1 at random, then computing $\overline{X}$, s, and $\sigma_{\overline{X}}$. Then one more Martian was selected and the computations done again. Then, a fourth, a fifth, and so on, always adding to the sample already drawn. Had we selected different random samples or the same samples in a different order, Fig. 2–10 would have been different.

was narrow indeed—4.56 to 5.44 L/min. These values describe the range which, with about 95 percent confidence, contains the mean cardiac output of the entire population from which the sample of 20 patients was drawn. (Chapter 7 discusses these ideas in detail.) In practice, one generally wants to compare a specific patient's cardiac output not only with the population mean but with the spread in the population taken as a whole.

SUMMARY

When a population follows a normal distribution, we can describe its location and variability completely with two parameters, the mean and standard deviation. When the population does not follow a normal distribution at least roughly, it is more informative to describe it with the median and other percentiles. Since one can rarely observe all members of a population, we will estimate these parameters from a sample drawn at random from the population. The standard error quantifies the precision of these estimates. For example, the standard error of the mean quantifies the precision with which the sample mean estimates the population mean.

In addition to being useful for describing a population or sample, these numbers can be used to estimate how compatible measurements are with clinical or scientific assertions that an intervention affected some variable. We now turn our attention to this problem.

PROBLEMS

2-1 Viral load of HIV-1 is a known risk factor for heterosexual transmission of HIV; people with higher viral loads of HIV-1 are significantly more likely to transmit the virus to their uninfected partners. Thomas Quinn and associates ("Viral Load and Heterosexual Transmission of Human Immunodeficiency Virus Type 1." *N. Engl. J. Med.,* **342:**921–929, 2000) studied this question by measuring the amount of HIV-1 RNA detected in blood serum. The following data represent HIV-1 RNA levels in the group whose partners seroconverted, which means that an initially uninfected partner became HIV positive during the course of the study; 79725, 12862, 18022, 76712, 256440, 14013, 46083, 6808, 85781, 1251, 6081, 50397, 11020, 13633, 1064, 496433, 25308, 6616, 11210, 13900 RNA copies/mL. Find the mean, median, standard deviation, and 25th and 75th percentiles of these concentrations. Do these data seem to be drawn from a normally distributed population? Why or why not?

2-2 When data are not normally distributed, researchers can sometimes *transform* their data to obtain values that more closely approximate a normal distribution. One approach to this is to take the logarithm of the observations. The following numbers represent the same data described in Prob. 2-1 following log (base 10) transformation: 4.90, 4.11, 4.26, 4.88, 5.41, 4.15, 4.66, 3.83, 4.93, 3.10, 3.78, 4.70, 4.04, 4.13, 3.03, 5.70, 4.40, 3.82, 4.05, 4.14. Find the mean, median, standard deviation, and 25th and 75th percentiles of these concentrations. Do these data seem to be drawn from a normally distributed population? Why or why not?

2-3 Polychlorinated biphenyls (PCBs) are a class of environmental chemicals associated with a variety of adverse health effects, including intellectual impairment in children exposed *in utero* while their mothers were pregnant. PCBs are also one of the most abundant contaminants found in human fat. Tu Binh Minh and colleagues analyzed PCB concentrations in the fat of a group of Japanese adults ("Occurrence of Tris (4-chlorophenyl)methane, Tris(4-chlorophenyl)methanol, and "Some Other Persistent Organochlorines in Japanese Human Adipose Tissue," *Environ. Health Perspect.,* **108:**599–603, 2000). They detected 1800, 1800, 2600, 1300, 520, 3200, 1700, 2500, 560, 930, 2300, 2300, 1700, 720 ng/g lipid weight of PCBs in the people they studied. Find the mean, median standard deviation, and 25th and 75th percentiles of these concentrations. Do these data seem to be drawn from a normally distributed population? Why or why not?

2-4 Sketch the distribution of all possible values of the number on the upright face of a die. What is the mean of this population of possible values?

2-5 Roll a *pair* of dice and note the numbers on each of the upright faces. These two numbers can be considered a sample of size 2 drawn from the population described in Prob. 2-4. This sample can be averaged. What does this average estimate? Repeat this procedure 20 times and plot the averages observed after each roll. What is this distribution? Compute its mean and standard deviation. What do they represent?

Chapter 3

How to Test for Differences between Groups

Statistical methods are used to summarize data and test hypotheses with those data. Chapter 2 discussed how to use the mean, standard deviation, median, and percentiles to summarize data and how to use the standard error of the mean to estimate the precision with which a sample mean estimates the population mean. Now we turn our attention to how to use data to test scientific hypotheses. The statistical techniques used to perform such tests are called *tests of significance;* they yield the highly prized *P value.* We now develop procedures to test the hypothesis that, on the average, different treatments all affect some variable identically. Specifically, we will develop a procedure to test the hypothesis that diet has no effect on the mean cardiac output of people living in a small town. Statisticians call this hypothesis of no effect the *null hypothesis.*

The resulting test can be generalized to analyze data obtained in experiments involving any number of treatments. In addition, it is the archetype for a whole class of related procedures known as *analysis of variance.*

THE GENERAL APPROACH

To begin our experiment, we randomly select four groups of seven people each from a small town with 200 healthy adult inhabitants. All participants give informed consent. People in the control group continue eating normally; people in the second group eat only spaghetti; people in the third group eat only steak; and people in the fourth group eat only fruit and nuts. After 1 month, each person has a cardiac catheter inserted and his or her cardiac output is measured.

As with most tests of significance, we begin with the hypothesis that all treatments (diets) have the same effect (on cardiac output). Since the study includes a control group (as experiments generally should), this hypothesis is equivalent to the hypothesis that diet has no effect on cardiac output. Figure 3–1 shows the distribution of cardiac outputs for the entire population, with each individual's cardiac output represented by a circle. The specific individuals who were randomly selected for each diet are indicated by shaded circles, with different shading for different diets. Figure 3–1 shows that the null hypothesis is, in fact, true. Unfortunately, as investigators we cannot observe the

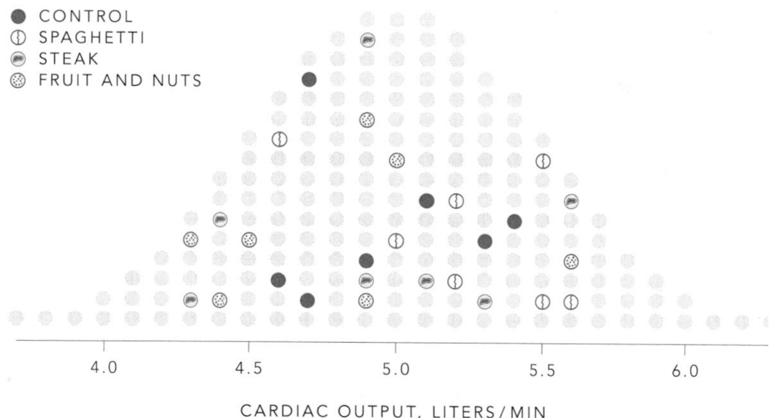

Figure 3–1 The values of cardiac output associated with all 200 members of the population of a small town. Since diet does not affect cardiac output, the four groups of seven people each selected at random to participate in our experiment (control, spaghetti, steak, fruit and nuts) simply represent four random samples drawn from a single population.

entire population and are left with the problem of deciding whether or not to reject the null hypothesis from the limited data shown in Fig. 3–2. There are obviously differences between the samples; the question is: *Are these differences due to the fact that the different groups of people ate differently or are these differences simply a reflection of the random variation in cardiac output between individuals?*

To use the data in Fig. 3–2 to address this question, we proceed under the assumption that the null hypothesis that diet has no effect on

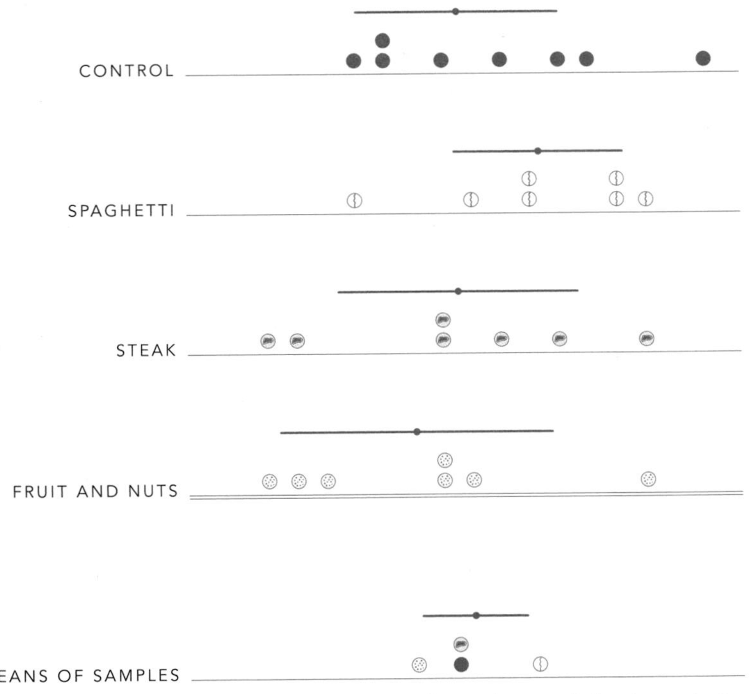

Figure 3–2 An investigator cannot observe the entire population but only the four samples selected at random for treatment. This figure shows the same four groups of individuals as in Fig. 3–1 with their means and standard deviations as they would appear to the investigator. The question facing the investigator is: Are the observed differences due to the different diets or simply random variation? The figure also shows the collection of sample means together with their standard deviation, which is an estimate of the standard error of the mean.

cardiac output is correct. Since we assume that it does not matter which diet any particular individual ate, we *assume* that the four experimental groups of seven people each are four random samples of size 7 *drawn from a single population* of 200 individuals. Since the samples are drawn at random from a population with some variance, we expect the samples to have different means and standard deviations, but *if our null hypothesis that the diet has no effect on cardiac output is true,* the observed differences are simply due to random sampling.

Forget about statistics for a moment. What is it about different samples that leads you to believe that they are representative samples drawn from different populations? Figures 3–2, 3–3, and 3–4 show three different possible sets of samples of some variable of interest. Simply looking at these pictures makes most people think that the four samples in Fig. 3–2 were all drawn from a single population, while the samples in Figs. 3–3 and 3–4 were not. Why? The variability within each sample, quantified with the standard deviation, is approximately the same. In Fig. 3–2, the variability in the mean values of the samples is consistent with the variability one observes within the individual samples. In contrast, in Figs. 3–3 and 3–4, the variability among sample means is much larger than one would expect from the variability within each sample. Notice that we reach this conclusion whether all (Fig. 3–3) or only one (Fig. 3–4) of the sample means appear to differ from the others.

Now let us formalize this analysis of variability to analyze our diet experiment. The standard deviation or its square, the variance, is a good measure of variability. We will use the variance to construct a procedure to test the hypothesis that diet does not affect cardiac output.

Chapter 2 showed that two population parameters—the mean and standard deviation (or, equivalently, the variance)—completely describe a normally distributed population. Therefore, we will use our raw data to compute these parameters and then base our analysis on their values rather than on the raw data directly. Since the procedures we will now develop are based on these parameters, they are called *parametric statistical methods.* Because these methods assume that the population from which the samples were drawn can be completely described by these parameters, they are valid only when the real population approximately follows the normal distribution. Other procedures, called

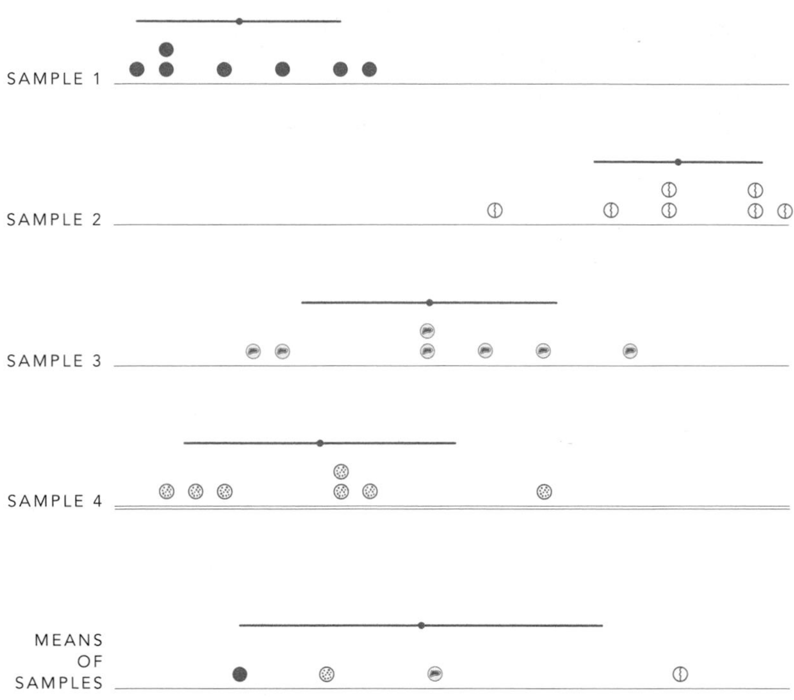

Figure 3–3 The four samples shown are identical to those in Fig. 3–2 except that the variability in the mean values has been increased substantially. The samples now appear to differ from each other because the variability between the sample means is larger than one would expect from the variability within each sample. Compare the relative variability in mean values with the variability within the sample groups with that seen in Fig. 3–2.

nonparametric statistical methods, are based on frequencies, ranks, or percentiles do not require this assumption.* Parametric methods generally provide more information about the treatment being studied and are more likely to detect a real treatment effect when the underlying population is normally distributed.

We will estimate the parameter population variance in two different ways: (1) The standard deviation or variance computed from each sample is an estimate of the standard deviation or variance of the entire population. Since each of these estimates of the population variance is computed

*We will study these procedures in Chaps. 5, 8, 10, and 11.

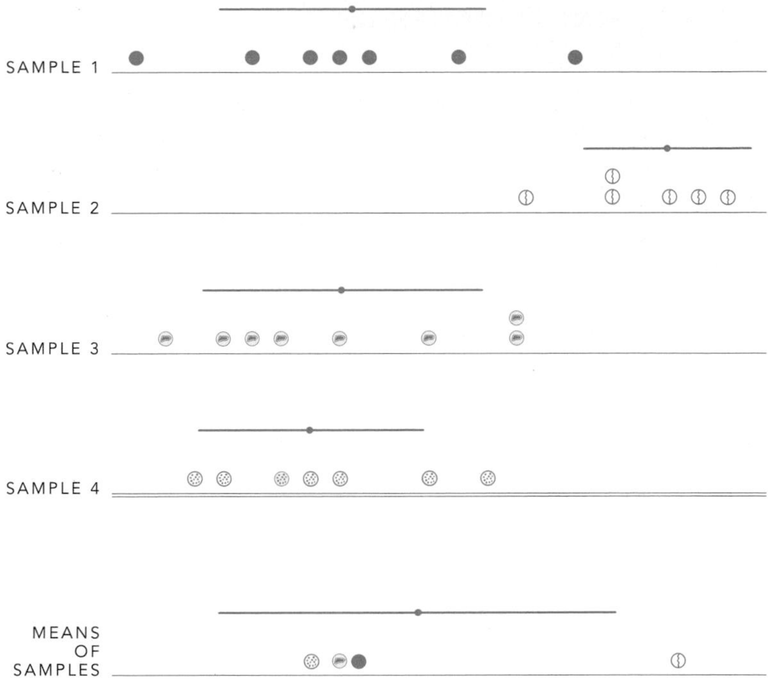

Figure 3–4 When the mean of even one of the samples (sample 2) differs substantially from the other samples, the variability computed from within the means is substantially larger than one would expect from examining the variability within the groups.

from within each sample group, the estimates will not be affected by any differences in the mean values of different groups. (2) We will use the values of the means of each sample to determine a second estimate of the population variance. In this case, the differences between the means will obviously affect the resulting estimate of the population variance. If all the samples were, in fact, drawn from the same population (i.e., the diet had no effect), these two different ways to estimate the population variance should yield approximately the same number. When they do, we will conclude that the samples were likely to have been drawn from a single population; otherwise, we will reject this hypothesis and conclude that at least one of the samples was drawn from a different population. In our experiment, rejecting the original hypothesis would lead to the conclusion that diet *does* alter cardiac output.

TWO DIFFERENT ESTIMATES OF THE POPULATION VARIANCE

How shall we estimate the population variance from the four sample variances? When the hypothesis that the diet does not affect cardiac output is true, the variances of each sample of seven people, regardless of what they ate, are equally good estimates of the population variance, so we simply average our four estimates of *variance within the treatment groups:*

> Average variance in cardiac output within treatment groups = 1/4 (variance in cardiac output of controls + variance in cardiac output of spaghetti eaters + variance in cardiac output of steak eaters + variance in cardiac output of fruit and nut eaters)

The mathematical equivalent is

$$s_{\text{wit}}^2 = \frac{1}{4}(s_{\text{con}}^2 + s_{\text{spa}}^2 + s_{\text{st}}^2 + s_{\text{f}}^2)$$

where s^2 represents variance. The variance of each sample is computed with respect to the mean of that sample. Therefore, the population variance estimated from within the groups, *the within-groups variance* s_{wit}^2, will be the same whether or not diet altered cardiac output.

Next we estimate the population variance from the means of the samples. Since we have hypothesized that all four samples were drawn from a single population, the standard deviation of the four sample means will approximate the standard error of the mean. Recall that the standard error of the mean $\sigma_{\overline{X}}$ is related to the sample size n (in this case 7) and the population standard deviation σ according to

$$\sigma_{\overline{X}} = \frac{\sigma}{\sqrt{n}}$$

Therefore, the true population variance σ^2 is related to the sample size and standard error of the mean according to

$$\sigma^2 = n\sigma_{\overline{X}}^2$$

We use this relationship to estimate the population variance from the variability between the sample means using

$$s_{\text{bet}}^2 = ns_{\bar{X}}^2$$

where s_{bet}^2 is the estimate of the population variance computed from between the sample means and $s_{\bar{X}}$ is the standard deviation of the means of the four sample groups, the standard error of the mean. This estimate of the population variance computed from between the group means is often called the *between-groups variance.*

If the null hypothesis that all four samples were drawn from the same population is true (i.e., that diet does not affect cardiac output), the within-groups variance and between-groups variance are both estimates of the same population variance and so should be about equal. Therefore, we will compute the following ratio, called the F-test statistic,

$$F = \frac{\text{population variance estimated from sample means}}{\begin{array}{c}\text{population variance estimated as average}\\ \text{of sample variances}\end{array}}$$

$$F = \frac{s_{\text{bet}}^2}{s_{\text{wit}}^2}$$

Since both the numerator and the denominator are estimates of the same population variance σ^2, F should be about $\sigma^2/\sigma^2 = 1$. For the four random samples in Fig. 3–2, F is about equal to 1, we conclude that the data in Fig. 3–2 are not inconsistent with the hypothesis that diet does not affect cardiac output and we continue to accept that hypothesis.

Now we have a rule for deciding when to reject the null hypothesis that all the samples were drawn from the same population:

> *If F is a big number, the variability between the sample means is larger than expected from the variability within the samples, so reject the null hypothesis that all the samples were drawn from the same population.*

This quantitative statement formalizes the qualitative logic we used when discussing Figs. 3–2 to 3–4. The F associated with Fig. 3–3 is 68.0, and that associated with Fig. 3–4 is 24.5.

WHAT IS A "BIG" F?

The exact value of F one computes depends on which individuals were drawn for the random samples. For example, Fig. 3–5 shows yet another set of four samples of seven people drawn from the population of 200 people in Fig. 3–1. In this example $F = 0.5$. Suppose we repeated our experiment 200 times on the same population. Each time

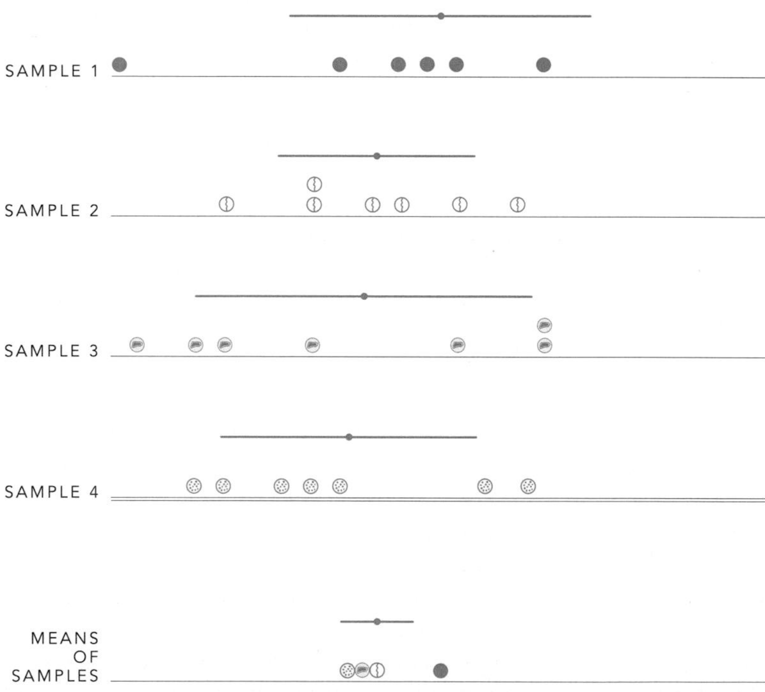

Figure 3–5 Four samples of seven members each drawn from the population shown in Fig. 3–1. Note that the variability in sample means is consistent with the variability within each of the samples, $F = 0.5$.

we would draw four different samples of people and—even if the diet had no effect on cardiac output—get slightly different values for F due to random variation. Figure 3–6*A* shows the result of this procedure, with the resulting F's rounded to one decimal place and represented with a circle; the two dark circles represent the values of F computed from the data in Figs. 3–2 and 3–5. The exact shape of the distribution of values of F depend on how many samples were drawn, the size of each sample, and the distribution of the population from which the samples were drawn.

As expected, most of the computed F's are around 1 (that is, between 0 and 2), but a few are much larger. Thus, even though most experiments will produce relatively small values of F, it is possible that, by sheer bad luck, one could select random samples that are not good representatives of the whole population. The result is an occasional relatively large value for F even though the treatment had no effect. Figure 3–6*B* shows, however, that such values are unlikely. Only 5 percent of the 200 experiments (10 experiments) produced F values equal to or greater than 3.0. We now have a tentative estimate of what to call a "big" value for F. Since F exceeded 3.0 only 10 out of 200 times *when all the samples were drawn from the same population,* we might decide that F is big when it exceeds 3.0 and reject the null hypothesis that all the samples were drawn from the same population (i.e., that the treatment had no effect). In deciding to reject the hypothesis of no effect when F is big, we accept the risk of erroneously rejecting this hypothesis 5 percent of the time because F will be 3.0 or greater about 5 percent of the time, even when the treatment does not alter mean response.

When we obtain such a "big" F, we reject the original null hypothesis that all the means are the same and report $P < .05$. $P < .05$ means that there is less than a 5 percent chance of getting a value of F as big or bigger than the computed value if the original hypothesis were true (i.e., diet did not affect cardiac output).

The critical value of F should be selected not on the basis of just 200 experiments but all 10^{42} possible experiments. Suppose we did all 10^{42} experiments and computed the corresponding F values, then plotted the results, just as we did for Fig. 3–6*B*. Figure 3–6*C* shows the results with grains of sand to represent each observed F value. The darker sand indicates the biggest 5 percent of the F values. Notice how similar it is to Fig. 3–6*B*. This similarity should not surprise you, since the results in panel *B* are just a random sample of the population in panel *C*. Finally, recall that everything so far has been based on an original population containing only 200 members. In reality, populations are usually much larger, so that there can be many more than 10^{42} possible values of *F*. Often, there are essentially an infinite number of possible experiments. In terms of Fig. 3–6*C*, it is as if all

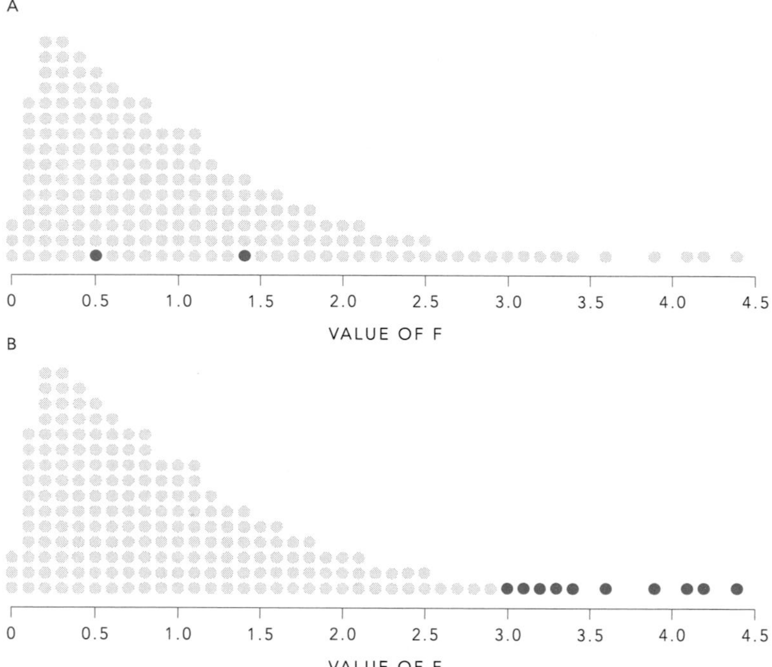

Figure 3–6 ***(A)*** Values of *F* computed from 200 experiments involving four samples, each of size 7, drawn from the population in Fig. 3–1. ***(B)*** We expect *F* to exceed 3.0 only 5 percent of the time when all samples were, in fact, drawn from a single population. ***(C)*** Results of computing the *F* ratio for all possible samples drawn from the original population. The 5 percent of most extreme *F* values are shown darker than the rest. ***(D)*** The *F* distribution one would obtain when sampling an infinite population. In this case, the cutoff value for considering *F* to be "big" is that value of *F* that subtends the upper 5 percent of the total area under the curve.

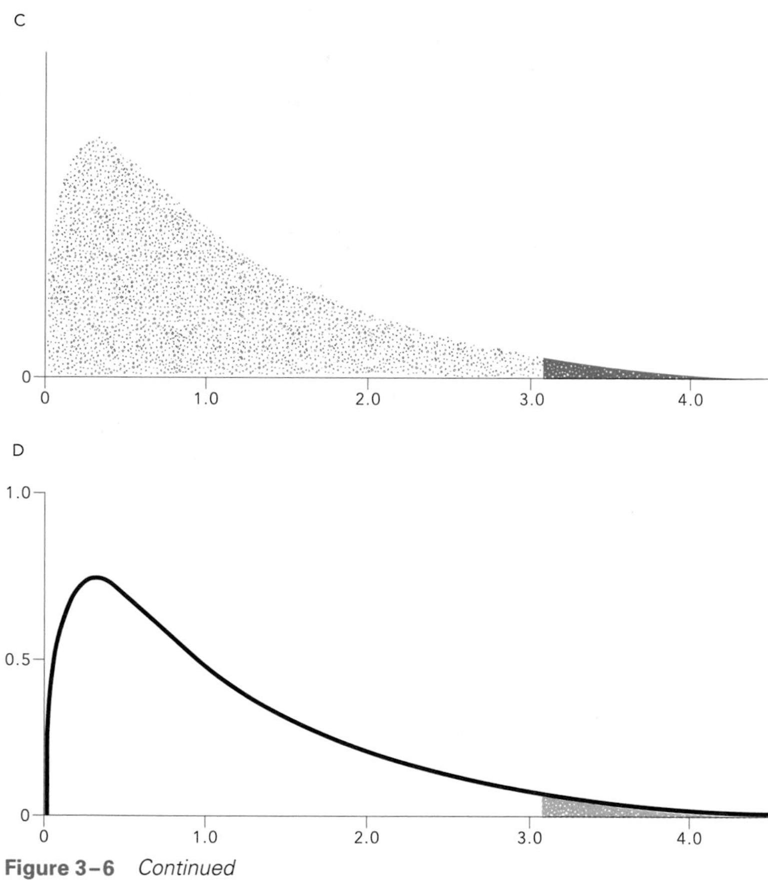

Figure 3–6 *Continued*

the grains of sand melted together to yield the continuous line in Fig. 3–6*D*.

Therefore, *areas under the curve* are analogous to the fractions of total number of circles or grains of sand in panels *B* and *C*. Since the shaded region in Fig. 3–6*D* represents 5 percent of the total area under the curve, it can be used to compute that the cutoff point for a "big" F with the number of samples and sample size in this study is 3.01. This and other cutoff values that correspond to $P < .05$ and $P < .01$ are listed in Table 3–1.

Table 3–1 Critical Values of F Corresponding to $P < .05$ (Lightface) and $P < .01$ (**Boldface**)

ν_d	ν_n 1	2	3	4	5	6	7	8	9	10	11	12	14	16	20	24	30	40	50	75	100	200	500	∞
1	161	200	216	225	230	234	237	239	241	242	243	244	245	246	248	249	250	251	252	253	253	254	254	254
	4052	**4999**	**5403**	**5625**	**5764**	**5859**	**5928**	**5981**	**6022**	**6056**	**6082**	**6106**	**6142**	**6169**	**6208**	**6234**	**6261**	**6286**	**6302**	**6323**	**6334**	**6352**	**6361**	**6366**
2	18.51	19.00	19.16	19.25	19.30	19.33	19.36	19.37	19.38	19.39	19.40	19.41	19.42	19.43	19.44	19.45	19.46	19.47	19.47	19.48	19.49	19.49	19.50	19.50
	98.49	**99.00**	**99.17**	**99.25**	**99.30**	**99.33**	**99.36**	**99.37**	**99.39**	**99.40**	**99.41**	**99.42**	**99.43**	**99.44**	**99.45**	**99.46**	**99.47**	**99.48**	**99.48**	**99.49**	**99.49**	**99.49**	**99.50**	**99.50**
3	10.13	9.55	9.28	9.12	9.01	8.94	8.88	8.84	8.81	8.78	8.76	8.74	8.71	8.69	8.66	8.64	8.62	8.60	8.58	8.57	8.56	8.54	8.54	8.53
	34.12	**30.82**	**29.46**	**28.71**	**28.24**	**27.91**	**27.67**	**27.49**	**27.34**	**27.23**	**27.13**	**27.05**	**26.92**	**26.83**	**26.69**	**26.60**	**26.50**	**26.41**	**26.35**	**26.27**	**26.23**	**26.18**	**26.14**	**26.12**
4	7.71	6.94	6.59	6.39	6.26	6.16	6.09	6.04	6.00	5.96	5.93	5.91	5.87	5.84	5.80	5.77	5.74	5.71	5.70	5.68	5.66	5.65	5.64	5.63
	21.20	**18.00**	**16.69**	**15.98**	**15.52**	**15.21**	**14.98**	**14.80**	**14.66**	**14.54**	**14.45**	**14.37**	**14.24**	**14.15**	**14.02**	**13.93**	**13.83**	**13.74**	**13.69**	**13.61**	**13.57**	**13.52**	**13.48**	**13.46**
5	6.61	5.79	5.41	5.19	5.05	4.95	4.88	4.82	4.78	4.74	4.70	4.68	4.64	4.60	4.56	4.53	4.50	4.46	4.44	4.42	4.40	4.38	4.37	4.36
	16.26	**13.27**	**12.06**	**11.39**	**10.97**	**10.67**	**10.45**	**10.29**	**10.15**	**10.05**	**9.96**	**9.89**	**9.77**	**9.68**	**9.55**	**9.47**	**9.38**	**9.29**	**9.24**	**9.17**	**9.13**	**9.07**	**9.04**	**9.02**
6	5.99	5.14	4.76	4.53	4.39	4.28	4.21	4.15	4.10	4.06	4.03	4.00	3.96	3.92	3.87	3.84	3.81	3.77	3.75	3.72	3.71	3.69	3.68	3.67
	13.74	**10.92**	**9.78**	**9.15**	**8.75**	**8.47**	**8.26**	**8.10**	**7.98**	**7.87**	**7.79**	**7.72**	**7.60**	**7.52**	**7.39**	**7.31**	**7.23**	**7.14**	**7.09**	**7.02**	**6.99**	**6.94**	**6.90**	**6.88**
7	5.59	4.74	4.35	4.12	3.97	3.87	3.79	3.73	3.68	3.63	3.60	3.57	3.52	3.49	3.44	3.41	3.38	3.34	3.32	3.29	3.28	3.25	3.24	3.23
	12.25	**9.55**	**8.45**	**7.85**	**7.46**	**7.19**	**7.00**	**6.84**	**6.71**	**6.62**	**6.54**	**6.47**	**6.35**	**6.27**	**6.15**	**6.07**	**5.98**	**5.90**	**5.85**	**5.78**	**5.75**	**5.70**	**5.67**	**5.65**
8	5.32	4.46	4.07	3.84	3.69	3.58	3.50	3.44	3.39	3.34	3.31	3.28	3.23	3.20	3.15	3.12	3.08	3.05	3.03	3.00	2.98	2.96	2.94	2.93
	11.26	**8.65**	**7.59**	**7.01**	**6.63**	**6.37**	**6.19**	**6.03**	**5.91**	**5.82**	**5.74**	**5.67**	**5.56**	**5.48**	**5.36**	**5.28**	**5.20**	**5.11**	**5.06**	**5.00**	**4.96**	**4.91**	**4.88**	**4.86**
9	5.12	4.26	3.86	3.63	3.48	3.37	3.29	3.23	3.18	3.13	3.10	3.07	3.02	2.98	2.93	2.90	2.86	2.82	2.80	2.77	2.76	2.73	2.72	2.71
	10.56	**8.02**	**6.99**	**6.42**	**6.06**	**5.80**	**5.62**	**5.47**	**5.35**	**5.26**	**5.18**	**5.11**	**5.00**	**4.92**	**4.80**	**4.73**	**4.64**	**4.56**	**4.51**	**4.45**	**4.41**	**4.36**	**4.33**	**4.31**
10	4.96	4.10	3.71	3.48	3.33	3.22	3.14	3.07	3.02	2.97	2.94	2.91	2.86	2.82	2.77	2.74	2.70	2.67	2.64	2.61	2.59	2.56	2.55	2.54
	10.04	**7.56**	**6.55**	**5.99**	**5.64**	**5.39**	**5.21**	**5.06**	**4.95**	**4.85**	**4.78**	**4.71**	**4.60**	**4.52**	**4.41**	**4.33**	**4.25**	**4.17**	**4.12**	**4.05**	**4.01**	**3.96**	**3.93**	**3.91**
11	4.84	3.98	3.59	3.36	3.20	3.09	3.01	2.95	2.90	2.86	2.82	2.79	2.74	2.70	2.65	2.61	2.57	2.53	2.50	2.47	2.45	2.42	2.41	2.40
	9.65	**7.20**	**6.22**	**5.67**	**5.32**	**5.07**	**4.88**	**4.74**	**4.63**	**4.54**	**4.46**	**4.40**	**4.29**	**4.21**	**4.10**	**4.02**	**3.94**	**3.86**	**3.80**	**3.74**	**3.70**	**3.66**	**3.62**	**3.60**
12	4.75	3.88	3.49	3.26	3.11	3.00	2.92	2.85	2.80	2.76	2.72	2.69	2.64	2.60	2.54	2.50	2.46	2.42	2.40	2.36	2.35	2.32	2.31	2.30
	9.33	**6.93**	**5.95**	**5.41**	**5.06**	**4.82**	**4.65**	**4.50**	**4.39**	**4.30**	**4.22**	**4.16**	**4.05**	**3.98**	**3.86**	**3.78**	**3.70**	**3.61**	**3.56**	**3.49**	**3.46**	**3.41**	**3.38**	**3.36**
13	4.67	3.80	3.41	3.18	3.02	2.92	2.84	2.77	2.72	2.67	2.63	2.60	2.55	2.51	2.46	2.42	2.38	2.34	2.32	2.28	2.26	2.24	2.22	2.21
	9.07	**6.70**	**5.74**	**5.20**	**4.86**	**4.62**	**4.44**	**4.30**	**4.19**	**4.10**	**4.02**	**3.96**	**3.85**	**3.78**	**3.67**	**3.59**	**3.51**	**3.42**	**3.37**	**3.30**	**3.27**	**3.21**	**3.18**	**3.16**
14	4.60	3.74	3.34	3.11	2.96	2.85	2.77	2.70	2.65	2.60	2.56	2.53	2.48	2.44	2.39	2.35	2.31	2.27	2.24	2.21	2.19	2.16	2.14	2.13
	8.86	**6.51**	**5.56**	**5.03**	**4.69**	**4.46**	**4.28**	**4.14**	**4.03**	**3.94**	**3.86**	**3.80**	**3.70**	**3.62**	**3.51**	**3.43**	**3.34**	**3.26**	**3.21**	**3.14**	**3.11**	**3.06**	**3.02**	**3.00**
15	4.54	3.68	3.29	3.06	2.90	2.79	2.70	2.64	2.59	2.55	2.51	2.48	2.43	2.39	2.33	2.29	2.25	2.21	2.18	2.15	2.12	2.10	2.08	2.07
	8.68	**6.36**	**5.42**	**4.89**	**4.56**	**4.32**	**4.14**	**4.00**	**3.89**	**3.80**	**3.73**	**3.67**	**3.56**	**3.48**	**3.36**	**3.29**	**3.20**	**3.12**	**3.07**	**3.00**	**2.97**	**2.92**	**2.89**	**2.87**

16	4.49	3.63	3.24	3.01	2.85	2.74	2.66	2.59	2.54	2.49	2.45	2.42	2.37	2.33	2.28	2.24	2.20	2.16	2.13	2.09	2.07	2.04	2.02	2.01
	8.53	**6.23**	**5.29**	**4.77**	**4.44**	**4.20**	**4.03**	**3.89**	**3.78**	**3.69**	**3.61**	**3.55**	**3.45**	**3.37**	**3.25**	**3.18**	**3.10**	**3.01**	**2.96**	**2.98**	**2.86**	**2.80**	**2.77**	**2.75**
17	4.45	3.59	3.20	2.96	2.81	2.70	2.62	2.55	2.50	2.45	2.41	2.38	2.33	2.29	2.23	2.19	2.15	2.11	2.08	2.04	2.02	1.99	1.97	1.96
	8.40	**6.11**	**5.18**	**4.67**	**4.34**	**4.10**	**3.93**	**3.79**	**3.68**	**3.59**	**3.52**	**3.45**	**3.35**	**3.27**	**3.16**	**3.08**	**3.00**	**2.92**	**2.86**	**2.79**	**2.76**	**2.70**	**2.67**	**2.65**
18	4.41	3.55	3.16	2.93	2.77	3.66	2.58	2.51	2.46	2.41	2.37	2.34	2.29	2.25	2.19	2.15	2.11	2.07	2.04	2.00	1.98	1.95	1.93	1.92
	8.28	**6.01**	**5.09**	**4.58**	**4.25**	**4.01**	**3.85**	**3.71**	**3.60**	**3.51**	**3.44**	**3.37**	**3.27**	**3.19**	**3.07**	**3.00**	**2.91**	**2.83**	**2.78**	**2.71**	**2.68**	**2.62**	**2.59**	**2.57**
19	4.38	3.52	3.13	2.90	2.74	2.63	2.55	2.48	2.43	2.38	2.34	2.31	2.26	2.21	2.15	2.11	2.07	2.02	2.00	1.96	1.94	1.91	1.90	1.88
	8.18	**5.93**	**5.01**	**4.50**	**4.17**	**3.94**	**3.77**	**3.63**	**3.52**	**3.43**	**3.36**	**3.30**	**3.19**	**3.12**	**3.00**	**2.92**	**2.84**	**2.76**	**2.70**	**2.63**	**2.60**	**2.54**	**2.51**	**2.49**
20	4.35	3.49	3.10	2.87	2.71	2.60	2.52	2.45	2.40	2.35	2.31	2.28	2.23	2.18	2.12	2.08	2.04	1.99	1.96	1.92	1.90	1.87	1.85	1.84
	8.10	**5.85**	**4.94**	**4.43**	**4.10**	**3.87**	**3.71**	**3.56**	**3.45**	**3.37**	**3.30**	**3.23**	**3.13**	**3.05**	**2.94**	**2.86**	**2.77**	**2.69**	**2.63**	**2.56**	**2.53**	**2.47**	**2.44**	**2.42**
21	4.32	3.47	3.07	2.84	2.68	2.57	2.49	2.42	2.37	2.32	2.28	2.25	2.20	2.15	2.09	2.05	2.00	1.96	1.93	1.89	1.87	1.84	1.82	1.81
	8.02	**5.78**	**4.87**	**4.37**	**4.04**	**3.81**	**3.65**	**3.51**	**3.40**	**3.31**	**3.24**	**3.17**	**3.07**	**2.99**	**2.88**	**2.80**	**2.72**	**2.63**	**2.58**	**2.51**	**2.47**	**2.42**	**2.38**	**2.36**
22	4.30	3.44	3.05	2.82	2.66	2.55	2.47	2.40	2.35	2.30	2.26	2.23	2.18	2.13	2.07	2.03	1.98	1.93	1.91	1.87	1.84	1.81	1.80	1.78
	7.94	**5.72**	**4.82**	**4.31**	**3.99**	**3.76**	**3.59**	**3.45**	**3.35**	**3.26**	**3.18**	**3.12**	**3.02**	**2.94**	**2.83**	**2.75**	**2.67**	**2.58**	**2.53**	**2.46**	**2.42**	**2.37**	**2.33**	**2.31**
23	4.28	3.42	3.03	2.80	2.64	2.53	2.45	2.38	2.32	2.28	2.24	2.20	2.14	2.10	2.04	2.00	1.96	1.91	1.88	1.84	1.82	1.79	1.77	1.76
	7.88	**5.66**	**4.76**	**4.26**	**3.94**	**3.71**	**3.54**	**3.41**	**3.30**	**3.21**	**3.14**	**3.07**	**2.97**	**2.89**	**2.78**	**2.70**	**2.62**	**2.53**	**2.48**	**2.41**	**2.37**	**2.32**	**2.28**	**2.26**
24	4.26	3.40	3.01	2.78	2.62	2.51	2.43	2.36	2.30	2.26	2.22	2.18	2.13	2.09	2.02	1.98	1.94	1.89	1.86	1.82	1.80	1.76	1.74	1.73
	7.82	**5.61**	**4.72**	**4.22**	**3.90**	**3.67**	**3.50**	**3.36**	**3.25**	**3.17**	**3.09**	**3.03**	**2.93**	**2.85**	**2.74**	**2.66**	**2.58**	**2.49**	**2.44**	**2.36**	**2.33**	**2.27**	**2.23**	**2.21**
25	4.24	3.38	2.99	2.76	2.60	2.49	2.41	2.34	2.28	2.24	2.20	2.16	2.11	2.06	2.00	1.96	1.92	1.87	1.84	1.80	1.77	1.74	1.72	1.71
	7.77	**5.57**	**4.68**	**4.18**	**3.86**	**3.63**	**3.46**	**3.32**	**3.21**	**3.13**	**3.05**	**2.99**	**2.89**	**2.81**	**2.70**	**2.62**	**2.54**	**2.45**	**2.40**	**2.32**	**2.29**	**2.23**	**2.19**	**2.17**
26	4.22	3.37	2.98	2.74	2.59	2.47	2.39	2.32	2.27	2.22	2.18	2.15	2.10	2.05	1.99	1.95	1.90	1.85	1.82	1.78	1.76	1.72	1.70	1.69
	7.72	**5.53**	**4.64**	**4.14**	**3.82**	**3.59**	**3.42**	**3.29**	**3.17**	**3.09**	**3.02**	**2.96**	**2.86**	**2.77**	**2.66**	**2.58**	**2.50**	**2.41**	**2.36**	**2.28**	**2.25**	**2.19**	**2.15**	**2.13**
27	4.21	3.35	2.96	2.73	2.57	2.46	2.37	2.30	2.25	2.20	2.16	2.13	2.08	2.03	1.97	1.93	1.88	1.84	1.80	1.76	1.74	1.71	1.68	1.67
	7.68	**5.49**	**4.60**	**4.11**	**3.79**	**3.56**	**3.39**	**3.26**	**3.14**	**3.06**	**2.98**	**2.93**	**2.83**	**2.74**	**2.63**	**2.55**	**2.47**	**2.38**	**2.33**	**2.25**	**2.21**	**2.16**	**2.12**	**2.10**
28	4.20	3.34	2.95	2.71	2.56	2.44	2.36	2.29	2.24	2.19	2.15	2.12	2.06	2.02	1.96	1.91	1.87	1.81	1.78	1.75	1.72	1.69	1.67	1.65
	7.64	**5.45**	**4.57**	**4.07**	**3.76**	**3.53**	**3.36**	**3.23**	**3.11**	**3.03**	**2.95**	**2.90**	**2.80**	**2.71**	**2.60**	**2.52**	**2.44**	**2.35**	**2.30**	**2.22**	**2.18**	**2.13**	**2.09**	**2.06**
29	4.18	3.33	2.93	2.70	2.54	2.43	2.35	2.28	2.22	2.18	2.14	2.10	2.05	2.00	1.94	1.90	1.85	1.80	1.77	1.73	1.71	1.68	1.65	1.64
	7.60	**5.42**	**4.54**	**4.04**	**3.73**	**3.50**	**3.33**	**3.20**	**3.08**	**3.00**	**2.92**	**2.87**	**2.77**	**2.68**	**2.57**	**2.49**	**2.41**	**2.32**	**2.27**	**2.19**	**2.15**	**2.10**	**2.06**	**2.03**
30	4.17	3.32	2.92	2.69	2.53	2.42	2.34	2.27	2.21	2.16	2.12	2.09	2.04	1.99	1.93	1.89	1.84	1.79	1.76	1.72	1.69	1.66	1.64	1.62
	7.56	**5.39**	**4.51**	**4.02**	**3.70**	**3.47**	**3.30**	**3.17**	**3.06**	**2.98**	**2.90**	**2.84**	**2.74**	**2.66**	**2.55**	**2.47**	**2.38**	**2.29**	**2.24**	**2.16**	**2.13**	**2.07**	**2.03**	**2.01**
32	4.15	3.30	2.90	2.67	2.51	2.40	2.32	2.25	2.19	2.14	2.10	2.07	2.02	1.97	1.91	1.86	1.82	1.76	1.74	1.69	1.67	1.64	1.61	1.59
	7.50	**5.34**	**4.46**	**3.97**	**3.66**	**3.42**	**3.25**	**3.12**	**3.01**	**2.94**	**2.86**	**2.80**	**2.70**	**2.62**	**2.51**	**2.42**	**2.34**	**2.25**	**2.20**	**2.12**	**2.08**	**2.02**	**1.98**	**1.96**
34	4.13	3.28	2.88	2.65	2.49	2.38	2.30	2.23	2.17	2.12	2.08	2.05	2.00	1.95	1.89	1.84	1.80	1.74	1.71	1.67	1.64	1.61	1.59	1.57
	7.44	**5.29**	**4.42**	**3.93**	**3.61**	**3.38**	**3.21**	**3.08**	**2.97**	**2.89**	**2.82**	**2.76**	**2.66**	**2.58**	**2.47**	**2.38**	**2.30**	**2.21**	**2.15**	**2.08**	**2.04**	**1.98**	**1.94**	**1.91**

(continued)

Table 3–1 Critical Values of F Corresponding to $P < .05$ (Lightface) and $P < .01$ (Boldface) (*Continued*)

ν_d	ν_n: 1	2	3	4	5	6	7	8	9	10	11	12	14	16	20	24	30	40	50	75	100	200	500	∞
36	4.11	3.26	2.86	2.63	2.48	2.36	2.28	2.21	2.15	2.10	2.06	2.03	1.98	1.93	1.87	1.82	1.78	1.72	1.69	1.65	1.62	1.59	1.56	1.55
	7.39	**5.25**	**4.38**	**3.89**	**3.58**	**3.35**	**3.18**	**3.04**	**2.94**	**2.86**	**2.78**	**2.72**	**2.62**	**2.54**	**2.43**	**2.35**	**2.26**	**2.17**	**2.12**	**2.04**	**2.00**	**1.94**	**1.90**	**1.87**
38	4.10	3.25	2.85	2.62	2.46	2.35	2.26	2.19	2.14	2.09	2.05	2.02	1.96	1.92	1.85	1.80	1.76	1.71	1.67	1.63	1.60	1.57	1.54	1.53
	7.35	**5.21**	**4.34**	**3.86**	**3.54**	**3.32**	**3.15**	**3.02**	**2.91**	**2.82**	**2.75**	**2.69**	**2.59**	**2.51**	**2.40**	**2.32**	**2.22**	**2.14**	**2.08**	**2.00**	**1.97**	**1.90**	**1.86**	**1.84**
40	4.08	3.23	2.84	2.61	2.45	2.34	2.25	2.18	2.12	2.07	2.04	2.00	1.95	1.90	1.84	1.79	1.74	1.69	1.66	1.61	1.59	1.55	1.53	1.51
	7.31	**5.18**	**4.31**	**3.83**	**3.51**	**3.29**	**3.12**	**2.99**	**2.88**	**2.80**	**2.73**	**2.66**	**2.56**	**2.49**	**2.37**	**2.29**	**2.20**	**2.11**	**2.05**	**1.97**	**1.94**	**1.88**	**1.84**	**1.81**
42	4.07	3.22	2.83	2.59	2.44	2.32	2.24	2.17	2.11	2.06	2.02	1.99	1.94	1.89	1.82	1.78	1.73	1.68	1.64	1.60	1.57	1.54	1.51	1.49
	7.27	**5.15**	**4.29**	**3.80**	**3.49**	**3.26**	**3.10**	**2.96**	**2.86**	**2.77**	**2.70**	**2.64**	**2.54**	**2.46**	**2.35**	**2.26**	**2.17**	**2.08**	**2.02**	**1.94**	**1.91**	**1.85**	**1.80**	**1.78**
44	4.06	3.21	2.82	2.58	2.43	2.31	2.23	2.16	2.10	2.05	2.01	1.98	1.92	1.88	1.81	1.76	1.72	1.66	1.63	1.58	1.56	1.52	1.50	1.48
	7.24	**5.12**	**4.26**	**3.78**	**3.46**	**3.24**	**3.07**	**2.94**	**2.84**	**2.75**	**2.68**	**2.62**	**2.52**	**2.44**	**2.32**	**2.24**	**2.15**	**2.06**	**2.00**	**1.92**	**1.88**	**1.82**	**1.78**	**1.75**
46	4.05	3.20	2.81	2.57	2.42	2.30	2.22	2.14	2.09	2.04	2.00	1.97	1.91	1.87	1.80	1.75	1.71	1.65	1.62	1.57	1.54	1.51	1.48	1.46
	7.21	**5.10**	**4.24**	**3.76**	**3.44**	**3.22**	**3.05**	**2.92**	**2.82**	**2.73**	**2.66**	**2.60**	**2.50**	**2.42**	**2.30**	**2.22**	**2.13**	**2.04**	**1.98**	**1.90**	**1.86**	**1.80**	**1.76**	**1.72**
48	4.04	3.19	2.80	2.56	2.41	2.30	2.21	2.14	2.08	2.03	1.99	1.96	1.90	1.86	1.79	1.74	1.70	1.64	1.61	1.56	1.53	1.50	1.47	1.45
	7.19	**5.08**	**4.22**	**3.74**	**3.42**	**3.20**	**3.04**	**2.90**	**2.80**	**2.71**	**2.64**	**2.58**	**2.48**	**2.40**	**2.28**	**2.20**	**2.11**	**2.02**	**1.96**	**1.88**	**1.84**	**1.78**	**1.73**	**1.70**
50	4.03	3.18	2.79	2.56	2.40	2.29	2.20	2.13	2.07	2.02	1.98	1.95	1.90	1.85	1.78	1.74	1.69	1.63	1.60	1.55	1.52	1.48	1.46	1.44
	7.17	**5.06**	**4.20**	**3.72**	**3.41**	**3.18**	**3.02**	**2.88**	**2.78**	**2.70**	**2.62**	**2.56**	**2.46**	**2.39**	**2.26**	**2.18**	**2.10**	**2.00**	**1.94**	**1.86**	**1.82**	**1.76**	**1.71**	**1.68**
60	4.00	3.15	2.76	2.52	2.37	2.25	2.17	2.10	2.04	1.99	1.95	1.92	1.86	1.81	1.75	1.70	1.65	1.59	1.56	1.50	1.48	1.44	1.41	1.39
	7.08	**4.98**	**4.13**	**3.65**	**3.34**	**3.12**	**2.95**	**2.82**	**2.72**	**2.63**	**2.56**	**2.50**	**2.40**	**2.32**	**2.20**	**2.12**	**2.03**	**1.93**	**1.87**	**1.79**	**1.74**	**1.68**	**1.63**	**1.60**
70	3.98	3.13	2.74	2.50	2.35	2.23	2.14	2.07	2.01	1.97	1.93	1.89	1.84	1.79	1.72	1.67	1.62	1.56	1.53	1.47	1.45	1.40	1.37	1.35
	7.01	**4.92**	**4.08**	**3.60**	**3.29**	**3.07**	**2.91**	**2.77**	**2.67**	**2.59**	**2.51**	**2.45**	**2.35**	**2.28**	**2.15**	**2.07**	**1.98**	**1.88**	**1.82**	**1.74**	**1.69**	**1.62**	**1.56**	**1.53**
80	3.96	3.11	2.72	2.48	2.33	2.21	2.12	2.05	1.99	1.95	1.91	1.88	1.82	1.77	1.70	1.65	1.60	1.54	1.51	1.45	1.42	1.38	1.35	1.32
	6.96	**4.88**	**4.04**	**3.56**	**3.25**	**3.04**	**2.87**	**2.74**	**2.64**	**2.55**	**2.48**	**2.41**	**2.32**	**2.24**	**2.11**	**2.03**	**1.94**	**1.84**	**1.78**	**1.70**	**1.65**	**1.57**	**1.52**	**1.49**
100	3.94	3.09	2.70	2.46	2.30	2.19	2.10	2.03	1.97	1.92	1.88	1.85	1.79	1.75	1.68	1.63	1.57	1.51	1.48	1.42	1.39	1.34	1.30	1.28
	6.90	**4.82**	**3.98**	**3.51**	**3.20**	**2.99**	**2.82**	**2.69**	**2.59**	**2.51**	**2.43**	**2.36**	**2.26**	**2.19**	**2.06**	**1.98**	**1.89**	**1.79**	**1.73**	**1.64**	**1.59**	**1.51**	**1.46**	**1.43**
120	3.92	3.07	2.68	2.45	2.29	2.18	2.09	2.02	1.96	1.91	1.87	1.84	1.78	1.73	1.66	1.61	1.56	1.50	1.46	1.39	1.37	1.32	1.28	1.25
	6.85	**4.79**	**3.95**	**3.48**	**3.17**	**2.96**	**2.79**	**2.66**	**2.56**	**2.47**	**2.40**	**2.34**	**2.23**	**2.15**	**2.03**	**1.95**	**1.86**	**1.76**	**1.70**	**1.61**	**1.56**	**1.48**	**1.42**	**1.38**
∞	3.84	2.99	2.60	2.37	2.21	2.09	2.01	1.94	1.88	1.83	1.79	1.75	1.69	1.64	1.57	1.52	1.46	1.40	1.35	1.28	1.24	1.17	1.11	1.00
	6.63	**4.60**	**3.78**	**3.32**	**3.02**	**2.80**	**2.64**	**2.51**	**2.41**	**2.32**	**2.24**	**2.18**	**2.07**	**1.99**	**1.87**	**1.79**	**1.69**	**1.59**	**1.52**	**1.41**	**1.36**	**1.25**	**1.15**	**1.00**

Note: ν_n = degrees of freedom for numerator; ν_d = degrees of freedom for denominator.
Source: Adapted from G. W. Snedecor and W. G. Cochran, *Statistical Methods*, Iowa State University Press, Arnes, 1978, pp. 560–563.

To construct these tables, mathematicians have assumed four things about the underlying population that must be at least approximately satisfied for the tables to be applicable to real data:

- *Each sample must be independent of the other samples.*
- *Each sample must be randomly selected from the population being studied.*
- *The populations from which the samples were drawn must be normally distributed.**
- *The variances of each population must be equal, even when the means are different, i.e., when the treatment has an effect.*

When the data suggest that these assumptions do not apply, one ought not to use the procedure we just developed, the analysis of variance. Since there is one factor (the diet) that distinguishes the different experimental groups, this is known as a *single-factor or one-way analysis of variance*. Other forms of analysis of variance (not discussed here) can be used to analyze experiments in which there is more than one experimental factor.

Since the distribution of possible F values depends on the size of each sample and number of samples under consideration, so does the exact value of F which corresponds to the 5 percent cutoff point. For example, in our diet study, the number of samples was 4 and the size of each sample was 7. This dependence enters into the mathematical formulas used to determine the value at which F gets "big" as two parameters known as *degree-of-freedom* parameters, often denoted ν (Greek nu). For this analysis, the between-groups degrees of freedom (also called the numerator degrees of freedom because the between-groups variance is in the numerator of F) is defined to be the number of samples m minus 1, or $\nu_n = m - 1$. The within-groups (or denominator) degrees of freedom is defined to be the number of samples times 1 less than the size of each sample, $\nu_d = m(n - 1)$. For our diet example, the numerator degrees of freedom are $4 - 1 = 3$, and the denominator degrees of freedom are $4(7 - 1) = 24$. Degrees of freedom often confuse and mystify people who are trying to work with

*This is another reason parametric statistical methods require data from normally distributed populations.

statistics. They simply represent the way *number of samples* and *sample size* enter the mathematical formulas used to construct all statistical tables.

THREE EXAMPLES

We now have the tools needed to form conclusions using statistical reasoning. We will examine examples, all based on results published in the medical literature. I have exercised some literary license with these examples for two reasons: (1) Medical and scientific authors usually summarize their raw data with descriptive statistics (like those developed in Chap. 2) rather than including the raw data. As a result, the "data from the literature" shown in this chapter—and the rest of the book—are usually my guess at what the raw data probably looked like based on the descriptive statistics in the original article.* (2) The analysis of variance as we developed it requires that each sample contain the same number of members. This is often not the case in reality, so I adjusted the sample sizes in the original studies to meet this restriction. We later generalize our statistical methods to handle experiments with different numbers of individuals in each sample or treatment group.

Glucose Levels in Children of Parents with Diabetes

Diabetes is a disease caused by abnormal carbohydrate metabolism and is characterized by excessive amounts of sugar in the blood and urine. Type I, or insulin-dependent diabetes mellitus (IDDM), occurs in children and young adults. Type II, or non-insulin-dependent diabetes mellitus (NIDDM), usually occurs in people over 40 years old and is often detected by elevated glucose levels rather than illness. Both types of diabetes tend to run in families, but because type II tends to occur in adults, few studies focus on determining when abnormalities in sugar regulation first appear in children and young adults. Gerald Berenson and colleagues† wanted to investigate whether abnormalities in

*Since authors often failed to include a complete set of descriptive statistics, I had to simulate them from the results of their hypothesis tests.

†G. S. Berenson, W. Bao, S. R. Srinivasan, "Abnormal Characteristics in Young Offspring of Parents with Non-Insulin-Dependent Diabetes Mellitus." *Am. J. Epidemiol.*, **144:**962–967, 1996.

carbohydrate metabolism could be detected in non-diabetic young adults whose parents had a history of type II diabetes. They identified parents who had a history of diabetes in Bogalusa, Louisiana in 1987 and 1988 from a survey of school age children. Next, in 1989 and 1991, they recruited children from these families, which they denoted the *cases*. Similarly aged offspring were recruited from families without a history of diabetes to serve as *controls*. Berenson and colleagues then measured many physiological variables that might be related to diabetes, including indicators of carbohydrate tolerance (fasting glucose, insulin, glucagon), blood pressure, cholesterol, weight, and body mass index.

This approach is called an *observational study* because the investigators obtained data by simply observing events without controlling them. Such studies are prone to two potentially serious problems. First, as discussed in Chap. 2 the groups may vary in ways the investigators do not notice or choose to ignore, and these differences—due to *confounding variables*—rather than the treatment itself, may account for the differences the investigators find. Second, such studies can be subject to bias in patient recall, investigator assessment, and selection of the treatment group or the control group.

Observational studies do, however, have advantages. First, they are relatively inexpensive because they are often based on reviews of existing information or information that is already being collected for other purposes (like medical records) and because they generally do not require direct intervention by the investigator. Second, ethical considerations or prevailing medical practice can make it impossible to carry out active manipulation of the variable under study.

Because of the potential difficulties in all observational studies, it is critical that the investigators explicitly specify the criteria they used for classifying each subject in the control or case group. Such specifications help minimize biases when the study is done as well as help you, as the consumer of the resulting information, judge whether the classification rules made sense.

Berenson and colleagues developed explicit criteria for including a person in their study, including the following.

- *Parental history of diabetes was verified by a physician through medical records to exclude possible type I diabetics.*
- *No child had parents who were both diabetic.*

- *The cases and control groups had similar ages (15.3 ± 4.5 SD and 15.1 ± 5.7 SD).*
- *All parents were white.*
- *Control offspring were matched according to age of parents from families with no history of diabetes in parents, grandparents, uncles, or aunts.*

A comparison of controls and cases found that the prevalence of potentially confounding lifestyle factors, such as smoking, drinking alcohol, and using oral contraceptives was similar between the two groups.

Figure 3–7 shows data for fasting glucose levels in the 25 offspring of parents with type II diabetes and 25 control offspring. On the average, the offspring of parents with type II diabetes had fasting

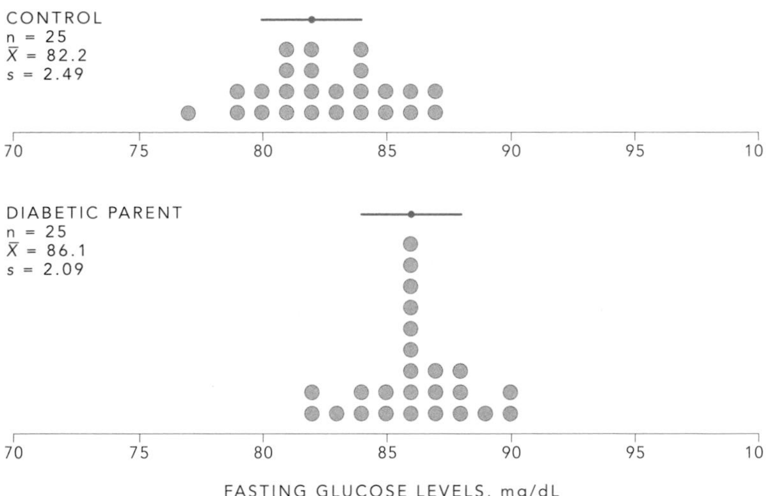

Figure 3–7 Results of a study comparing fasting glucose levels in children of parents who have type II diabetes and children of parents without type II diabetes. Each child's fasting glucose level is indicated by a circle at the appropriate glucose level. The average fasting glucose level for children of diabetic parents is higher than the average glucose level in children whose parents did not have diabetes. The statistical question is to assess whether or not the difference is due simply to random sampling or to an actual effect of the differences in parental history.

glucose levels of 86.1 mg/dL, whereas the control offspring had glucose levels of 82.2 mg/dL. There was not much variability in either group's fasting glucose levels. The standard deviations in glucose levels were 2.09 and 2.49 mg/dL, respectively.

How consistent are these data with the null hypothesis that fasting glucose levels do not differ in children of parents with type II diabetes compared to children of parents without a history of type II diabetes? In other words, how likely are the differences between the two samples of offspring shown in Fig. 3–7 to be due to random sampling rather than the difference based on parental history of diabetes?

To answer this question, we perform an analysis of variance.

We begin by estimating the within-groups variance by averaging the variances of the two groups of children.

$$s^2_{\text{wit}} = \frac{1}{2}(s^2_{\text{diabetes}} + s^2_{\text{control}})$$

$$= \frac{1}{2}(2.09^2 + 2.49^2) = 5.28\ (\text{mg/dL})^2$$

We then go on to calculate the between-groups variance. The first step is to estimate the standard error of the mean by computing the standard deviation of the two sample means. The mean of the two sample means is

$$\overline{X} = \frac{1}{2}(\overline{X}_{\text{diabetes}} + \overline{X}_{\text{control}})$$

$$= \frac{1}{2}(86.1 + 82.2) = 84.2\ \text{mg/dL}$$

Therefore the standard deviation of the sample means is

$$s_{\overline{X}} = \sqrt{\frac{(\overline{X}_{\text{diabetes}} - \overline{X})^2 + (\overline{X}_{\text{control}} - \overline{X})^2}{m - 1}}$$

$$= \sqrt{\frac{(86.1 - 84.2)^2 + (82.2 - 84.2)^2}{2 - 1}} = 2.76\ \text{mg/dL}$$

Since the sample size n is 25, the estimation of the population variance from between the groups is

$$s^2_{\text{bet}} = ns^2_{\bar{X}} = 25(2.76^2) = 190.13\ (\text{mg/dL})^2$$

Finally, the ratio of these two different estimates of the population variance is

$$F = \frac{s^2_{\text{bet}}}{s^2_{\text{wit}}} = \frac{190.13}{5.28} = 36.01$$

The degrees of freedom for the numerator are the number of groups minus 1, and so $\nu_n = 2 - 1 = 1$, and the degrees of freedom for the denominator are the number of groups times 1 less than the sample size, or $\nu_d = 2(25 - 1) = 48$. Look in the column headed 1 and the row headed 48 in Table 3–1. The resulting entry indicates that there is less than a 1 percent chance of F exceeding 7.19; we therefore conclude that the value of F associated with our observations is "big" and we reject the null hypothesis that there is no difference in the average glucose level in the two groups of children shown in Fig. 3–7.

By rejecting the null hypothesis of no difference, we conclude that there are higher levels of fasting glucose in children of diabetics than in children of nondiabetics.

Halothane versus Morphine for Open-Heart Surgery

Halothane is a popular drug to induce general anesthesia because it is potent, nonflammable, easy to use, and very safe. Since halothane can be carried with oxygen, it can be vaporized and administered to the patient with the same equipment used to ventilate the patient. The patient absorbs and releases it through the lungs, making it possible to change anesthetic states more rapidly than would be possible with drugs that have to be administered intravenously. It does, however, lessen the heart's ability to pump blood directly by depressing the myocardium (heart muscle) itself and indirectly by increasing peripheral venous capacity. Some anesthesiologists believed that these effects could produce complications in people with cardiac problems and suggested using morphine as an anesthetic agent in these patients because it has little effect on cardiac performance in supine individuals. Conahan and colleagues* directly compared these two anesthetic agents in a large number of patients during routine surgery for cardiac valve repair or replacement.

To obtain two similar samples of patients who differed only in the type of anesthesia used, they selected the anesthesia at random for each patient who was suitable for the study.

During the operation, they recorded many hemodynamic variables, such as blood pressures before induction of anesthesia, after anesthesia but before incision, and during other important periods during the operation. They also recorded information relating to length of stay in the postsurgical intensive care unit, total length of hospitalization, and any deaths that occurred during this period. We will analyze these latter data after we have developed the necessary statistical tools in Chap. 5. For now, we will focus on a representative pressure measurement, the lowest mean arterial blood pressure between the start of anesthesia and the time of incision. This variable is thought to be a good measure of depression of the cardiovascular system before any surgical stimulation occurs. Specifically, we will investigate the null hypothesis that, on the average, there was no difference in patients anesthetized with halothane or morphine.

Figure 3–8 shows the lowest mean arterial blood pressure observed from the start of anesthesia until the time of incision for 122 patients, half of whom were anesthetized with each agent. Pressures were rounded to the nearest even number, and each patient's pressure is represented by a circle. On the average, patients anesthetized with halothane had pressures 6.3 mmHg below those anesthetized with morphine. There is quite a bit of overlap in the pressures observed in the two different groups because of biological variability in how different people respond to anesthesia. The standard deviations in pressures are 12.2 and 14.4 mmHg for the people anesthetized with halothane and morphine, respectively. Given these results, is the 6.3 mmHg difference large enough to assert that halothane produced lower lowest mean arterial pressures?

*T. J. Conahan III, A. J. Ominsky, H. Wollman, and R. A. Stroth, "A Prospective Random Comparison of Halothane and Morphine for Open-Heart Anesthesia: One Year's Experience," *Anesthesiology,* **38:**528–535, 1973.

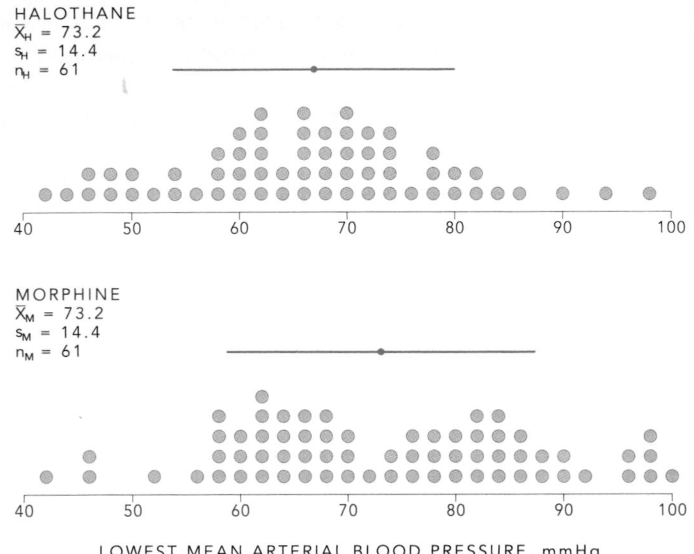

Figure 3–8 Lowest mean arterial blood pressure between the beginning of anesthesia and the incision in patients during open-heart surgery for patients anesthetized with halothane and morphine. Are the observed differences consistent with the hypothesis that, on the average, anesthetic did not affect blood pressure?

To answer this question, we perform an analysis of variance exactly as we did to compare length of hospitalizations in the study of glucose levels in children of parents with diabetes. We estimate the within-groups variance by averaging the estimates of the variance obtained from the two samples:

$$s_{\text{wit}}^2 = \tfrac{1}{2}\,(s_{\text{hlo}}^2 + s_{\text{mor}}^2) = \tfrac{1}{2}\,(12.2^2 + 14.4^2) = 178.1 \text{ mmHg}^2$$

Since this estimate of the population variance is computed from the variances of the separate samples, it does not depend on whether or not the means are different.

Next, we estimate the population variance by assuming that the null hypothesis that halothane and morphine produce the same effect on arterial blood pressure is true. In that case, the two groups of patients in Fig. 3–8 are simply two random samples drawn from a single population. As a result, the standard deviation of the sample means is an estimate of the standard error of the mean. The mean of the two samples means is

$$\bar{X} = \frac{1}{2}(\bar{X}_{\text{hlo}} + \bar{X}_{\text{mor}}) = \frac{1}{2}(66.9 + 73.2) = 70 \text{ mmHg}$$

The standard deviation of the $m = 2$ sample means is

$$s_{\bar{X}} = \sqrt{\frac{(\bar{X}_{\text{hlo}} - \bar{X})^2 + (\bar{X}_{\text{mor}} - \bar{X})^2}{m - 1}}$$

$$= \sqrt{\frac{(66.9 - 70.0)^2 + (73.2 - 70.0)^2}{2 - 1}} = 4.46 \text{ mmHg}$$

Since the sample size n is 61, the estimate of the population variance computed from the variability in the sample means is

$$s^2_{\text{bet}} = ns^2_{\bar{X}} = 61(4.46^2) = 1213 \text{ mmHg}^2$$

To test whether these two estimates are compatible, we compute

$$F = \frac{s^2_{\text{bet}}}{s^2_{\text{wit}}} = \frac{1213}{178.1} = 6.81$$

The degrees of freedom for the numerator are $\nu_n = m - 1 = 2 - 1 = 1$, and the degrees of freedom for the denominator are $\nu_d = m(n - 1) = 2(61 - 1) = 120$. Since $F = 6.81$ is greater than the critical value of 3.92 from (interpolating in) Table 3–1, we conclude that there is less than a 5 percent chance that our data were all drawn from a single population. In other words, we conclude that halothane produced lower lowest mean arterial blood pressures than morphine did, on the average.

Given the variability in response among patients to each drug (quantified by the standard deviations), do you expect this *statistically* significant result to be *clinically significant*? We will return to this question later.

Menstrual Dysfunction in Distance Runners

Infrequent or suspended menstruation can be a symptom of serious metabolic disorders, such as anorexia nervosa (a psychological disorder that leads people to stop eating, then waste away) or tumors of the pituitary gland. Infrequent or suspended menstruation can also frustrate a woman's wish to have children. It can also be a side effect of birth control pills or indicate that a woman is pregnant or entering menopause. Gynecologists see many women who complain about irregular menstrual cycles and must decide how to diagnose and perhaps treat this possible problem. In addition to these potential explanations, there is evidence that strenuous exercise, perhaps by changing the percentage of body fat, may affect the ovulation cycle. Since jogging and long-distance running have become popular, Edwin Dale and colleagues* decided to investigate whether there is a relationship between the frequency of menstruation and the amount of jogging young women do, as well as to look for possible effects on body weight, fat, and levels of circulating hormones that play an important role in the menstrual cycle.

They did an observational study of three groups of women. The first two groups were volunteers who regularly engaged in some form of running, and the third, a control group, consisted of women who did not run but were otherwise similar to the other two groups. The runners were divided into *joggers* who jog "slow and easy" 5 to 30 miles per week, and *runners* who run more than 30 miles per week and combine long, slow distance with speed work. The investigators used a survey to show that the three groups were similar in the amount of physical activity (aside from running), distribution of ages, heights, occupations, and type of birth control methods being used.

Figure 3–9 shows the number of menstrual periods per year for the 26 women in each experimental group. The women in the control group averaged 11.5 menses per year, the joggers averaged 10.1 menses per year, and the runners averaged 9.1 menses per year. Are these

*E. Dale, D. H. Gerlach, and A. L. Wilhite, "Menstrual Dysfunction in Distance Runners," *Obstet. Gynecol.*, **54**:47–53, 1979.

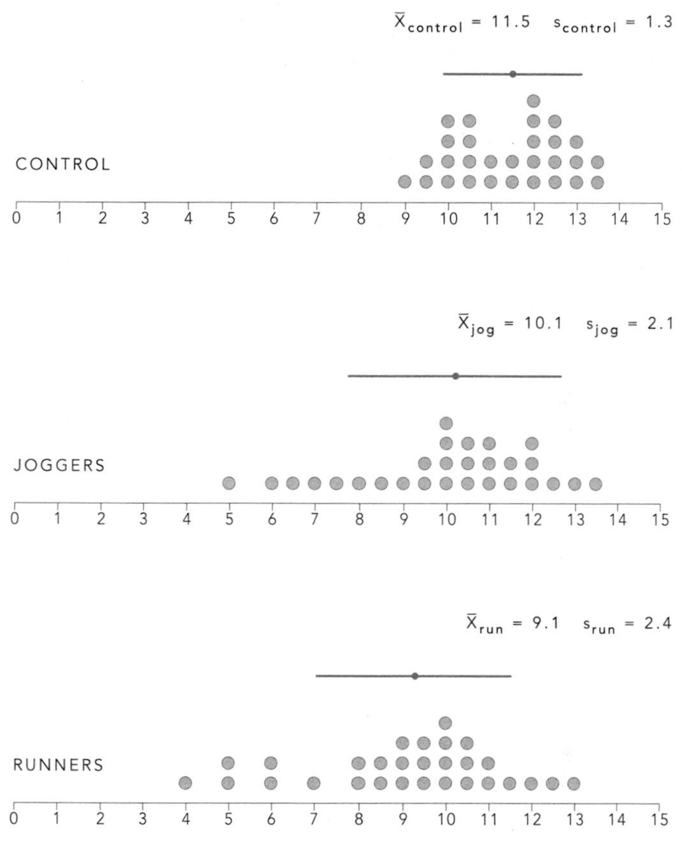

Figure 3–9 The number of menstrual cycles per year in women who were sedentary, joggers, and long-distance runners. The mean values of the three samples of women were different. Is this variation beyond what would be expected from random sampling, i.e., that the amount of running one does has no effect on the number of menstrual cycles, or is it compatible with the view that jogging affects menstruation? Furthermore, if there is an effect, is there a different effect for joggers and long-distance runners?

differences in mean number of menses compatible with what one would expect from the variability within each group?

To answer this question, we first estimate the population variance by averaging the variance from within the groups

$$s^2_{\text{wit}} = \frac{1}{3}(s^2_{\text{con}} + s^2_{\text{jog}} + s^2_{\text{run}})$$

$$= \frac{1}{3}(1.3^2 + 2.1^2 + 2.4^2) = 3.95 \text{ (menses/year)}^2$$

To estimate the population variance from the variability in the sample means, we must first estimate the standard error of the mean by computing the standard deviation of the means of the three samples. Since the mean of the three means is

$$\overline{X} = \frac{1}{3}(\overline{X}_{\text{con}} + \overline{X}_{\text{jog}} + \overline{X}_{\text{run}})$$

$$= \frac{1}{3}(11.5 + 10.1 + 9.1) = 10.2 \text{ menses/year}$$

Our estimate of the standard error is

$$s_{\overline{X}} = \sqrt{\frac{(\overline{X}_{\text{con}} - \overline{X})^2 + (\overline{X}_{\text{jog}} - \overline{X})^2 + (\overline{X}_{\text{run}} - \overline{X})^2}{m - 1}}$$

$$= \sqrt{\frac{(11.5 - 10.2)^2 + (10.1 - 10.2)^2 + (9.1 - 10.2)^2}{3 - 1}}$$

$$= 1.206 \text{ menses/year}$$

The sample size n is 26, and so the estimate of the population variance from the variability in the means is

$$s^2_{\text{bet}} = ns^2_{\overline{X}} = 26(1.206^2) = 37.79 \text{ (menses/year)}^2$$

Finally,

$$F = \frac{s^2_{\text{bet}}}{s^2_{\text{wit}}} = \frac{37.79}{3.95} = 9.56$$

The numerator has $m - 1 = 3 - 1 = 2$ degrees of freedom and the denominator has $m(n - 1) = 3(26 - 1) = 75$ degrees of freedom. Interpolating in Table 3–1, we find that F will exceed 4.90 only

1 percent of the time when all the groups are drawn from a single population; we conclude that jogging or running has an effect on the frequency of menstruation.

When a woman comes to her gynecologist complaining about irregular or infrequent periods, the physician should not only look for biochemical abnormalities but also ask whether or not she jogs.

One question remains: Which of the three groups differed from the others? Does one have to be a marathon runner to expect menstrual dysfunction, or does it accompany less strenuous jogging? Or is the effect graded, becoming more pronounced with more strenuous exercise? We will have to defer answering these questions until we develop another statistical tool, the *t* test, in Chap. 4.

PROBLEMS

3-1 In order to study the cellular changes in people with tendencies to develop diabetes, Kitt Petersen and her colleagues ("Impaired mitochondrial activity in the insulin-resistant offspring of patients with Type 2 diabetes," *N. Engl. J. Med.* **350:**664–671, 2004) studied the ability of muscle cells in normal children and insulin-resistant children to convert glucose into adenosine triphosphate (ATP), the "energy molecule" muscle cells produce to power contraction. The body produces insulin to permit cells to process glucose and muscle cells of insulin-resistant people do not respond normally to process glucose. They measured the amount of ATP produced per gram of muscle tissue after giving the study participants a dose of glucose. Persons in the control group produced 7.3 μmol/g of muscle/min) of ATP (standard deviation 2.3 μmol/g of muscle/min) and insulin-resistant persons produced 5.0 μmol/g of muscle/min (standard deviation 1.9 μmol/g of muscle/min). There were 15 children in each test group. Is there a difference in the rate of ATP production in these two groups of people?

3-2 It is generally believed that infrequent and short-term exposure to pollutants in tobacco, such as carbon monoxide, nicotine, benzo[*a*]pyrene, and oxides of nitrogen, will not permanently alter lung function in healthy adult nonsmokers. To investigate this hypothesis, James White and Herman Froeb ("Small-Airways Dysfunction in Nonsmokers Chronically Exposed to Tobacco Smoke," *N. Engl. J. Med.,* **302:**720–723, 1980, used by permission) measured lung function in cigarette smokers and nonsmokers during a "physical fitness profile" at the University of California, San Diego. They measured how rapidly a person could force air from the lungs (mean forced midexpiratory flow). Reduced forced midexpiratory flow is associated with small-airways disease of the lungs. For the women they tested White and Froeb found:

		Mean forced midexpiratory flow, L/s	
Group	No. of subjects	Mean	SD
Nonsmokers			
Worked in smokefree environment	200	3.17	0.74
Worked in smoky environment	200	2.72	0.71
Light smokers	200	2.63	0.73
Moderate smokers	200	2.29	0.70
Heavy smokers	200	2.12	0.72

Is there evidence that the presence of small-airways disease, as measured by this test, is any different among the different experimental groups?

3-3 Elevated levels of plasma high-density-lipoprotein (HDL) cholesterol may be associated with a lowered risk of coronary heart disease. Several studies have suggested that vigorous exercise may result in increased levels of HDL. To investigate whether or not jogging is associated with an increase in the plasma HDL concentration, G. Harley Hartung and colleagues ("Relation of Diet to High-Density-Lipoprotein Cholesterol in Middle-Aged Marathon Runners, Joggers, and Inactive Men," *N. Engl. J. Med.,* **302:**357–361, 1980, used by permission) measured HDL concentrations in middle-aged (35 to 66 years old) marathon runners, joggers, and inactive men. The mean HDL concentration observed in the inactive men was 43.3 mg/dL with a standard deviation of 14.2 mg/dL. The mean and standard deviation of the HDL concentration for the joggers and marathon runners were 58.0 and 17.7 mg/dL and 64.8 and 14.3 mg/dL, respectively. If there were 70 men in each group, test the hypothesis that there is no difference in the average HDL concentration between these groups of men.

3-4 If heart muscle is briefly deprived of oxygen—a condition known as ischemia—the muscle stops contracting and, if the ischemia is long enough or severe enough, the muscle dies. When the muscle dies, the person has a myocardial infarction (heart attack). Surprisingly, when the heart muscle is subjected to a brief period of ischemia before a major ischemic episode, the muscle is more able to survive the major ischemic episode. This phenomenon is known as ischemic preconditioning. This protective effect of ischemic preconditioning is known to involve activation of adenosine A1 receptors, which stimulate protein kinase C (PKC), a protein involved in many cellular processes including proliferation, migration, secretion, and cell death. Akihito Tsuchida and colleagues ("α_1-Adrenergic Agonist Precondition Rabbit Ischemic Myocardium Independent of Adenosine by Direct Activation of Protein Kinase C," *Circ. Res.*, **75:**576–585, 1994) hypothesized that α_1-adrenergic receptors might have an independent rule in this process. To address this question, Tsuchida and colleagues subjected isolated rabbit hearts to a brief 5-min ischemia or exposed the hearts to a variety of adenosine and α_1-adrenergic agonists and antagonists. In any case, following a 10-min recovery period, the heart was subject to ischemia for 30 min and the size of the resulting infarct measured. The control group was only subjected to 30 min of ischemia. If each group included 7 rabbit hearts, is there evidence that pretreatment with ischemia or a pharmacological agent affected infarct size, measured as the volume of heart muscle that dies?

	Infarct size, cm^3	
Group	Mean	SEM
Control	0.233	0.024
Ischemic preconditioning (PC)	0.069	0.015
α_1-Adrenergic receptor agonist (Phenylephrine)	0.065	0.008
Adenosine receptor antagonist (8-p-[sulfophenyl] theophylline)	0.240	0.033
α_1-Adrenergic receptor antagonist (Phenoxybenzamine)	0.180	0.033
Protein kinase C inhibitor (Polymyxin B)	0.184	0.038

3-5 Men and women differ in risk of spinal fracture. Men are at increased risk for all types of bone fractures until approximately 45 years of age, an effect probably due to the higher overall trauma rate in men during this time. However, after age 45, women are at increased risk for spinal fracture, most likely due to age-related increases in osteoporosis, a disease characterized by decreased bone density. S. Kudlacek and colleagues ("Gender Differences in Fracture Risk and Bone Mineral Density," *Maturitas,* **36:**173–180, 2000) wanted to investigate the relationship between gender and bone density in a group of older adults who have had a vertebral bone fracture. Their data are presented below. Are there differences in vertebral bone density between similarly aged men and women who have had a vertebral bone fracture?

	Vertebral bone density (mg/cm^3)		
Group	n	Mean	SEM
Women with bone fractures	50	70.3	2.55
Men with bone fractures	50	76.2	3.11

3-6 Burnout is a term that loosely describes a condition of fatigue, frustration, and anger manifested as a lack of enthusiasm for and feeling of entrapment in one's job. This situation can arise when treating people who have serious diseases. In recent years, AIDS has joined the list of diseases that may have a negative impact on professionals serving people suffering from this disease. To investigate whether there were differences in burnout associated with caring for people who have AIDS compared with other people who have serious diseases, J. López-Castillo and coworkers ("Emotional distress and occupational burnout in health care professionals serving HIV-infected patients: A comparison with oncology and internal medicine services," *Psychother. Psychosom.* **68:**348–356, 1999) administered the Maslach Burnout Inventory questionnaire to health professionals working in four clinical units: infectious disease, hemophilia, oncology, and internal medicine in Spain. (Ninety percent of the people in the infectious disease and 60 percent of the people in the hemophilia unit were HIV-positive.) Are there differences in burnout scores between health professionals working in these different units?

	Infectious Disease	Hemophilia	Oncology	Internal Medicine
Mean	46.1	35.0	44.4	47.9
Standard deviation	16.1	11.1	15.6	18.2
Sample size	25	25	25	25

3-7 High doses of estrogen interfere with male fertility in many animals, including mice. However, there may be significant differences in the response to estrogen in different mouse strains. To compare estrogen responsiveness in different strains of mice, Spearow and colleagues ("Genetic Variation in Susceptibility to Endocrine Disruption by Estrogen in Mice," *Science,* **285:**1259–1261, 1999) implanted capsules containing 1 μg of estrogen into four different strains of juvenile male mice. After 20 days, they measured their testicular weight. They found:

Mouse strain	*n*	Testes weight (mg)	
		Mean	SEM
CD-1	13	142	6
S15/Jls	16	82	3
C17/Jls	17	60	5
B6	15	38	3

Is there sufficient evidence to conclude that any of these strains differ in response to estrogen? (The formulas for analysis of variance with unequal sample sizes are in Appendix A.)

3-8 Several studies suggest that schizophrenic patients have lower IQ scores measured before the onset of schizophrenia (premorbid IQ) than would be expected based on family and environmental variables. These deficits can be detected during childhood and increase with age. Catherine Gilvarry and colleagues ("Premorbid IQ in Patients with Functional Psychosis and Their First-Degree Relatives," *Schizophr. Res.* **41:**417–429, 2000) investigated whether this was also the case with patients diagnosed with affective psychosis, which encompasses schizoaffective disorder, mania, and major depression. In addition, they also wanted to assess whether any IQ deficits could be detected in first-degree relatives (parents, siblings, and children) of patients with affective psychosis. They administered the National Adult Reading Test (NART), which is an indicator of premorbid IQ, to a set of patients with affective psychosis, their first-degree relatives, and a group of normal subjects without any psychiatric history. Gilvarry and colleagues also considered whether there was an obstetric complication (OC) during the birth of the psychotic patient, which is another risk factor for impaired intellectual development. Is there any evidence that NART scores differ among these groups of people? (The formulas for analysis of variance with unequal sample sizes are in Appendix A.)

Group	*n*	NART score	
		Mean	SD
Controls	50	112.7	7.8
Psychotic patients (no obstetric complications)	28	111.6	10.3
Relatives of psychotic patients (no obstetric complications)	25	114.3	12.1
Psychotic patients with obstetric complications	13	110.4	10.1
Relatives of psychotic patients with obstetric complications	19	116.4	8.8

Chapter 4

The Special Case of Two Groups: The *t* Test

As we have just seen in Chapter 3, many investigations require comparing only two groups. In addition, as the last example in Chapter 3 illustrated, when there are more than two groups, analysis of variance allows you to conclude only that the data are not consistent with the hypothesis that all the samples were drawn from a single population. It does not help you decide which one or ones are most likely to differ from the others. To answer these questions, we now develop a procedure that is specifically designed to test for differences in two groups: the *t test* or *Student's t test.* While we will develop the t test from scratch, we will eventually show that it is just a different way of doing an analysis of variance. In particular, we will see that $F = t^2$ when there are two groups.

The t test is the most common statistical procedure in the medical literature; you can expect it to appear in more than half the papers you read in the general medical literature. In addition to being used to compare two group means, it is widely applied incorrectly to compare multiple groups, by doing all the pairwise comparisons, for example, by comparing more than one intervention with a control condition or the state of a patient at different times following an intervention. Figure 4–1 shows the results of an analysis of the use of *t* tests for the clinical journal *Circulation;* 54 percent of all the papers used the *t* test, more often than not to analyze experiments for which it is not appropriate. As we will see, this incorrect use increases the chances of rejecting the null hypothesis of no effect above the nominal level, say 5 percent, used to select the cutoff value for a "big" value of the test statistic *t*. In practical terms, this boils down to increasing the chances of reporting that some therapy had an effect when the evidence does not support this conclusion.

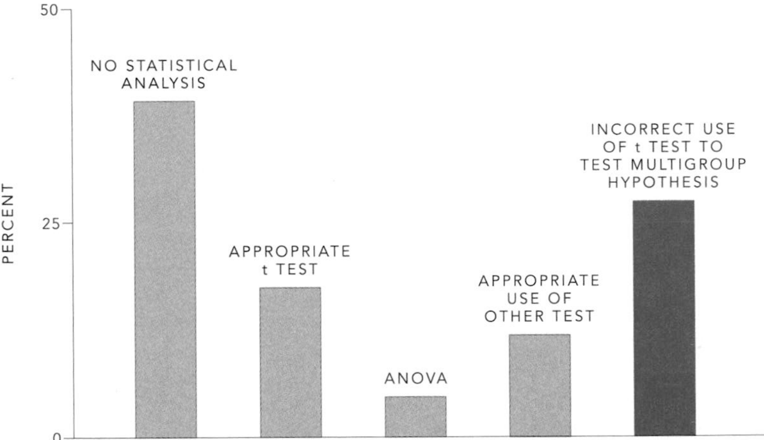

Figure 4–1 Of 142 original articles published in Vol. 56 of *Circulation* (excluding radiology, clinicopathologic, and case reports), 39 percent did not use statistics; 34 percent used a *t* test appropriately to compare two groups, analysis of variance (ANOVA), or other methods; and 27 percent used the *t* test incorrectly to compare more than two groups with each other. Twenty years later, misuse of the *t* test to compare more than two groups remained a common error in the biomedical literature. *(From S. A. Glantz, "How to Detect, Correct, and Prevent Errors in the Medical Literature,"* Circulation, ***61:****1–7, 1980. By permission of the American Heart Association, Inc.)*

THE GENERAL APPROACH

Suppose we wish to test a new drug that may be an effective diuretic. We assemble a group of 10 people and divide them at random into two groups, a control group that receives a placebo and a treatment group that receives the drug; then we measure their urine production for 24 h. Figure 4–2*A* shows the resulting data. The average urine production of the group receiving the diuretic is 240 mL higher than that of the group receiving the placebo. Simply looking at Fig. 4–2*A*, however, does not provide very convincing evidence that this difference is due to anything more than random sampling.

Nevertheless, we pursue the problem and give the placebo or drug to another 30 people to obtain the results shown in Fig. 4–2*B*. The mean responses of the two groups of people, as well as the standard deviations, are almost identical to those observed in the smaller samples shown in Fig. 4–2*A*. Even so, most observers are more confident in claiming that the diuretic increased average urine output from the data in Fig. 4–2*B* than the data in Fig. 4–2*A*, even though the samples in each case are good representatives of the underlying population. Why?

As the sample size increases, most observers become more confident in their estimates of the population means, so they can begin to discern a difference between the people taking the placebo or the drug. Recall that the standard error of the mean quantifies the uncertainty of the estimate of the true population mean based on a sample. Furthermore, as the sample size increases, the standard error of the mean decreases according to

$$\sigma_{\overline{X}} = \frac{\sigma}{\sqrt{n}}$$

where n is the sample size and σ is the standard deviation of the population from which the sample was drawn. As the sample size increases, the uncertainty in the estimate of the difference of the means between the people who received placebo and the patients who received the drug decreases relative to the difference of the means. As a result, we become more confident that the drug actually has an effect. More precisely, we become less confident in the hypothesis that the drug had no effect, in which case, the two samples of patients could be considered two samples drawn from a single population.

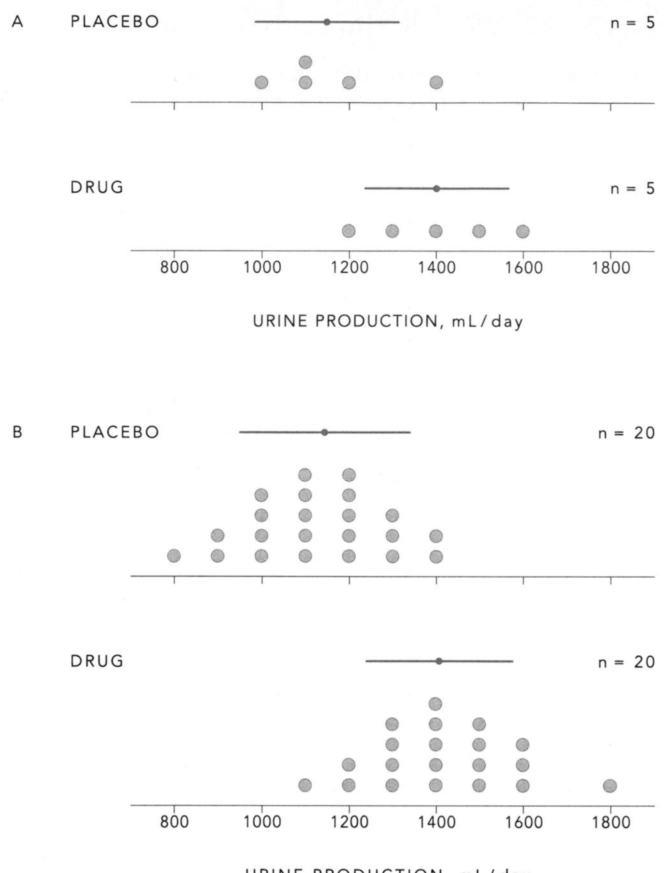

Figure 4–2 ***(A)*** Results of a study in which five people were treated with a placebo and five people were treated with a drug thought to increase daily urine production. On the average, the five people who received the drug produced more urine than the placebo group. Are these data convincing evidence that the drug is an effective diuretic? ***(B)*** Results of a similar study with 20 people in each treatment group. The means and standard deviations associated with the two groups are similar to the results in panel ***A***. Are these data convincing evidence that the drug is an effective diuretic? If you changed your mind, why did you do it?

To formalize this logic, we will examine the ratio

$$t = \frac{\text{difference in sample means}}{\text{standard error of difference of sample means}}$$

When this ratio is small, we will conclude that the data are compatible with the hypothesis that both samples were drawn from a single population. When this ratio is large, we will conclude that it is unlikely that the samples were drawn from a single population and assert that the treatment (e.g., the diuretic) produced an effect.

This logic, while differing in emphasis from that used to develop the analysis of variance, is essentially the same. In both cases, we are comparing the relative magnitude of the differences in the sample means with the amount of variability that would be expected from looking within the samples.

To compute the t ratio we need to know two things: the difference of the sample means and the standard error of this difference. Computing the difference of the sample means is easy; we simply subtract. Computing an estimate for the standard error of this difference is a bit more involved. We begin with a slightly more general problem, that of finding the standard deviation of the difference of two numbers drawn at random from the same population.

THE STANDARD DEVIATION OF A DIFFERENCE OR A SUM

Figure 4–3*A* shows a population with 200 members. The mean is 0, and the standard deviation is 1. Now, suppose we draw two samples at random and compute their difference. Figure 4–3*B* shows this result for the two members indicated by solid circles in panel *A*. Drawing five more pairs of samples (indicated by different symbols in panel *A*) and computing their differences yields the corresponding shaded points in panel *B*. Note that there seems to be more variability in the differences of the samples than in the samples themselves. Figure 4–3*C* shows the results of panel *B*, together with the results of drawing another 50 pairs of numbers at random and computing

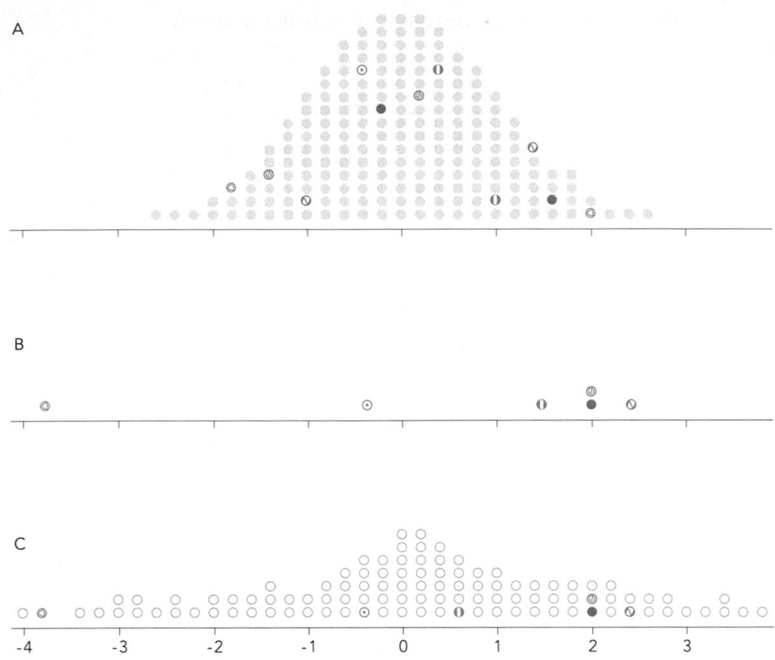

Figure 4–3 If one selects pairs of members of the population in panel ***A*** at random and computes the difference, the population of differences, shown in panel ***B***, has a wider variance than the original population. Panel ***C*** shows another 100 values for differences of pairs of members selected at random from the population in ***A*** to make this point again.

their differences. The standard deviation of the population of differences is about 40 percent larger than the standard deviation of the population from which the samples were drawn.

In fact, it is possible to demonstrate mathematically that *the variance of the difference (or sum) of two variables selected at random equals the sum of the variances of the two populations from which the samples were drawn.* In other words, if X is drawn from a population with standard deviation σ_X and Y is drawn from a population with standard deviation σ_Y, the distribution of all possible values of $X - Y$ (or $X + Y$) will have variance

$$\sigma^2_{X-Y} = \sigma^2_{X+Y} = \sigma^2_X + \sigma^2_Y$$

This result should seem reasonable to you because when you select pairs of values that are on opposite (the same) sides of the population mean and compute their difference (sum), the result will be even farther from the mean. Returning to the example in Fig. 4–3, we can observe that both the first and second numbers were drawn from the same population, whose variance was 1, and so the variance of the difference should be

$$\sigma^2_{X-Y} = \sigma^2_X + \sigma^2_Y = 1 + 1 = 2$$

Since the standard deviation is the square root of the variance, the standard deviation of the population of differences will be $\sqrt{2}$ times the standard deviation of the original population, or about 40 percent bigger, confirming our earlier subjective impression.*

When we wish to estimate the variance in the difference or sum of members of two populations based on the observations, we simply

*The fact that the sum of randomly selected variables has a variance equal to the sum of the variances of the individual numbers explains why the standard error of the mean equals the standard deviation divided by $\sqrt{n}$. Suppose we draw n numbers at random from a population with standard deviation σ. The mean of these numbers will be

$$\overline{X} = \frac{1}{n}(X_1 + X_2 + X_3 + \cdots + X_n)$$

so

$$n\overline{X} = X_1 + X_2 + X_3 + \cdots + X_n$$

Since the variance associated with each of the X_i's is a σ^2, the variance of $n\overline{X}$ will be

$$\sigma^2_{n\overline{X}} = \sigma^2 + \sigma^2 + \sigma^2 + \cdots + \sigma^2 = n\sigma^2$$

and the standard deviation will be

$$\sigma_{n\overline{X}} = \sqrt{n}\sigma$$

But we want the standard deviation of $\overline{X}$, which is $n\overline{X}/n$, therefore

$$\sigma_{\overline{X}} = \sqrt{n}\sigma/n = \sigma/\sqrt{n}$$

which is the formula for the standard error of the mean. Note that we made no assumptions about the population from which the sample was drawn. (In particular, we did *not* assume that it had a normal distribution.)

replace the population variances σ^2 in the equation above with the estimates of the variances computed from our samples.

$$s^2_{X-Y} = s^2_X + s^2_Y$$

The standard error of the mean is just the standard deviation of the population of all possible sample means of samples of size *n,* and so we can find the standard error of the difference of two means using the equation above. Specifically,

$$s^2_{\overline{X}-\overline{Y}} = s^2_{\overline{X}} + s^2_{\overline{Y}}$$

in which case

$$s_{\overline{X}-\overline{Y}} = \sqrt{s^2_{\overline{X}} + s^2_{\overline{Y}}}$$

Now we are ready to construct the *t* ratio from the definition in the last section.

USE OF *t* TO TEST HYPOTHESES ABOUT TWO GROUPS

Recall that we decided to examine the ratio

$$t = \frac{\text{difference in sample means}}{\text{standard error of difference of sample means}}$$

We can now use the result of the last section to translate this definition into the equation

$$t = \frac{\overline{X}_1 - \overline{X}_2}{\sqrt{\overline{X}_1 - \overline{X}_2}}$$

$$= \frac{\overline{X}_1 - \overline{X}_2}{\sqrt{s^2_{\overline{X}_1} + s^2_{\overline{X}_2}}}$$

Alternatively, we can write t in terms of the sample standard deviations rather than the standard errors of the mean

$$t = \frac{\bar{X}_1 - \bar{X}_2}{\sqrt{(s_1^2/n) + (s_2^2/n)}}$$

in which n is the size of each sample.

If the hypothesis that the two samples were drawn from the same population is true, the variances s_1^2 and s_2^2 computed from the two samples are both estimates of the same population variance σ^2. Therefore, we replace the two different estimates of the population variance in the equation above with a single estimate, s^2, that is obtained by averaging these two separate estimates

$$s^2 = \tfrac{1}{2}(s_1^2 + s_2^2)$$

This is called the *pooled-variance estimate* since it is obtained by pooling the two estimates of the population variance to obtain a single estimate. The t-test statistic based on the pooled-variance estimate is

$$t = \frac{\bar{X}_1 - \bar{X}_2}{\sqrt{(s^2/n) + (s^2/n)}}$$

The specific value of t one obtains from any two samples depends not only on whether or not there actually is a difference in the means of the populations from which the samples were drawn but also on which specific individuals happened to be selected for the samples. Thus, as for F, there will be a range of possible values that t can have, even when both samples are drawn from the same population. Since the means computed from the two samples will generally be close to the mean of the population from which they were drawn, the value of t will tend to be small when the two samples are drawn from the same population. Therefore, we will use the same procedure to test hypotheses with t as we did with F in Chapter 3. Specifically, we will compute t from the data, then reject the assertion that the two samples were drawn from the same population if the resulting value of t is "big."

Let us return to the problem of assessing the value of the diuretic we were discussing earlier. Suppose the entire population of interest contains 200 people. In addition, we will assume that the diuretic had no effect, so that the two groups of people being studied can be considered to represent two samples drawn from a single population. Figure 4–4*A* shows this population, together with two samples of 10 people each selected at random for study. The people who received the placebo

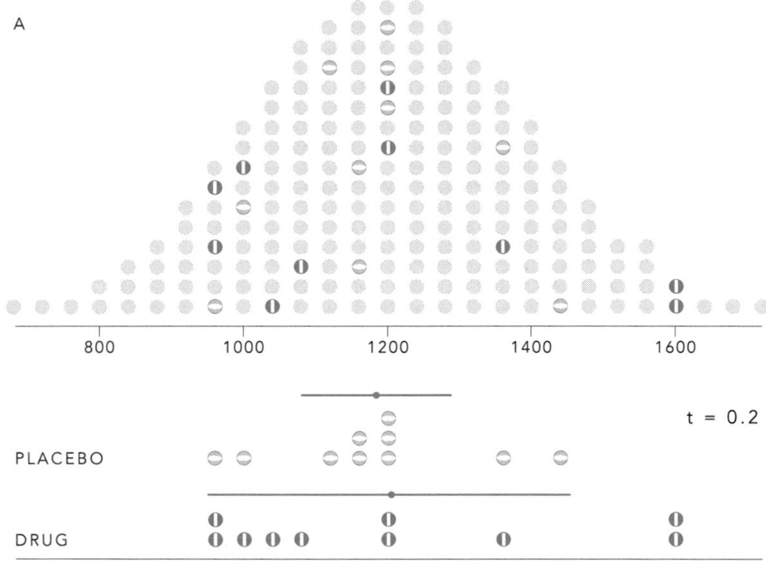

Figure 4–4 A population of 200 individuals and two groups selected at random for study of a drug designed to increase urine production but which is totally ineffective. The people shown as dark circles received the placebo and those with the lighter circles received the drug. An investigator would not see the entire population but just the information as reflected in the lower part of panel ***A***; nevertheless, the two samples show very little difference, and it is unlikely that one would have concluded that the drug had an effect on urine production. Of course, there is nothing special about the two random samples shown in panel ***A***, and an investigator could just as well have selected the two groups of people in panel ***B*** for study. There is more difference between these two groups than the two shown in panel ***A***, and there is a chance that the investigator would think that this difference is due to the drug's effect on urine production rather than simple random sampling. Panel ***C*** shows yet another pair of random samples the investigator might have drawn for the study.

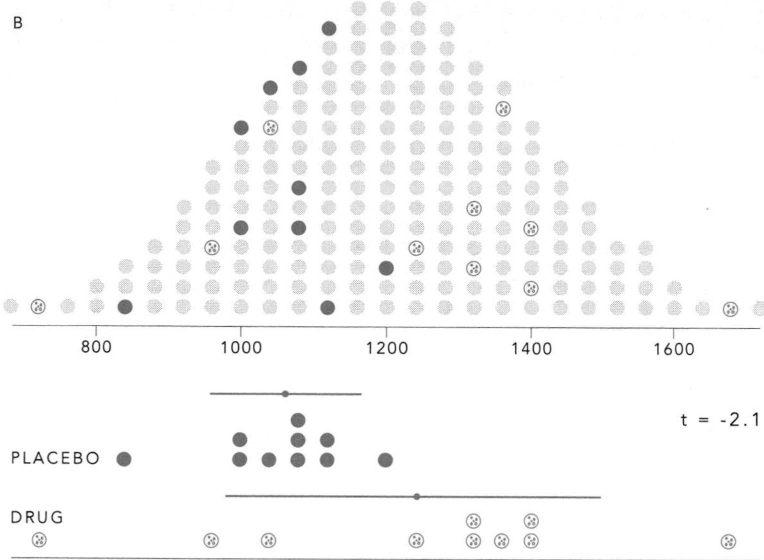

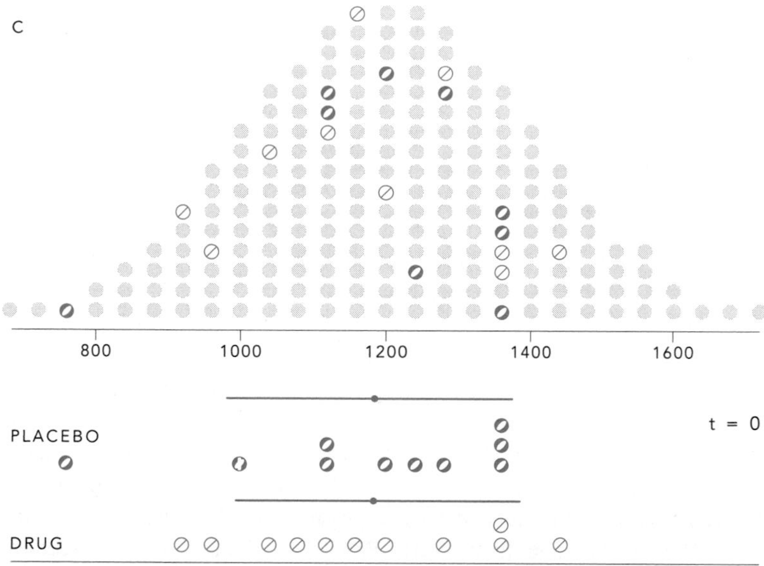

Figure 4–4 *Continued*

are shown as dark circles, and the people who received the diuretic are shown as lighter circles. The lower part of panel *A* shows the data as they would appear to the investigator, together with the mean and standard deviations computed from each of the two samples. Looking at these data certainly does not suggest that the diuretic had any effect. The value of t associated with these samples is -0.2.

Of course, there is nothing special about these two samples, and we could just as well have selected two different groups of people to study. Figure 4–4*B* shows another collection of people that could have been selected at random to receive the placebo (dark circles) or diuretic (light circles). Not surprisingly, these two samples differ from each other as well as the samples selected in panel *A*. Given only the data in the lower part of panel *B*, we might think that the diuretic increases urine production. The t value associated with these data is -2.1. Panel *C* shows yet another pair of samples. They differ from each other and the other samples considered in panels *A* and *B*. The samples in panel *C* yield a value of 0 for t.

We could continue this process for quite a long time since there are more than 10^{27} different pairs of samples of 10 people each that we could draw from the population of 200 individuals shown in Fig. 4–4*A*. We can compute a value of t for each of these 10^{27} different pairs of samples. Figure 4–5 shows the values of t associated with 200 different pairs of random samples of 10 people each drawn from the original population, including the three specific pairs of samples shown in Fig. 4–4. The distribution of possible t values is symmetrical about $t = 0$ because it does not matter which of the two samples we subtract from the other. As predicted, most of the resulting values of t are close to zero; t rarely is below about -2 or above $+2$.

Figure 4–5 allows us to determine what a "big" t is. Panel *B* shows that t will be less than -2.1 or greater than $+2.1$ 10 out of 200, or 5 percent of the time. In other words, there is only a 5 percent chance of getting a value of t more extreme than -2.1 or $+2.1$ when the two samples are drawn from the same population. Just as with the F distribution, the number of possible t values rapidly increases beyond 10^{27} as the population size grows, and the distribution of possible t values approaches a smooth curve. Figure 4–5*C* shows the result of this limiting process. We define the cutoff values for t that are large enough to be called "big" on the basis of the total area in the two tails. Panel *C* shows that only 5 percent of the possible values of t will lie beyond -2.1 or $+2.1$ when the two samples are drawn from a single population. When the data are associated

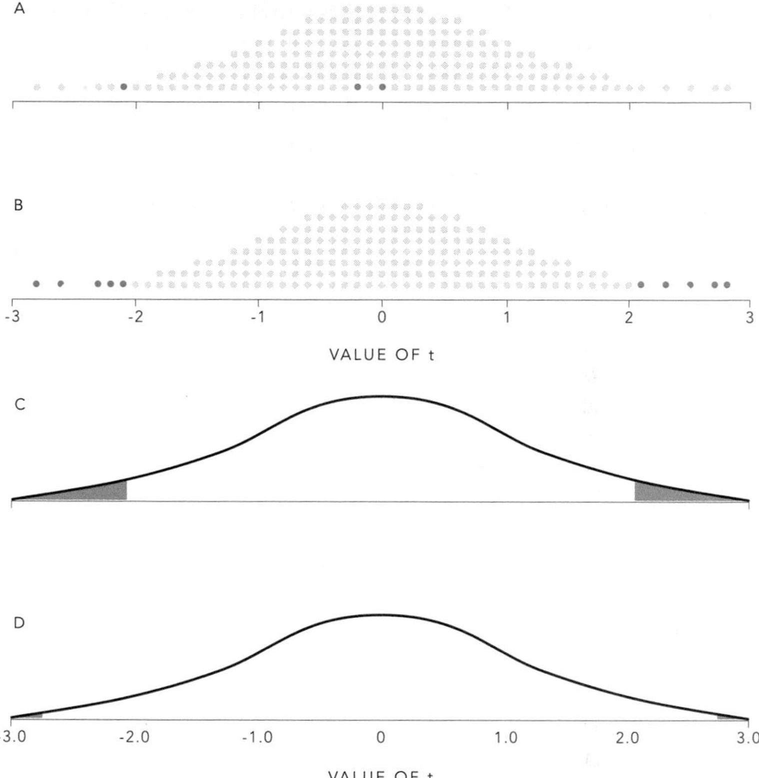

Figure 4–5 The results of 200 studies like that described in Fig. 4–4; the three specific studies from Fig. 4–4 are indicated in panel ***A***. Note that most values of the *t* statistic cluster around 0, but it is possible for some values of *t* to be quite large, exceeding 1.5 or 2. Panel ***B*** shows that there are only 5 chances in 100 of *t* exceeding 2.1 in magnitude if the two samples were drawn from the same population. If one continues examining all possible samples drawn from the population and our pairs of samples drawn from the same population, one obtains a distribution of all possible *t* values which becomes the smooth curve in panel ***C***. In this case, one defines the critical value of *t* by saying that it is unlikely that this value of *t* statistic was observed under the hypothesis that the drug had no effect by taking the 5 percent most extreme error areas under the tails of distribution and selecting the *t* value corresponding to the beginning of this region. Panel ***D*** shows that if one required a more stringent criterion for rejecting the hypothesis for no difference by requiring that *t* be in the most extreme 1 percent of all possible values, the cutoff value of *t* is 2.878.

with a value of t beyond this range, it is customary to conclude that the data are inconsistent with the null hypothesis of no difference between the two samples and report that there was a difference in treatment.

The extreme values of t that lead us to reject the hypothesis of no difference lie in both tails of the distribution. Therefore, the approach we are taking is sometimes called a *two-tailed t test.* Occasionally, people use a one-tailed t test, and there are indeed cases where this is appropriate. One should be suspicious of such one-tailed tests, however, because the cutoff value for calling t "big" for a given value of P is smaller. In reality, people are almost always looking for a *difference* between the control and treatment groups, and a two-tailed test is appropriate. This book always assumes a two-tailed test.

Note that the data in Fig. 4–4*B* are associated with a t value of -2.1, which we have decided to consider "big." If all we had were the data shown in Fig. 4–5*B*, we would conclude that the observations were inconsistent with the hypothesis that the diuretic had no effect and report that it *increased* urine production, and even though we did the statistical analysis correctly, *our conclusion about the drug would be wrong.*

Reporting $P < .05$ means that if the treatment had no effect, there is less than a 5 percent chance of getting a value of t from the data as far or farther from 0 as the critical value for t to be called "big." It does not mean it is impossible to get such a large value of t when the treatment has no effect. We could, of course, be more conservative and say that we will reject the hypothesis of no difference between the populations from which the samples were drawn if t is in the most extreme 1 percent of possible values. Figure 4–5*D* shows that this would require t to be beyond -2.88 or $+2.88$ in this case, so we would not erroneously conclude that the drug had an effect on urine output in any of the specific examples shown in Fig. 4–4. In the long run, however, we will make such errors about 1 percent of the time. The price of this conservatism is decreasing the chances of concluding that there is a difference when one really exists. Chapter 6 discusses this trade-off in more detail.

The critical values of t, like F, have been tabulated and depend not only on the level of confidence with which one rejects the hypothesis of no difference—the P value—but also on the sample size. As with the F distribution, this dependence on sample size enters the table as the *degrees of freedom* ν, which is equal to $2(n - 1)$ for this t test, where n is the size of each sample. As the sample size increases, the value of t needed to reject the hypothesis of no difference decreases. In other words, as sample size increases, it becomes possible to detect smaller differences with a given level of confidence. Reflecting on Fig. 4–2 should convince you that this is reasonable.

WHAT IF THE TWO SAMPLES ARE NOT THE SAME SIZE?

It is easy to generalize the t test to handle problems in which there are different numbers of members in the two samples being studied. Recall that t is defined by

$$t = \frac{\bar{X}_1 - \bar{X}_2}{\sqrt{s_{\bar{X}_1}^2 + s_{\bar{X}_2}^2}}$$

in which $s_{\bar{X}_1}$ and $s_{\bar{X}_2}$ are the standard errors of the means of the two samples. If the first sample is of size n_1 and the second sample contains n_2 members,

$$s_{\bar{X}_1}^2 = \frac{s_1^2}{n_1} \quad \text{and} \quad s_{\bar{X}_2}^2 = \frac{s_2^2}{n_2}$$

in which s_1 and s_2 are the standard deviations of the two samples. Use these definitions to rewrite the definition of t in terms of the sample standard deviations

$$t = \frac{\bar{X}_1 - \bar{X}_2}{\sqrt{(s_1^2/n_1) + (s_2^2/n_2)}}$$

When the two samples are different sizes, the pooled estimate of the variance is given by

$$s^2 = \frac{(n_1 - 1)s_1^2 + (n_2 - 1)s_2^2}{n_1 + n_2 - 2}$$

so that

$$t = \frac{\bar{X}_1 - \bar{X}_2}{\sqrt{(s^2/n_1) + (s^2/n_2)}}$$

This is the definition of t for comparing two samples of unequal size. There are $\nu = n_1 + n_2 - 2$ degrees of freedom.

Notice that this result reduces to our earlier results when the two sample sizes are equal, that is, when $n_1 = n_2 = n$.

THE EXAMPLES REVISITED

We can now use the t test to analyze the data from the examples we discussed in Chap. 3 to illustrate analysis of variance. The conclusions will be no different from those obtained with analysis of variance because, as already stated, the t test is just a special case of analysis of variance.

Glucose Levels in Children of Parents with Diabetes

From Fig. 3–7, the 25 children of parents with type II diabetes had an average fasting glucose level of 86.1 mg/dL and the 25 children of parents without diabetes had an average fasting glucose level of 82.2 mg/dL. The standard deviations for both these groups were 2.09 and 2.49 mg/dL, respectively. Since the sample sizes are equal, the pooled estimate for the variance is $s^2 = 1/2\,(2.09^2 + 2.49^2) = 5.28\ (\text{mg/dL})^2$.

$$t = \frac{86.1 - 82.2}{\sqrt{(5.28/25) + (5.28/25)}} = 6.001$$

with $\nu = 2(n - 1) = 2(25 - 1) = 48$. Table 4–1 shows that, for 48 degrees of freedom, the magnitude of t will exceed 2.011 only 5 percent of the time, and 2.682 only 1 percent of the time when the two samples are drawn from the same population. Since the magnitude of t associated with our data exceed 2.682, we conclude that the children of parents with type II diabetes have significantly higher fasting glucose levels than children of parents without type II diabetes ($P < .01$).

Halothane versus Morphine for Open-Heart Surgery

Figure 3–8 showed that the lowest mean arterial blood pressure between the start of anesthesia and the beginning of the incision was 66.9 mmHg in the 61 patients anesthetized with halothane and 73.2 in the 61 patients anesthetized with morphine. The standard deviations of the blood pressures in the two groups of patients was 12.2 and 14.4 mmHg, respectively. Thus,

$$s^2 = \tfrac{1}{2}(12.2^2 + 14.4^2) = 178.1 \text{ mmHg}^2$$

and

$$t = \frac{66.9 - 73.2}{\sqrt{(178.1/61) + (178.1/61)}} = -2.607$$

with $\nu = 2(n - 1) = 2(61 - 1) = 120$ degrees of freedom. Table 4–1 shows that the magnitude to t should exceed 2.358 only 2 percent of the time when the two samples are drawn from a single population, as they would be if halothane and morphine both affected patients' blood pressure similarly. Since the magnitude of the value of t associated with the observations exceeds this value, we conclude that halothane is associated with a lower lowest mean arterial pressure than morphine, on the average.

Conahan and colleagues also measured the amount of blood being pumped by the heart in some of the patients they anesthetized to obtain another measure of how the two anesthetic agents affected cardiac function in people having heart-valve replacement surgery. To normalize the measurements to account for the fact that patients are different sizes and hence have different-sized hearts and blood flows, they computed the cardiac index, which is defined as the rate at which the heart pumps blood (the cardiac output) divided by body surface area. Table 4–2 reproduces some of their results. Morphine seems to produce lower cardiac indexes than halothane, but is this difference large enough to reject the hypothesis that the difference reflects random sampling rather than an actual physiological difference?

From the information in Table 4–2, the pooled estimate of the variance is

$$s^2 = \frac{(9 - 1)(1.05^2) + (16 - 1)(.88^2)}{9 + 16 - 2} = 0.89$$

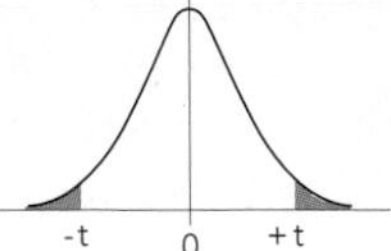

Table 4–1 Critical Values of *t* (Two-Tailed)

ν	Probability of greater value, *P*								
	0.50	0.20	0.10	0.05	0.02	0.01	0.005	0.002	0.001
1	1.000	3.078	6.314	12.706	31.821	63.657	127.321	318.309	636.619
2	0.816	1.886	2.920	4.303	6.965	9.925	14.089	22.327	31.599
3	0.765	1.638	2.353	3.182	4.541	5.841	7.453	10.215	12.924
4	0.741	1.533	2.132	2.776	3.747	4.604	5.598	7.173	8.610
5	0.727	1.476	2.015	2.571	3.365	4.032	4.773	5.893	6.869
6	0.718	1.440	1.943	2.447	3.143	3.707	4.317	5.208	5.959
7	0.711	1.415	1.895	2.365	2.998	3.449	4.029	4.785	5.408
8	0.706	1.397	1.860	2.306	2.896	3.355	3.833	4.501	5.041
9	0.703	1.383	1.833	2.262	2.821	3.250	3.690	4.297	4.781
10	0.700	1.372	1.812	2.228	2.764	3.169	3.581	4.144	4.587
11	0.697	1.363	1.796	2.201	2.718	3.106	3.497	4.025	4.437
12	0.695	1.356	1.782	2.179	2.681	3.055	3.428	3.930	4.318
13	0.694	1.350	1.771	2.160	2.650	3.012	3.372	3.852	4.221
14	0.692	1.345	1.761	2.145	2.624	2.977	3.326	3.787	4.140
15	0.691	1.341	1.753	2.131	2.602	2.947	3.286	3.733	4.073
16	0.690	1.337	1.746	2.120	2.583	2.921	3.252	3.686	4.015
17	0.689	1.333	1.740	2.110	2.567	2.898	3.222	3.646	3.965
18	0.688	1.330	1.734	2.101	2.552	2.878	3.197	3.610	3.922
19	0.688	1.328	1.729	2.093	2.539	2.861	3.174	3.579	3.883
20	0.687	1.325	1.725	2.086	2.528	2.845	3.153	3.552	3.850
21	0.686	1.323	1.721	2.080	2.518	2.831	3.135	3.527	3.819
22	0.686	1.321	1.717	2.074	2.508	2.819	3.119	3.505	3.792
23	0.685	1.319	1.714	2.069	2.500	2.807	3.104	3.485	3.768
24	0.685	1.318	1.711	2.064	2.492	2.797	3.091	3.467	3.745
25	0.684	1.316	1.708	2.060	2.485	2.787	3.078	3.450	3.725
26	0.684	1.315	1.706	2.056	2.479	2.779	3.067	3.435	3.707
27	0.684	1.314	1.703	2.052	2.473	2.771	3.057	3.421	3.690
28	0.683	1.313	1.701	2.048	2.467	2.763	3.047	3.408	3.674
29	0.683	1.311	1.699	2.045	2.462	2.756	3.038	3.396	3.659
30	0.683	1.310	1.697	2.042	2.457	2.750	3.030	3.385	3.646
31	0.682	1.309	1.696	2.040	2.453	2.744	3.022	3.375	3.633
32	0.682	1.309	1.694	2.037	2.449	2.738	3.015	3.365	3.622
33	0.682	1.308	1.692	2.035	2.445	2.733	3.008	3.356	3.611
34	0.682	1.307	1.691	2.032	2.441	2.728	3.002	3.348	3.601
35	0.682	1.306	1.690	2.030	2.438	2.724	2.996	3.340	3.591

(*continued*)

Table 4–1 Critical Values of *t* (Two-Tailed) (*Continued*)

	Probability of greater value, *P*								
ν	0.50	0.20	0.10	0.05	0.02	0.01	0.005	0.002	0.001
36	0.681	1.306	1.688	2.028	2.434	2.719	2.990	3.333	3.582
37	0.681	1.305	1.687	2.026	2.431	2.715	2.985	3.326	3.574
38	0.681	1.304	1.686	2.024	2.429	2.712	2.980	3.319	3.566
39	0.681	1.304	1.685	2.023	2.426	2.708	2.976	3.313	3.558
40	0.681	1.303	1.684	2.021	2.423	2.704	2.971	3.307	3.551
42	0.680	1.302	1.682	2.018	2.418	2.698	2.963	3.296	3.538
44	0.680	1.301	1.680	2.015	2.414	2.692	2.956	3.286	3.526
46	0.680	1.300	1.679	2.013	2.410	2.687	2.949	3.277	3.515
48	0.680	1.299	1.677	2.011	2.407	2.682	2.943	3.269	3.505
50	0.679	1.299	1.676	2.009	2.403	2.678	2.937	2.261	3.496
52	0.679	1.298	1.675	2.007	2.400	2.674	2.932	3.255	3.488
54	0.679	1.297	1.674	2.005	2.397	2.670	2.927	3.248	3.480
56	0.679	1.297	1.673	2.003	2.395	2.667	2.923	3.242	3.473
58	0.679	1.296	1.672	2.002	2.392	2.663	2.918	3.237	3.466
60	0.679	1.296	1.671	2.000	2.390	2.660	2.915	3.232	3.460
62	0.678	1.295	1.670	1.999	2.388	2.657	2.911	3.227	3.454
64	0.678	1.295	1.669	1.998	2.386	2.655	2.908	3.223	3.449
66	0.678	1.295	1.668	1.997	2.384	2.652	2.904	3.218	3.444
68	0.678	1.294	1.668	1.995	2.382	2.650	2.902	3.214	3.439
70	0.678	1.294	1.667	1.994	2.381	2.648	2.899	3.211	3.435
72	0.678	1.293	1.666	1.993	2.379	2.646	2.896	3.207	3.431
74	0.678	1.293	1.666	1.993	2.378	2.644	2.894	3.204	3.427
76	0.678	1.293	1.665	1.992	2.376	2.642	2.891	3.201	3.423
78	0.678	1.292	1.665	1.991	2.375	2.640	2.889	3.198	3.420
80	0.678	1.292	1.664	1.990	2.374	2.639	2.887	3.195	3.416
90	0.677	1.291	1.662	1.987	2.368	2.632	2.878	3.183	3.402
100	0.677	1.290	1.660	1.984	2.364	2.626	2.871	3.174	3.390
120	0.677	1.289	1.658	1.980	2.358	2.617	2.860	3.160	3.373
140	0.676	1.288	1.656	1.977	2.353	2.611	2.852	3.149	3.361
160	0.676	1.287	1.654	1.975	2.350	2.607	2.846	3.142	3.352
180	0.676	1.286	1.653	1.973	2.347	2.603	2.842	3.136	3.345
200	0.676	1.286	1.653	1.972	2.345	2.601	2.839	3.131	3.340
∞	0.6745	1.2816	1.6449	1.9600	2.3263	2.5758	2.8070	3.0902	3.2905
Normal	0.6745	1.2816	1.6449	1.9600	2.3263	2.5758	2.8070	3.0902	3.2905

Source: Adapted from J. H. Zar, *Biostatistical Analysis* (2 ed.), Prentice-Hall, Englewood Cliffs, N.J., 1984, pp. 484–485, table B.3. Used by permission.

Table 4–2 Comparison of Anesthetic Effects on the Cardiovascular System

	Halothane ($n = 9$)		Morphine ($n = 16$)	
	Mean	SD	Mean	SD
Best cardiac index, induction to bypass, $L/m^2 \cdot min$	2.08	1.05	1.75	.88
Mean arterial blood pressure at time of best cardiac index, mmHg	76.8	13.8	91.4	19.6
Total peripheral resistance associated with best cardiac index, $dyn \cdot s/cm^5$	2210	1200	2830	1130

Source: Adapted from T. J. Conahan et al., "A Prospective Random Comparison of Halothane and Morphine for Open-Heart Anesthesia," *Anesthesiology*, **38:**528–535, 1973.

and so

$$t = \frac{2.08 - 1.75}{\sqrt{(.89/9) + (.89/16)}} = 0.84$$

which does not exceed the 5 percent critical value of 2.069 for $\nu = n_{hlo} + n_{mor} - 2 = 9 + 16 - 2 = 23$ degrees of freedom. Hence, we do not have strong enough evidence to assert that there is really a difference in cardiac index with the two anesthetics. Does this *prove* that there really was not a difference? No. It just means that we do not have strong enough evidence to reject the null hypothesis of no difference.

THE t TEST IS AN ANALYSIS OF VARIANCE*

The t test we just developed and analysis of variance we developed in Chapter 3 are really two different ways of doing the same thing. Since few people recognize this, we will prove that when comparing the

*This section represents the only mathematical proof in this book and as such is a bit more technical than everything else. The reader can skip this section with no loss of continuity.

means of two groups, $F = t^2$. In other words, the *t* test is simply a special case of analysis of variance applied to two groups.

We begin with two samples, each of size *n*, with means and standard deviations $\overline{X}_1$ and $\overline{X}_2$ and s_1 and s_2, respectively.

To form the *F* ratio used in analysis of variance, we first estimate the population variance as the average of the variances computed for each group

$$s^2_{\text{wit}} = \tfrac{1}{2}(s_1^2 + s_2^2)$$

Next, we estimate the population variance from the sample means by computing the standard deviation of the sample means with

$$s_{\overline{X}} = \sqrt{\frac{(\overline{X}_1 - \overline{X})^2 + (\overline{X}_2 - \overline{X})^2}{2 - 1}}$$

Therefore

$$s^2_{\overline{X}} = (\overline{X}_1 - \overline{X})^2 + (\overline{X}_2 - \overline{X})^2$$

in which $\overline{X}$ is the mean of the two sample means

$$\overline{X} = \tfrac{1}{2}(\overline{X}_1 + \overline{X}_2)$$

Eliminate $\overline{X}$ from the equation for $s^2_{\overline{X}}$ to obtain

$$s^2_{\overline{X}} = [\overline{X}_1 - \tfrac{1}{2}(\overline{X}_1 + \overline{X}_2)]^2 + [\overline{X}_2 - \tfrac{1}{2}(\overline{X}_1 + \overline{X}_2)]^2$$

$$= (\tfrac{1}{2}\overline{X}_1 - \tfrac{1}{2}\overline{X}_2)^2 + (\tfrac{1}{2}\overline{X}_2 - \tfrac{1}{2}\overline{X}_1)^2$$

Since the square of a number is always positive, $(a - b)^2 = (b - a)^2$ and the equation above becomes

$$s_{\bar{X}}^2 = (\tfrac{1}{2}\,\bar{X}_1 - \tfrac{1}{2}\,\bar{X}_2)^2 + (\tfrac{1}{2}\,\bar{X}_1 - \tfrac{1}{2}\,\bar{X}_2)^2$$

$$= 2[\tfrac{1}{2}\,(\bar{X}_1 - \bar{X}_2)]^2 = \tfrac{1}{2}\,(\bar{X}_1 - \bar{X}_2)^2$$

Therefore, the estimate of the population variance from between the groups is

$$s_{\text{bet}}^2 = n s_{\bar{X}}^2 = (n/2)(\bar{X}_1 - \bar{X}_2)^2$$

Finally, F is the ratio of these two estimates of the population variance

$$F = \frac{s_{\text{bet}}^2}{s_{\text{wit}}^2} = \frac{(n/2)(\bar{X}_1 - \bar{X}_2)^2}{\tfrac{1}{2}\,(s_1^2 + s_2^2)} = \frac{(\bar{X}_1 - \bar{X}_2)^2}{(s_1^2/n) + (s_2^2/n)}$$

$$= \left[\frac{\bar{X}_1 - \bar{X}_2}{\sqrt{(s_1^2/n) + (s_2^2/n)}}\right]^2$$

The quantity in the brackets is t, hence

$$F = t^2$$

The degrees of freedom for the numerator of F equals the number of groups minus 1, that is, $2 - 1 = 1$ for all comparisons of two groups. The degrees of freedom for the denominator equals the number of groups times 1 less than the sample size of each group, $2(n - 1)$, which is the same as the degrees of freedom associated with the t test.

In sum, the t test and analysis of variance are just two different ways of looking at the same test for two groups. Of course, if there are more than two groups, one cannot use the t-test form of analysis of variance but must use the more general form we developed in Chapter 3.

COMMON ERRORS IN THE USE OF THE *t* TEST AND HOW TO COMPENSATE FOR THEM

The *t* test is used to compute the probability of being wrong, the *P* value, when asserting that the mean values of *two* treatment groups are different, when, in fact, they were drawn from the same population. We have already seen (Fig. 4–1) that it is also used widely but erroneously to test for differences between more than two groups by comparing all possible pairs of means with *t* tests.

For example, suppose an investigator measured blood sugar under control conditions, in the presence of drug A, and in the presence of drug B. It is common to perform three *t* tests on these data: one to compare control versus drug A, one to compare control versus drug B, and one to compare drug A versus drug B. This practice is incorrect because the true probability of erroneously concluding that the drug affected blood sugar is actually higher than the nominal level, say 5 percent, used when looking up the "big" cutoff value of the *t* statistic in a table.

To understand why, reconsider the experiment described in the last paragraph. Suppose that if the value of the *t* statistic computed in one of the three comparisons just described is in the most extreme 5 percent of the values that would occur if the drugs really had no effect, we will reject that assumption and assert that the drugs changed blood sugar. We will be satisfied if $P < .05$; in other words, in the long run we are willing to accept the fact that 1 statement in 20 will be wrong. Therefore, when we test control versus drug A, we can expect erroneously to assert a difference 5 percent of the time. Similarly, when testing control versus drug B, we expect erroneously to assert a difference 5 percent of the time, and when testing drug A versus drug B, we expect erroneously to assert a difference 5 percent of the time. Therefore, when considering the three tests together, we expect to conclude that at least one pair of groups differs about 5 percent + 5 percent + 5 percent = 15 percent of the time, even if in reality the drugs did not affect blood sugar (*P* actually equals 14 percent). If there are not too many comparisons, simply adding the *P* values obtained in multiple tests produces a realistic and conservative estimate of the true *P* value for the set of comparisons.

In the example above, there were three *t* tests, so the effective *P* value was about $3(.05) = .15$, or 15 percent. When comparing four groups, there are six possible *t* tests (1 versus 2, 1 versus 3, 1 versus 4, 2 versus 3, 2 versus 4, 3 versus 4); so if the author concludes that there is a difference and reports $P < .05$, the effective P value is about $6(.05) = .30$; there is about a 30 percent chance of at least one incorrect statement if the author concludes that the treatments had an effect!

In Chapter 2, we discussed random samples of Martians to illustrate the fact that different samples from the same population yield different estimates of the population mean and standard deviation. Figure 2–8 showed three such samples of the heights of Martians, all drawn from a single population. Suppose we chose to study how these Martians respond to human hormones. We draw three samples at random, give one group a placebo, one group testosterone, and one group estrogen. Suppose that these hormones have no effect on the Martians' heights. Thus, the three groups shown in Fig. 2–8 represent three samples drawn at random from the same population.

Figure 4–6 shows how these data would probably appear in a typical medical journal. The large vertical bars denote the value of the mean responses, and the small vertical bars denote 1 standard error of the mean above or below the sample means. (Showing 1 standard deviation would be the appropriate way to describe variability in the samples.) Most authors would analyze these data by performing three t tests: placebo against testosterone, placebo against estrogen, and testosterone against estrogen. These three tests yield t values of 2.39, 0.93, and 1.34, respectively. Since each test is based on 2 samples of 10 Martians each, there are $2(10 - 1) = 18$ degrees of freedom. From Table 4–1, the critical value of t with a 5 percent chance of erroneously concluding that a difference exists is 2.101. Thus, the author would conclude that testosterone produced shorter Martians than placebo, whereas estrogen did not differ significantly from placebo, and that the two hormones did not produce significantly different results.

Think about this result for a moment. What is wrong with it? If testosterone produced results not detectably different from those of estrogen and estrogen produced results not detectably different from those of placebo, how can testosterone have produced results different from placebo? Far from alerting medical researchers that there is something wrong with their analysis, this illogical result usually leads to a very creatively written "Discussion" section in their paper.

An analysis of variance of these data yields $F = 2.74$ [with numerator degrees of freedom $= m - 1 = 3 - 1 = 2$ and denominator degrees of

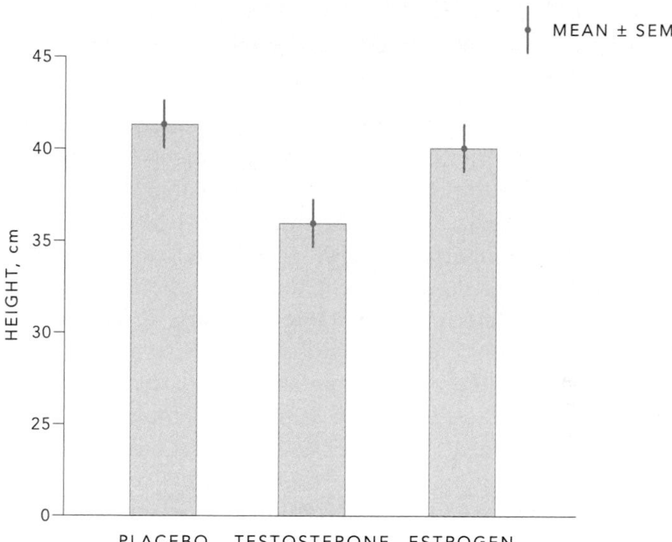

Figure 4–6 Results of a study of human hormones on Martians as it would be commonly presented in the medical literature. Each large bar has a height equal to the mean of the group; the small vertical bars indicate 1 standard error of the mean on either side of the mean (not 1 standard deviation).

freedom $m(n - 1) = 3(10 - 1) = 27$], which is below the critical value of 3.35 we have decided is required to assert that the data are incompatible with the hypothesis that all three treatments acted as placebos.

Of course, performing an analysis of variance does not ensure that we will not reach a conclusion that is actually wrong, but it will make it less likely.

We end our discussion of common errors in the use of the *t* test with three rules of thumb.

- *The* t *test can be used to test the hypothesis that two group means are not different.*
- *When the experimental design involves multiple groups, analysis of variance should be used.*
- *When* t *tests are used to test for differences between multiple groups, you can estimate the true* P *value by multiplying the reported* P *value times the number of possible* t *tests.*

HOW TO USE *t* TESTS TO ISOLATE DIFFERENCES BETWEEN GROUPS IN ANALYSIS OF VARIANCE

The last section demonstrated that when presented with data from experiments with more than two groups of subjects, one must do an analysis of variance to determine how inconsistent the observations are with the hypothesis that all the treatments had the same effect. Doing pairwise comparisons with t tests increases the chances of erroneously reporting an effect above the nominal value, say 5 percent, used to determine the value of a "big" t. The analysis of variance, however, only tests the global hypothesis that *all* the samples were drawn from a single population. In particular, it does not provide any information on which sample or samples differed from the others.

There are a variety of methods, called *multiple-comparison procedures,* that can be used to provide information on this point. All are essentially based on the t test but include appropriate corrections for the fact that we are comparing more than one pair of means. We will develop several approaches, beginning with the *Bonferroni t test.* The general approach we take is first to perform an analysis of variance to see whether *anything* appears different, then use a multiple-comparison procedure to isolate the treatment or treatments producing the different results.*

The Bonferroni *t* Test

In the last section, we saw that if one analyzes a set of data with three t tests, each using the 5 percent critical value for concluding that there is a difference, there is about a 3(5) = 15 percent chance of finding it. This result is a special case of a formula called the *Bonferroni inequality,* which states that if k statistical tests are performed with the cutoff value for the test statistics, for example, t or F, at the α level, the likelihood of observing a value of the test statistic exceeding the cutoff

*Some statisticians believe that this approach is too conservative and that one should skip the analysis of variance and proceed directly to the multiple comparisons of interest. For an introductory treatment from this perspective, see Byron W. Brown, Jr., and Myles Hollander, *Statistics: A Biomedical Introduction,* Wiley, New York, 1977, chap. 10, "Analysis of k-Sample Problems."

value at least once when the treatments did not produce an effect is no greater than k times α. Mathematically, the Bonferroni inequality states

$$\alpha_T < k\alpha$$

where α_T is the true probability of erroneously concluding a difference exists at least once. α_T is the error rate we want to control. From the equation above,

$$\frac{\alpha_T}{k} < \alpha$$

Thus, if we do *each* of the t tests using the critical value of t corresponding to α_T / k, the error rate for *all* the comparisons taken as a group will be at most α_T. For example, if we wish to do three comparisons with t tests while keeping the probability of making at least one false-positive error to less than 5 percent, we use the t value corresponding to $.05/3 = 1.6$ percent for each of the individual comparisons. This procedure is called the *Bonferroni t test* because it is based on the Bonferroni inequality.

This procedure works reasonably well when there are only a few groups to compare, but as the number of comparisons k increases above 3 or 4, the value of t required to conclude that a difference exists becomes much larger than it really needs to be and the method becomes overconservative. Other multiple-comparison procedures, such as the Holm test (discussed in the next section), are less conservative. All, however, are similar to the Bonferroni t test in that they are essentially modifications of the t test to account for the fact that we are making multiple comparisons.

One way to make the Bonferroni t test less conservative is to use the estimate of the population variance computed from within the groups in the analysis of variance. Specifically, recall that we defined t as

$$t = \frac{\bar{X}_1 - \bar{X}_2}{\sqrt{(s^2/n_1) + (s^2/n_2)}}$$

where s^2 is an estimate of the population variance. We will replace this estimate with the population variance estimated from within the groups as part of the analysis of variance, s^2_{wit}, to obtain

$$t = \frac{\bar{X}_1 - \bar{X}_2}{\sqrt{(s^2_{\text{wit}}/n_1) + (s^2_{\text{wit}}/n_2)}}$$

When the sample sizes are equal, the equation becomes

$$t = \frac{\bar{X}_1 - \bar{X}_2}{\sqrt{2s^2_{\text{wit}}/n}}$$

The degrees of freedom for this test are the same as the denominator degrees of freedom for the analysis of variance and will be higher than for a simple t test based on the two samples being compared.* Since the critical value of t decreases as the degrees of freedom increase, it will be possible to detect a difference with a given confidence with smaller absolute differences in the means.

More on Menstruation and Jogging

In Chapter 3 we analyzed the data in Fig. 3–9 and concluded that they were inconsistent with the hypothesis that a control group, a group of joggers, and a group of runners had on the average the same number of menstrual periods per year. At the time, however, we were unable to isolate where the difference came from. Now we can use our Bonferroni t test to compare the three groups pairwise.

Recall that our best estimate of the within-groups variance s^2_{wit} is 3.95 (menses/year)^2. There are $m = 3$ samples, each containing $n = 26$ women. Therefore, there are $m(n - 1) = 3(26 - 1) = 75$ degrees of freedom associated with the estimate of the within-groups variance. [By comparison, if we just used the pooled variance from the two samples, there would be only $2\ (n - 1) = 2(26 - 1) = 50$ degrees of

*The number of degrees of freedom is the same if there are only two groups.

freedom.] Therefore, we can compare the three different groups by computing three values of t. To compare control with the joggers, we compute

$$t = \frac{\bar{X}_{\text{jog}} - \bar{X}_{\text{con}}}{\sqrt{2s_{\text{wit}}^2/n}} = \frac{10.1 - 11.5}{\sqrt{2(3.95)/26}} = -2.54$$

To compare the control group with the runners, we compute

$$t = \frac{\bar{X}_{\text{run}} - \bar{X}_{\text{con}}}{\sqrt{2s_{\text{wit}}^2/n}} = \frac{9.1 - 11.5}{\sqrt{2(3.95)/26}} = -4.35$$

To compare the joggers with the runners, we compute

$$t = \frac{\bar{X}_{\text{jog}} - \bar{X}_{\text{run}}}{\sqrt{2s_{\text{wit}}^2/n}} = \frac{10.1 - 9.1}{\sqrt{2(3.95)/26}} = 1.81$$

There are three comparisons, so to have an overall error rate of less than 5 percent we compare each of these values of t with the critical value of t associated with the $.05/3 = 1.6$ percent level and 75 degrees of freedom. Interpolating* in Table 4–1 shows this value to be about 2.45.

Thus, we have sufficient evidence to conclude that both jogging and running decrease the frequency of menstruation, but we do not have evidence that running decreases menstruation any more than simply jogging.

A Better Approach to Multiple Comparisons: The Holm *t* Test

There have been several refinements of the Bonferroni t test designed to maintain the computational simplicity while avoiding the excessive caution that the Bonferroni correction brings, beginning with the *Holm t test.*†

*Appendix A describes how to interpolate.

†S. Holm, "A Simple Sequentially Rejective Multiple Test Procedure," *Scand. J. Stat.*, **6**:65–70, 1979.

The Holm test is nearly as easy to compute as the Bonferroni t test, but is more powerful.* The Holm test is a so-called sequentially rejective, or step-down, procedure because it applies an accept/reject criterion to a set of ordered null hypotheses, starting with the smallest P value, and proceeding until it fails to reject a null hypothesis.

To perform the Holm t test, we compute the family of pairwise comparisons of interest (with t tests using the pooled variance estimate from the analysis of variance as we did with the Bonferroni t test) and determine the *unadjusted P* value for each test in the family. We then compare these P values (or the corresponding t values) to critical values that have been adjusted to allow for the fact that we are doing multiple comparisons. In contrast to the Bonferroni correction, however, we take into account how many tests we have already done and become less conservative with each subsequent comparison. We begin with a correction just as conservative as the Bonferroni correction, then take advantage of the conservatism of the earlier tests and become less cautious with each subsequent comparison.

Suppose we wish to make k pairwise comparisons.† Order these k uncorrected P values from smallest to largest, with the smallest uncorrected P value considered first in the sequential step-down test procedure. P_1 is the smallest P value in the sequence and P_k is the largest. For the jth hypothesis test in this ordered sequence, Holm's test applies the Bonferroni criterion in a step-down manner that depends on k and j, beginning with $j = 1$, and proceeding until we fail to reject the null hypothesis or run out of comparisons to do. Specifically, the uncorrected P value for the jth test is compared to $\alpha_j = \alpha_T/(k - j + 1)$. For the first comparison, $j = 1$, and the uncorrected

*J. Ludbrook, "Multiple Comparison Procedures Updated," *Clin. Exp. Pharmacol. Physiol.,* **25:**1032–1037 1998; M. Aickin and H. Gensler, "Adjusting for Multiple Testing When Reporting Research Results: The Bonferroni vs. Holm Methods" *Am. J. Public Health,* **86:**726–728, 1996; B. Levin, "Annotation: On the Holm, Simes, and Hochberg Multiple Test Procedures," *Am. J. Public Health,* **86:**628–629, 1996; B. W. Brown and K. Russel, "Methods for Correcting for Multiple Testing: Operating Characteristics," *Stat. Med.* **16:**2511–2528, 1997. T. Morikawa, A. Terao, and M. Iwasaki, "Power Evaluation of Various Modified Bonferroni Procedures by a Monte Carlo Study," *J. Biopharm. Stat.,* **6:**343–359, 1996.

†Like the Bonferroni correction, the Holm procedure can be applied to any family of hypothesis tests, not just multiple pairwise comparisons.

P value needs to be smaller than $\alpha_1 = \alpha_T/(k - 1 + 1) = \alpha_T/k$, the same as the Bonferroni correction. If this smallest observed P value is less than α_1, we reject that null hypothesis and then compare the next smallest uncorrected P value with $\alpha_2 = \alpha_T/(k - 2 + 1) = \alpha_T/(k - 1)$, which is a larger cutoff than we would obtain just using the Bonferroni correction. Because this critical value is larger, the test is less conservative and has higher power.

In the example of the relationship between menstruation and jogging that we have been studying, the t values for control versus joggers, control versus runners, and joggers versus runners were −2.54, −4.35, and 1.81, respectively, each with 75 degrees of freedom. The corresponding uncorrected P values are .013, .001, and .074. The ordered P values, from smallest to largest are:

.001	.013	.074
control vs. runners	control vs. joggers	joggers vs. runners
$j = 1$	$j = 2$	$j = 3$

We have $k = 3$ null hypothesis tests of interest, which led to these three P values. The rejection criterion for the test of the first of these ordered hypotheses ($j = 1$) is $P \leq \alpha_1 = 0.05/(3 - 1 + 1) = 0.05/3 = .0167$, which is identical to the Bonferroni critical level we applied previously to each of the members of this family of three tests. The computed P, .001, is less than this critical α, and so we reject the null hypothesis that there is no difference between runners and controls. Because the null hypothesis was rejected at this step, we proceed to the next step, $j = 2$, using as a rejection criterion for this second test $P \leq \alpha_2 = 0.05/(3 - 2 + 1) = 0.05/2 = .025$. Note that this is a less restrictive criterion than in the Bonferroni procedure we applied previously. The computed P, .013, is less than this critical value, and so we reject the null hypothesis that there is no difference in cortisol level between joggers and controls. Because the null hypothesis was rejected at this second step, we proceed to the third and, in this example, final step, $j = 3$, using as a rejection criterion for this third test $P \leq \alpha_3 = 0.05/(3 - 3 + 1) = 0.05/1 = .05$. Note that this rejection criteria is even less restrictive than in the Bonferroni procedure we applied previously, and is, in fact, equal to the criterion for an unadjusted t test. The computed P, .074, is greater than this critical value, and so we do not reject the null hypothesis that there is no difference in cortisol level between joggers and runners.

An alternative, and equivalent, approach is to compute the critical values of t corresponding to 0.0167, 0.025, and 0.05, and compare the observed values of the t test statistic for these comparisons with these critical t values. For 75 degrees of freedom, the corresponding critical values of the t test statistic are 2.45, 2.29, and 1.99. Therefore, like the Bonferroni t test, the Holm test requires the test statistic to exceed 2.45 for the comparison showing the largest difference (smallest P value), but this value drops to 2.29 for the second of the ordered comparisons, and finally to 1.99 for the last of the three ordered comparisons (largest P value, corresponding to smallest mean difference).

In this example, we reached the same conclusion that we did when using the regular, single-step Bonferroni, procedure. However, you can see from the progressively less conservative α at each step in the sequence that this collection of tests makes it easier to reject the null hypothesis for all but the first pairwise comparison than the traditional single-step Bonferroni procedure.* Because of the improved power while controlling the overall false-positive error for the family of comparisons at the desired level, we recommend the Holm test over the Bonferroni test.

The Holm-Sidak Test†

As noted earlier, the Bonferroni inequality, which forms the basis for the Bonferroni t test and, indirectly, the Holm test, gives a reasonable

*There are several other sequential tests, all of which operate in this manner, but apply different criteria. Some of these other tests are computationally more difficult, and less well understood, than Holm's test. Some, like Hochberg's test (Y. Hochberg, "A Sharper Bonferroni Procedure for Multiple Tests of Significance," *Biometrika* **75:**800–802, 1988), are step-up rather than step-down procedures in that they use a reverse stepping logic, starting with the kth (i.e., largest) P value in the ordered list of k P values, and proceeding until the first rejection of a null hypothesis, after which no more testing is done and all smaller P values are considered significant. Hochberg's test is exactly like the Holm test except that it applies the sequentially stepping Bonferroni criterion in this reverse, step-up order. Although Hochberg's test is claimed to be slightly more powerful than Holm's test, it is less well studied and so for the time being it is probably best to use one of the Holm tests, it is less well studied and so for the time being it is probably best to use one of the Holm tests (B. Levin, "Annotation: On the Holm, Simes, and Hochberg Multiple Test Procedures," *Am. J. Public Health,* **86:**628–629, 1996).

†This section can be skipped without any loss of continuity.

approximation for the total risk of a false-positive in a family of k comparisons when the number of comparisons is not too large, around 3 or 4. The actual probability of at least one false-positive conclusion (when the null hypothesis of no difference is true) is given by the formula

$$\alpha_T = 1 - (1 - \alpha)^k$$

When there are $k = 3$ comparisons, each done at the $\alpha = 0.05$ level, the Bonferroni inequality says that the total risk of at least one false-positive is less than $k\alpha = 3 \times 0.05 = .150$. This probability is reasonably close to the actual risk of at least one false-positive statement given by the equation above, $1 - (1 - 0.05)^3 = .143$. As the number of comparisons increases, the Bonferroni inequality more and more overestimates the true false-positive risk. For example, if there are $k = 6$ comparisons, $k\alpha = 6 \times 0.05 = .300$ compared with the actual probability of at least one false-positive of .265, nearly 10 percent lower. If there are 12 comparisons, the Bonferroni inequality says that the risk of at least one false-positive is below $12 \times 0.05 = .600$, 25 percent above the true risk of .460.

The *Holm-Sidak test** is a further refinement of the Holm test that is based on the exact formula for α_T rather than the Bonferroni inequality. The Holm-Sidak test works just like the Holm test, except that the criteria for rejecting the jth hypothesis test in an ordered sequence of k tests is an uncorrected P value below $1 - (1 - \alpha_T)^{1/(k-j+1)}$ rather than the $\alpha_T/(k - j + 1)$ used in the Holm test. This further refinement makes the Holm-Sidak test slightly more powerful than the Holm test. The differences between these two formulas is small. For example, if there are $k = 20$ comparisons, the differences between the resulting threshold values of P are in the fourth decimal place.

While we will use the Holm test in this book because of its computational simplicity, most computer programs report the results of the slightly better Holm-Sidak test. The logic of both tests is the same (as, in most cases, are the results).

*Z. Sidak, "Rectangular Confidence Regions for the Means of Multivariate Normal Distributions," *J. Am. Stat. Assoc.* **62:**626–633, 1967.

OTHER APPROACHES TO MULTIPLE COMPARISON TESTING: THE STUDENT-NEWMAN-KEULS TEST*

As noted in the previous section, the Bonferroni t test is overly conservative when there are more than a few group means to compare. This section presents the *Student-Newman-Keuls (SNK) test.* The SNK test statistic q is constructed similarly to the t test statistic, but the sampling distribution used to determine the critical values is based on a more sophisticated mathematical model of the multiple-comparison problem than does the simple Bonferroni inequality. This more sophisticated model gives rise to a more realistic estimate of the total true probability of erroneously concluding a difference exists, α_T, than does the Bonferroni t test.

The first step in the analysis is to complete an analysis of variance on all the data to test the global hypothesis that all the samples were drawn from a single population. If this test yields a significant value of F, arrange all the means in increasing order and compute the SNK test statistic q according to

$$q = \frac{\bar{X}_A - \bar{X}_B}{\sqrt{\dfrac{s_{\text{wit}}^2}{2}\left(\dfrac{1}{n_A} + \dfrac{1}{n_B}\right)}}$$

where $\bar{X}_A$ and $\bar{X}_B$ are the two means being compared, s_{wit}^2 is the variance within the treatment groups estimated from the analysis of variance, and n_{A} and n_{B} are the sample sizes of the two samples being compared.

This value of q is then compared with the table of critical values (Table 4–3). This critical value depends on α_T, the total risk of erroneously asserting a difference for all comparisons combined, ν_d, the denominator degrees of freedom from the analysis of variance, and a parameter p,

*This material is important for people who are using this book as a guide for analysis of their data; it can be skipped in a course on introductory biostatistics without interfering with the presentation of the rest of the material in this book. For a complete discussion of these (and other) multiple comparison procedures, see S. E. Maxwell and H. D. Delaney, *Designing Experiments and Analyzing Data: A Model Comparison Perspective,* 2nd ed. Mahwah NJ: Lawrence Erlbaum Associates, 2004, chapter 5. "Testing Several Contrasts: The Multiple Comparison Problem."

which is the number of means being tested. For example, when comparing the largest and smallest of four means, $p = 4$; when comparing the second smallest and smallest means, $p = 2$.

The conclusions reached by multiple-comparisons testing depend on the order that the pairwise comparisons are made. The proper procedure is to compare first the largest mean with the smallest, then the largest with the second smallest, and so on, until the largest has been compared with the second largest. Next, compare the second largest with the smallest, the second largest with the next smallest, and so forth. For example, after ranking four means in ascending order, the sequence of comparisons should be: 4 versus 1, 4 versus 2, 4 versus 3, 3 versus 1, 3 versus 2, 2 versus 1.

Another important procedural rule is that if no significant difference exists between two means, then conclude that no difference exists between any means enclosed by the two without testing for them. Thus, in the preceding example, if we failed to find a significant difference between means 3 and 1, we would not test for a difference between means 3 and 2 or means 2 and 1.

Still More on Menstruation and Jogging

To illustrate the SNK procedure, we once again analyze the data in Fig. 3–9, which presents the number of menses per year in women runners, joggers, and sedentary controls. The women in the control group had an average of 11.5 menses per year, the joggers had an average of 10.1 menses per year, and the runners had an average of 9.1 menses per year. We begin by ordering these means in descending order (which is how they happen to be listed). Next, we compute the change in means between the largest and smallest (control versus runners), the largest and the next smallest (control versus joggers), and the second largest and the smallest (joggers versus runners). Finally, we use the estimate of the variance from within the groups in the analysis of variance, $s^2_{\text{wit}} = 3.95$ (menses/year)^2 with $\nu_d = 75$ degrees of freedom, and the fact that each test group contained 26 women to complete the computation of each value of q.

To compare the controls with the runners, we compute

$$q = \frac{\bar{X}_{\text{con}} - \bar{X}_{\text{run}}}{\sqrt{\dfrac{s^2_{\text{wit}}}{2}\left(\dfrac{1}{n_{\text{con}}} + \dfrac{1}{n_{\text{run}}}\right)}} = \frac{11.5 - 9.1}{\sqrt{\dfrac{3.95}{2}\left(\dfrac{1}{26} + \dfrac{1}{26}\right)}} = 6.157$$

Table 4–3 Critical Values of q

				$\alpha_T = 0.05$					
ν_d	$p = 2$	3	4	5	6	7	8	9	10
1	17.97	26.98	32.82	37.08	40.41	43.12	45.40	47.36	49.07
2	6.085	8.331	9.798	10.88	11.74	12.44	13.03	13.54	13.99
3	4.501	5.910	6.825	7.502	8.037	8.478	8.853	9.177	9.462
4	3.927	5.040	5.757	6.287	6.707	7.053	7.347	7.602	7.826
5	3.635	4.602	5.218	5.673	6.033	6.330	6.582	6.802	6.995
6	3.461	4.339	4.896	5.305	5.628	5.895	6.122	6.319	6.493
7	3.344	4.165	4.681	5.060	5.359	5.606	5.815	5.998	6.158
8	3.261	4.041	4.529	4.886	5.167	5.399	5.597	5.767	5.918
9	3.199	3.949	4.415	4.756	5.024	5.244	5.432	5.595	5.739
10	3.151	3.877	4.327	4.654	4.912	5.124	5.305	5.461	5.599
11	3.113	3.820	4.256	4.574	4.823	5.028	5.202	5.353	5.487
12	3.082	3.773	4.199	4.508	4.751	4.950	5.119	5.265	5.395
13	3.055	3.735	4.151	4.453	4.690	4.885	5.049	5.192	5.318
14	3.033	3.702	4.111	4.407	4.639	4.829	4.990	5.131	5.254
15	3.014	3.674	4.076	4.367	4.595	4.782	4.940	5.077	5.198
16	2.998	3.649	4.046	4.333	4.557	4.741	4.897	5.031	5.150
17	2.984	3.628	4.020	4.303	4.524	4.705	4.858	4.991	5.108
18	2.971	3.609	3.997	4.277	4.495	4.673	4.824	4.956	5.071
19	2.960	3.593	3.977	4.253	4.469	4.645	4.794	4.924	5.038
20	2.950	3.578	3.958	4.232	4.445	4.620	4.768	4.896	5.008
24	2.919	3.532	3.901	4.166	4.373	4.541	4.684	4.807	4.915
30	2.888	3.486	3.845	4.102	4.302	4.464	4.602	4.720	4.824
40	2.858	3.442	3.791	4.039	4.232	4.389	4.521	4.635	4.735
60	2.829	3.399	3.737	3.977	4.163	4.314	4.441	4.550	4.646
120	2.800	3.356	3.685	3.917	4.096	4.241	4.363	4.468	4.560
∞	2.772	3.314	3.633	3.858	4.030	4.170	4.286	4.387	4.474

(continued)

This comparison spans three means, so $p = 3$. From Table 4–3, the critical value of q for $\alpha_T = .05$, $\nu_d = 75$ (from the analysis of variance), and $p = 3$ is 3.385. Since the value of q associated with this comparison, 6.157, exceeds this critical value, we conclude that there is a significant difference between the controls and the runners. Since this result is significant, we go on to the next comparison.

Table 4–3 Critical Values of *q* (*Continued*)

$\alpha_T = 0.01$

ν_d	$p = 2$	3	4	5	6	7	8	9	10
1	90.03	135.0	164.3	185.6	202.2	215.8	227.2	237.0	245.6
2	14.04	19.02	22.29	24.72	26.63	28.20	29.53	30.68	31.69
3	8.261	10.62	12.17	13.33	14.24	15.00	15.64	16.20	16.69
4	6.512	8.120	9.173	9.958	10.58	11.10	11.55	11.93	12.27
5	5.702	6.976	7.804	8.421	8.913	9.321	9.669	9.972	10.24
6	5.243	6.331	7.033	7.556	7.973	8.318	8.613	8.869	9.097
7	4.949	5.919	6.543	7.005	7.373	7.679	7.939	8.166	8.368
8	4.746	5.635	6.204	6.625	6.960	7.237	7.474	7.681	7.863
9	4.596	5.428	5.957	6.348	6.658	6.915	7.134	7.325	7.495
10	4.482	5.270	5.769	6.136	6.428	6.669	6.875	7.055	7.213
11	4.392	5.146	5.621	5.970	6.247	6.476	6.672	6.842	6.992
12	4.320	5.046	5.502	5.836	6.101	6.321	6.507	6.670	6.814
13	4.260	4.964	5.404	5.727	5.981	6.192	6.372	6.528	6.667
14	4.210	4.895	5.322	5.634	5.881	6.085	6.258	6.409	6.543
15	4.168	4.836	5.252	5.556	5.796	5.994	6.162	6.309	6.439
16	4.131	4.786	5.192	5.489	5.722	5.915	6.079	6.222	6.349
17	4.099	4.742	5.140	5.430	5.659	5.847	6.007	6.147	6.270
18	4.071	4.703	5.094	5.379	5.603	5.788	5.944	6.081	6.201
19	4.046	4.670	5.054	5.334	5.554	5.735	5.889	6.022	6.141
20	4.024	4.639	5.018	5.294	5.510	5.688	5.839	5.970	6.087
24	3.956	4.546	4.907	5.168	5.374	5.542	5.685	5.809	5.919
30	3.889	4.455	4.799	5.048	5.242	5.401	5.536	5.653	5.756
40	3.825	4.367	4.696	4.931	5.114	5.265	5.392	5.502	5.559
60	3.762	4.282	4.595	4.818	4.991	5.133	5.253	5.356	5.447
120	3.702	4.200	4.497	4.709	4.872	5.005	5.118	5.214	5.299
∞	3.643	4.120	4.403	4.603	4.757	4.882	4.987	5.078	5.157

Source: H. L. Harter, *Order Statistics and Their Use in Testing and Estimation*, Vol. I: *Tests Based on Range and Studentized Range of Samples from a Normal Population*, U.S. Government Printing Office, Washington, D.C., 1970.

To compare the controls with the joggers, we compute

$$q = \frac{\bar{X}_{\text{con}} - \bar{X}_{\text{jog}}}{\sqrt{\dfrac{s_{\text{wit}}^2}{2}\left(\dfrac{1}{n_{\text{con}}} + \dfrac{1}{n_{\text{jog}}}\right)}} = \frac{11.5 - 10.1}{\sqrt{\dfrac{3.95}{2}\left(\dfrac{1}{26} + \dfrac{1}{26}\right)}} = 3.592$$

For this comparison, α_T and ν_d are the same as before, but $p = 2$. From Table 4–3, the critical value of q is 2.822. The value of 3.592 associated with this comparison also exceeds the critical value, so we conclude that controls are also significantly different from joggers.

To compare the joggers with the runners, we compute

$$q = \frac{\bar{X}_{\text{con}} - \bar{X}_{\text{run}}}{\sqrt{\frac{s^2_{\text{wit}}}{2}\left(\frac{1}{n_{\text{jog}}} + \frac{1}{n_{\text{run}}}\right)}} = \frac{10.1 - 9.1}{\sqrt{\frac{3.95}{2}\left(\frac{1}{26} + \frac{1}{26}\right)}} = 2.566$$

The value of q associated with this comparison, 2.566, is less than the critical value of 2.822 required to assert that there is a difference between joggers and runners. (The values of ν_d and p are the same as before, so the critical value of q is too.)

Tukey Test

The *Tukey test* is computed identically to the SNK test; the only difference is the critical value used to test whether a given difference is significant. (In fact, the SNK test is actually derived from the Tukey test.) In the SNK test, the value of the parameter p used to determine the critical value of q is the number of means spanned in the comparison being considered. As a result, completing a family of comparisons with the SNK test involves changing values of the critical value of q, depending on which comparison is being made. In the Tukey test, the parameter p is set to m, the number of groups in the study, for all comparisons.

Had we used the Tukey test for multiple comparisons in the example of the effect of jogging on menstruation discussed previously, we would have used $m = 3$ for p, and so compared the observed values of q with a critical value of 3.385 for *all* the comparisons. Despite the fact that the critical value for the last two comparisons in the example would be larger than the critical values used in the SNK test, we would draw the same conclusions from the Tukey test as the SNK test; that is, the joggers and runners are not significantly different from each other, and both are significantly different from the control group.

The Tukey and SNK tests, however, do not always yield the same results. The Tukey test controls the error rate for *all* comparisons simultaneously, whereas the SNK test controls the error rate for all comparisons that involve spanning p means. As a result, the Tukey test is more conservative (i.e., less likely to declare a difference significant) than SNK. People who like the Tukey test use it because it controls the overall error rate for all multiple comparisons. People who like the SNK test observe that the test is done *after* doing an analysis of variance, and they depend on the analysis of variance to control the overall error rate. They argue that because the SNK test is done only after the analysis of variance finds a significant difference, they need not worry about excess false positives from the SNK test that are the price of the increased power. Some believe that the Tukey test is overly conservative because it requires that all groups be tested as though they were separated by the maximum number of steps, whereas the SNK procedure allows each comparison to be made with reference to the exact number of steps that separate the two means actually being compared.

WHICH MULTIPLE COMPARISON PROCEDURE SHOULD YOU USE?

There is no strong consensus among statisticians about which multiple comparison test is preferred, and part of the choice is philosophic. For example, some would choose to be more conservative so that they only follow up avenues of inquiry that are more strongly suggested by their data.

Unadjusted t tests (also known as Fisher's Protected Least Significant Difference Test) are too liberal and the Bonferroni t test is too conservative for all possible comparisons. The SNK test tends to over-report significant differences between means because it controls the error rate among all comparisons spanning a fixed number of means rather than all pairwise comparisons. The Tukey test tends to under-report significant differences. The Holm test is less conservative than Tukey or Bonferroni, while at the same time controlling the overall risk of a false-positive conclusion at the nominal level for the entire family of pairwise tests (not just all tests spanning a given number of means). We recommend the Holm test (or, better yet, the Holm-Sidak test) as the first line procedure for most multiple comparison testing.

MULTIPLE COMPARISONS AGAINST A SINGLE CONTROL*

In addition to all pairwise comparisons, the need sometimes arises to compare the values of multiple treatment groups to a single control group. One alternative would be to use Bonferroni *t*, SNK, or Tukey tests to do all pairwise comparisons, then only consider the ones that involve the control group. The problem with this approach is that it requires many more comparisons than are actually necessary, with the result that each individual comparison is done much more conservatively than is necessary based on the actual number of comparisons of interest. We now present three techniques specifically designed for the situation of multiple comparisons against a single control: additional *Bonferroni* and Holm *t tests* and *Dunnett's test.* As with all pairwise multiple comparisons, use these tests *after* finding significant differences among all the groups with an analysis of variance.

Bonferroni *t* Test

The Bonferroni *t* test can be used for multiple comparisons against a single control group. The *t* test statistic and adjustment of the critical value to control the total error, α_T, proceed as before. The only difference is that the number of comparisons, *k*, is smaller because comparisons are being done against the control group only.

Suppose that we had only wanted to compare menstruation patterns in joggers and runners with the controls, but not with each other. Because we are only making comparisons against control, there are a total of $k = 2$ comparisons (as opposed to 3 when making all pairwise comparisons). To keep the total error rate at or below $\alpha_T = .05$ with these two comparisons, we do *each* of the *t* tests using the critical value of *t* corresponding to $\alpha_T/k = .05/2 = .025$. There are 75 degrees of freedom associated with the within-groups variance, so, interpolating† in Table 4–1, the critical value of *t* for each of the comparisons is 2.29. (This value compares with 2.45 for all possible comparisons. The lower critical value of *t* for comparisons

*This material is important for people who are using this book as a guide for analysis of their data; it can be skipped in a course on introductory biostatistics without interfering with the presentation of the rest of the material in this book.

†Appendix A includes the formulas for interpolating.

against control means that it is easier to identify a difference against control than when making all possible comparisons.) From the previous section, the observed values of t for the comparisons of joggers with controls and runners with controls are −2.54 and −4.35, respectively. The magnitudes of both these values exceed the critical value of 2.29, so we conclude that both joggers and runners differ significantly from control. *No statement can be made about the comparison of joggers with runners.*

Holm *t* Test

Just as it is possible to use Bonferroni t tests for multiple comparisons against a single control group, it is possible to use Holm t tests (or Holm Sidak tests). In the menstruation example, there are $k = 2$ comparisons, so using the Holm test, the critical value of t for the first comparison is that corresponding to $\alpha_1 = \alpha_T/(k - j + 1) = .05/(2 - 1 + 1) = .025$, 2.29. From the previous section, the observed value of t for the comparison of runners with controls is −4.35, which exceeds the 2.29 critical value, so we reject the null hypothesis of no difference. For the second comparison, $\alpha_2 = \alpha_T/(k - j + 1) = .05/(2 - 2 + 1) = .05$, 1.99. The value of t for the comparison of joggers with controls is −2.54, which exceeds this value. Therefore, we again conclude that both joggers and runners are significantly different from controls.

Dunnett's Test

The analog of the SNK test for multiple comparisons against a single control group is *Dunnett's test.* Like the SNK test statistic, the Dunnett q' test statistic is defined analogously to the t test statistic:

$$q' = \frac{\bar{X}_{\text{con}} - \bar{X}_A}{\sqrt{s^2_{\text{wit}}\left(\dfrac{1}{n_{\text{con}}} + \dfrac{1}{n_A}\right)}}$$

The smaller number of comparisons in multiple comparisons against a single control group compared with all possible comparisons is reflected in the sampling distribution of the q' test statistic, which is in turn reflected in the table of critical values (Table 4–4). As with the

Table 4–4 Critical Values of q'

ν_d	$\alpha_T = 0.05$ $\rho = 2$	3	4	5	6	7	8	9	10	11	12	13	16	21
5	2.57	3.03	3.29	3.48	3.62	3.73	3.82	3.90	3.97	4.03	4.09	4.14	4.26	4.42
6	2.45	2.86	3.10	3.26	3.39	3.49	3.57	3.64	3.71	3.76	3.81	3.86	3.97	4.11
7	2.36	2.75	2.97	3.12	3.24	3.33	3.41	3.47	3.53	3.58	3.63	3.67	3.78	3.91
8	2.31	2.67	2.88	3.02	3.13	3.22	3.29	3.35	3.41	3.46	3.50	3.54	3.64	3.76
9	2.26	2.61	2.81	2.95	3.05	3.14	3.20	3.26	3.32	3.36	3.40	3.44	3.53	3.65
10	2.23	2.57	2.76	2.89	2.99	3.07	3.14	3.19	3.24	3.29	3.33	3.36	3.45	3.57
11	2.20	2.53	2.72	2.84	2.94	3.02	3.08	3.14	3.19	3.23	3.27	3.30	3.39	3.50
12	2.18	2.50	2.68	2.81	2.90	2.98	3.04	3.09	3.14	3.18	3.22	3.25	3.34	3.45
13	2.16	2.48	2.65	2.78	2.87	2.94	3.00	3.06	3.10	3.14	3.18	3.21	3.29	3.40
14	2.14	2.46	2.63	2.75	2.84	2.91	2.97	3.02	3.07	3.11	3.14	3.18	3.26	3.36
15	2.13	2.44	2.61	2.73	2.82	2.89	2.95	3.00	3.04	3.08	3.12	3.15	3.23	3.33
16	2.12	2.42	2.59	2.71	2.80	2.87	2.92	2.97	3.02	3.06	3.09	3.12	3.20	3.30
17	2.11	2.41	2.58	2.69	2.78	2.85	2.90	2.95	3.00	3.03	3.07	3.10	3.18	3.27
18	2.10	2.40	2.56	2.68	2.76	2.83	2.89	2.94	2.98	3.01	3.05	3.08	3.16	3.25
19	2.09	2.39	2.55	2.66	2.75	2.81	2.87	2.92	2.96	3.00	3.03	3.06	3.14	3.23
20	2.09	2.38	2.54	2.65	2.73	2.80	2.86	2.90	2.95	2.98	3.02	3.05	3.12	3.22
24	2.06	2.35	2.51	2.61	2.70	2.76	2.81	2.86	2.90	2.94	2.97	3.00	3.07	3.16
30	2.04	2.32	2.47	2.58	2.66	2.72	2.77	2.82	2.86	2.89	2.92	2.95	3.02	3.11
40	2.02	2.29	2.44	2.54	2.62	2.68	2.73	2.77	2.81	2.85	2.87	2.90	2.97	3.06
60	2.00	2.27	2.41	2.51	2.58	2.64	2.69	2.73	2.77	2.80	2.83	2.86	2.92	3.00
120	1.98	2.24	2.38	2.47	2.55	2.60	2.65	2.69	2.73	2.76	2.79	2.81	2.87	2.95
∞	1.96	2.21	2.35	2.44	2.51	2.57	2.61	2.65	2.69	2.72	2.74	2.77	2.83	2.91

						$\alpha_T = 0.01$								
ν_d	$\rho = 2$	3	4	5	6	7	8	9	10	11	12	13	16	21
5	4.03	4.63	4.98	5.22	5.41	5.56	5.69	5.80	5.89	5.98	6.05	6.12	6.30	6.52
6	3.71	4.21	4.51	4.71	4.87	5.00	5.10	5.20	5.28	5.35	5.41	5.47	5.62	5.81
7	3.50	3.95	4.21	4.39	4.53	4.64	4.74	4.82	4.89	4.95	5.01	5.06	5.19	5.36
8	3.36	3.77	4.00	4.17	4.29	4.40	4.48	4.56	4.62	4.68	4.73	4.78	4.90	5.05
9	3.25	3.63	3.85	4.01	4.12	4.22	4.30	4.37	4.43	4.48	4.53	4.57	4.68	4.82
10	3.17	3.53	3.74	3.88	3.99	4.08	4.16	4.22	4.28	4.33	4.37	4.42	4.52	4.65
11	3.11	3.45	3.65	3.79	3.89	3.98	4.05	4.11	4.16	4.21	4.25	4.29	4.30	4.52
12	3.05	3.39	3.58	3.71	3.81	3.89	3.96	4.02	4.07	4.12	4.16	4.19	4.29	4.41
13	3.01	3.33	3.52	3.65	3.74	3.82	3.89	3.94	3.99	4.04	4.08	4.11	4.20	4.32
14	2.98	3.29	3.47	3.59	3.69	3.76	3.83	3.88	3.93	3.97	4.01	4.05	4.13	4.24
15	2.95	3.25	3.43	3.55	3.64	3.71	3.78	3.83	3.88	3.92	3.95	3.99	4.07	4.18
16	2.92	3.22	3.39	3.51	3.60	3.67	3.73	3.78	3.83	3.87	3.91	3.94	4.02	4.13
17	2.90	3.19	3.36	3.47	3.56	3.63	3.69	3.74	3.79	3.83	3.86	3.90	3.98	4.08
18	2.88	3.17	3.33	3.44	3.53	3.60	3.66	3.71	3.75	3.79	3.83	3.86	3.94	4.04
19	2.86	3.15	3.31	3.42	3.50	3.57	3.63	3.68	3.72	3.76	3.79	3.83	3.90	4.00
20	2.85	3.13	3.29	3.40	3.48	3.55	3.60	3.65	3.69	3.73	3.77	3.80	3.87	3.97
24	2.80	3.07	3.22	3.32	3.40	3.47	3.52	3.57	3.61	3.64	3.68	3.70	3.78	3.87
30	2.75	3.01	3.15	3.25	3.33	3.39	3.44	3.49	3.52	3.56	3.59	3.62	3.69	3.78
40	2.70	2.95	3.09	3.19	3.26	3.32	3.37	3.41	3.44	3.48	3.51	3.53	3.60	3.68
60	2.66	2.90	3.03	3.12	3.19	3.25	3.29	3.33	3.37	3.40	3.42	3.45	3.51	3.59
120	2.62	2.85	2.97	3.06	3.12	3.18	3.22	3.26	3.29	3.32	3.35	3.37	3.43	3.51
∞	2.58	2.79	2.92	3.00	3.06	3.11	3.15	3.19	3.22	3.25	3.27	3.29	3.35	2.42

Source: Reprinted from C. W. Dunnett, "New Tables for Multiple Comparisons with a Control," *Biometrics*, 20:482–491, 1964.

SNK test, first order the means, then do the comparisons from the largest to smallest difference. In contrast to the SNK test, the parameter p is the same for all comparisons, equal the number of means in the study. The number of degrees of freedom is the number of degrees of freedom associated with the denominator in the analysis of variance F test statistic.

To repeat the analysis of the effect of running on menstruation using Dunnett's test, we first compare the runners with controls (the largest difference) by computing

$$q' = \frac{\bar{X}_{\text{con}} - \bar{X}_{\text{run}}}{\sqrt{s^2_{\text{wit}}\left(\dfrac{1}{n_{\text{con}}} + \dfrac{1}{n_{\text{run}}}\right)}} = \frac{11.5 - 9.1}{\sqrt{3.95\left(\dfrac{1}{26} + \dfrac{1}{26}\right)}} = 4.35$$

There are three means, so $p = 3$, and there are 75 degrees of freedom associated with the within-groups variance estimate. From Table 4–4 the critical value of q' for $\alpha_T = .05$ is 2.26, so we conclude that there is a difference between the runners and controls ($P < .05$). Next, we compare the joggers with controls by computing

$$q' = \frac{\bar{X}_{\text{con}} - \bar{X}_{\text{jog}}}{\sqrt{s^2_{\text{wit}}\left(\dfrac{1}{n_{\text{con}}} + \dfrac{1}{n_{\text{jog}}}\right)}} = \frac{11.5 - 10.1}{\sqrt{3.95\left(\dfrac{1}{26} + \dfrac{1}{26}\right)}} = 2.54$$

As before, there are three means, so $p = 3$; from Table 4–4, the critical value of q' remains 2.26, so we conclude that there is a significant difference between the joggers and controls ($P < .05$). Our overall conclusion is that there is a significant difference in menstruation patterns between both the runners and the joggers and the controls. No statement can be made concerning the differences between the runners and the joggers.

In sum, we conclude that runners and joggers have significantly fewer menses per year than women in the control group, but that there is not a significant difference between the runners and the joggers. Since we only did a small number of comparisons (three), this is the same conclusion we drew using the Bonferroni and Holm t tests to conduct the multiple comparisons. Had we had an experiment with more test groups (and hence many more comparisons), we would see that Dunnett's test was capable of detecting differences that the Bonferroni t test missed because of the large values of t (i.e., small values of P) required to assert a statistically significant difference in any individual pairwise comparison. Dunnett's test is more sensitive than the Bonferroni t test because it uses a more sophisticated mathematical model to estimate the probability of erroneously concluding a difference.

It is less clear whether to recommend the Holm test over Dunnett's test for multiple comparisons against a control group. Theoretically, the sequentially rejective step-down Holm test should be more powerful than the single-step Dunnett's test, but there have been no comprehensive studies of the relative power of Holm's versus Dunnett's tests. You can get a simplified idea of the relative power by considering the running example that we have been considering. The critical value of Dunnett's q' (for $p = 3$, $\nu = 75$, and $\alpha = 0.05$) for each of the two groups of runners versus controls (runners versus controls and joggers versus controls) is 2.26. The Holm test applied to this family of two comparisons would require critical values of 2.29 for the first test and 1.99 for the second test. Thus, it would be slightly harder to reject the null hypothesis of no difference for the first comparison and slightly easier for the second.

THE MEANING OF P

Understanding what P means requires understanding the logic of statistical hypothesis testing. For example, suppose an investigator wants to test whether or not a drug alters body temperature. The obvious experiment is to select two similar groups of people, administer a placebo to one and the drug to the other, measure body temperature in both groups, then compute the mean and standard deviation of the temperatures measured in each group. The mean responses of the two groups will probably be different, regardless of whether the drug has an effect or not for the same reason that different random samples drawn from the same population yield different estimates for the mean. Therefore, the question becomes: Is the observed difference in mean temperature of the two groups likely to be due to random variation associated with the allocation of individuals to the two experimental groups or due to the drug?

To answer this question, statisticians first quantify the observed difference between the two samples with a single number, called *a test statistic,* such as F, t, q or q'. These statistics, like most test statistics, have the property that the greater the difference between the samples, the greater their value. If the drug has no effect, the test statistic will be a small number. But what is "small"?

To find the boundary between "small" and "big" values of the test statistic, statisticians assume that the drug does *not* affect temperature (the *null hypothesis*). If this assumption is correct, the two groups of people are simply random samples from a single population, all of whom received a placebo (because the drug is, in effect, a placebo). Now, in theory, the statistician repeats the experiment using all possible samples of people and computes the test statistic for each hypothetical experiment. Just as random variation produced different values for means of different samples, this procedure will yield a range of values for the test statistic. Most of these values will be relatively small, but sheer bad luck requires that there be a few samples that are not representative of the entire population. These samples will yield relatively large values of the test statistic *even if the drug had no effect.* This exercise produces only a few of the possible values of the test statistic, say 5 percent of them, above some cutoff point. The test statistic is "big" if it is larger than this cutoff point.

Having determined this cutoff point, we execute an experiment on a drug with unknown properties and compute the test statistic. It is "big." Therefore, we conclude that *there is less than a 5 percent chance of observing data which led to the computed value of the test statistic on the assumption that the drug has had no effect was true.* Traditionally, if the chances of observing the computed test statistic when the intervention has no effect are below 5 percent, one rejects the working assumption that the drug has no effect and asserts that the drug *does* have an effect. There is, of course, a chance that this assertion is wrong: about 5 percent. This 5 percent is known as the *P value* or *significance level.*

Precisely,

> *The P value is the probability of obtaining a value of the test statistic as large as or larger than the one computed from the data when in reality there is no difference between the different treatments.*

As a result of this logic, if we are willing to assert a difference when $P < .05$, we are tacitly agreeing to accept the fact that, over the long run, we expect 1 assertion of a difference in 20 to be wrong.

Statistical versus Real (Clinical) Thinking

As we have said several times, statistical hypothesis testing as presented in this book and generally practiced is an argument by contradiction. One begins with the null hypothesis of no difference and estimates the probability of obtaining the observed data assuming that the null hypothesis is true. If that probability is low, we reject the null hypothesis. Even though this formalism is widely used, the simple fact is that investigators rarely begin a study actually *expecting* the null hypothesis to be true. Quite the contrary, generally one expects that some alternative hypothesis—that the treatment or observational factor being studied—*does* have an effect.

Indeed, in terms of practical thinking, if the results of the study reject the null hypothesis of no effect, it actually reinforces the "real" hypothesis that there was an effect, which is what motivated the study in the first place. If, on the other hand, you fail to reject the null hypothesis of no effect, that fact is evidence that the "real" hypothesis is not correct. This use of information in an incremental way, which involves beginning with some prior expectation of what the underlying relationship between the treatment (or observational factor) and the outcome is, then modifying that belief on the basis of the experimental data is how scientific and clinical decision making is actually done.

There is a branch of statistical reasoning called *Baysian decision making,* based on simple probability calculations known as *Bayes' rule,**

*Bayes' Rule states:

$$\left(\begin{array}{c}\textit{Posterior Odds}\\ \textit{of Null Hypothesis}\end{array}\right) = \left(\begin{array}{c}\textit{Prior Odds}\\ \textit{of Null Hypothesis}\end{array}\right) \times \frac{\Pr(\textit{Data, given the null hyphothesis})}{\Pr(\textit{Data, given the alternative hyphothesis})}$$

where *Pr* means the probability of the stated situation. For a detailed discussion of the application of this formulation of Bayes' Rule to biomedical data, see S. N. Goodman, "Toward Evidence-Based Medical Statistics, 2: The Bayes Factor," *Ann. Intern. Med.* **130:**1005–1013, 1999.

that allows you to use the results of an experiment to modify, in a quantitative way, your prior expectations of the relationship you are studying.

Bayes' rule allows you to begin with a *prior* distribution of possible outcomes (each with a probability attached to it, much like the F and t sampling distributions we have already discussed) then mathematically modify that distribution based on the information obtained in your study to obtain your *posterior* distribution of probabilities associated with different possible outcomes. Indeed, at a qualitative level, that is the process that people use to integrate new information in making decisions—be they scientific, clinical, or personal.

Many statisticians,* especially those concerned with clinical decision making, have argued that the simple null hypothesis approach to statistical decision making both oversimplifies the process of using data to make clinical and scientific decisions and leads to being overly reluctant to conclude that the treatment actually had an effect.

There are two reasons for this view. First, traditional statistical hypothesis testing based on the null hypothesis of no effect is equivalent to saying that at the outset of the study you do not believe that there is any evidence to support the possibility that the treatment actually had an effect, which is, as discussed above, rarely the case. Second, each hypothesis is tested without taking in to account anything else you know about the likely effects of the intervention. These two factors combine to lead you to implicitly underestimate the prior probability that the treatment has an effect, which makes it harder to conclude that there is an effect than the data may warrant.

They are correct. Why, then, do people persist in using the classic approach to statistical decision making described in this book?

*For a discussion of the Bayesian approach, with a comparison to the frequentist approach used in this book and several clinical examples, see W. S. Browner and T. B. Newman, "Are All Significant *P* Values Created Equal? The Analogy between Diagnostic Tests and Clinical Research," *JAMA* **257:**2459–2463, 1987; J. Brophy and L. Joseph, "Placing Trials in Context Using Bayesian Analysis: GUSTO Revisited by Reverend Bayes," *JAMA,* **273:**871–875, 1995; S. N. Goodman, "Toward Evidence-Based Medical Statistics, 1: The P Value Fallacy," *Ann. Intern. Med.* **130:** 995–1004, 1999; S. N. Goodman, "Toward Evidence-Based Medical Statistics, 2: The Bayes Factor," *Ann. Intern. Med.* **130:** 1005–1013, 1999; G. A. Diamond and S. Kaul, "Baysian Approaches to the Analysis and Interpretation of Clinical Megatrends," *J. Am. Coll. Cardiol.* **43:** 1929–1939, 2004.

The primary reason is the difficulty in obtaining good estimates of the prior probabilities of the possible outcomes before the experiment was conducted. Indeed, despite repeated entreaties to use Baysian decision making by its enthusiasts, they can point to few examples where it has been used in routine clinical or scientific research because of the difficulties in obtaining meaningful prior probability distributions.

Nevertheless, it is worth keeping in mind this process and recognizing that the results of classic statistical hypothesis testing—embodied as the P value—need to be integrated into the larger collection of knowledge that creators and consumers of scientific and clinical results possess in order to further refine their understanding of the problems at hand. From this perspective, the P value is not the arbiter of truth but rather an assistant in making evolving judgments as to what the truth is.

Why $P < .05$?

The convention of considering a difference "statistically significant" when $P < .05$ is widely accepted. In fact, it came from an arbitrary decision by one person, Ronald A. Fisher, who invented much of modern parametric statistics (including the F statistic, which is named for him). In 1926, Fisher published a paper* describing how to assess whether adding manure to a field would increase crop yields which introduced the idea of statistical significance and established the 5 percent standard.
He said:

> To an acre of ground the manure is applied; a second acre, sown with similar seed and treated in all other ways like the first, receives none of the manure. When the produce is weighed, it is found that the acre which received the manure has yielded a crop larger indeed by, say, 10 percent. The manure has scored a success, but the confidence with which such

*R. A. Fisher. "The Arrangement of Field Experiments," *J. Ministry Ag.* **33:** 503–513, 1926. For a discussion of this paper in its historical context, including evidence that the logic of hypothesis testing dates back to Blaise Pascal and Pierre Fermat, in 1964, see M. Cowles and C. Davis, "On the Origins of the .05 Level of Statistical Significance, *Am. Psychol.* **37:** 533–558, 1982.

> a result should be received by the purchasing public depends wholly on the manner in which the experiment was carried out.
>
> First, if the experimenter could say that in twenty years of experience with uniform treatment the difference in favour of the acre treated with manure had never before touched 10 percent, the evidence would have reached a point which may be called the verge of significance; for it is convenient to draw the line at about the level at which we can say: "Either there is something in the treatment, or a coincidence has occurred such as does not occur more than one in twenty trials." This level, which we may call the 5 percent point, would be indicated, though very roughly, by the greatest chance deviation observed in twenty successive trials. To locate the 5 percent point with any accuracy we should need about 500 years' experience, for we could then, supposing no progressive changes in fertility were in progress, count out the 25 largest deviations and draw the line between the 25th and 26th largest deviation. If the difference between the two acres in our experimental year exceeded this value, we should have reasonable grounds for calling this value significant.
>
> If one in 20 does not seem high enough odds, we may, if we prefer it, draw the line at 1 in 50 (the 2 percent point) or 1 in 100 (the 1 percent point.) *Personally, the writer prefers to set a low standard of significance at the 5 percent point, and ignore entirely all results which fails to reach this level.* [emphasis added]

Although $P < .05$ is widely accepted, and you will certainly not generate controversy if you use it, a more sensible approach is to consider the P value in making decisions about how to interpret your results without slavishly considering 5 percent a rigid criterion for "truth."

It is commonly believed that the P value is the probability of making a mistake. There are obviously two ways an investigator can reach a mistaken conclusion based on the data, reporting that the treatment had an effect when in reality it did not or reporting that the treatment did not have an effect when in reality it did. As noted above, the P value only quantifies the probability of making the first kind of error (called a *Type I* or α *error*), that of erroneously concluding that the treatment had an effect when in reality it did not. It gives no information about the probability of making the second kind of error (called a *Type II* or β *error*), that of concluding that the treatment had no effect when in reality it did. Chapter 6 discusses how to estimate the probability of making Type II errors.

PROBLEMS

4-1 Conahan and associates also measured the mean arterial pressure and total peripheral resistance (a measure of how hard it is to produce a given flow through the arterial bed) in 9 patients who were anesthetized with halothane and 16 patients who were anesthetized with morphine. The results are summarized in Table 4–2. Is there evidence that these two anesthetic agents are associated with differences in either of these two variables?

4-2 Cocaine has many adverse effects on the heart, to the point that when people under 40 years of age appear in an emergency room with a heart attack, it is a good guess that it was precipitated by cocaine. In experiments, cocaine has been shown to constrict coronary arteries and reduce blood flow to the heart muscle as well as depress the overall mechanical function of the heart. A class of drugs know as calcium channel blockers has been used to treat problems associated with coronary artery vasoconstriction in other contexts, so Sharon Hale and colleagues ("Nifedipine Protects the Heart from the Acute Deleterious Effects of Cocaine if Administered Before but Not After Cocaine," *Circulation*, **83:**1437–1443, 1991) hypothesized that the calcium channel blocker nifedipine could prevent coronary artery vasoconstriction and the attendant reduction in blood flow to the heart and mechanical function. If true, nifedipine might be useful for treating people who had heart problems brought on by cocaine use. They measured mean arterial pressure in two groups of dogs after administering cocaine, one of whom was treated with nifedipine and the other of which received a placebo.

Mean Arterial Pressure (mmHg) after Receiving Cocaine

Placebo	Nifedipine
156	73
171	81
133	103
102	88
129	130
150	106
120	106
110	111
112	122
130	108
105	99

Does treatment with nifedipine after administering cocaine affect mean arterial pressure?

4-3 Hale and her colleagues also directly measured the diameter of coronary arteries in dogs after receiving cocaine, and then being treated with a placebo or nifedipine. Based on the following data, did the nifedipine affect the diameters of the coronary arteries?

Diameter of Coronary Artery (mm)

Placebo	Nifedipine
2.5	2.5
2.2	1.7
2.6	1.5
2.0	2.5
2.1	1.4
1.8	1.9
2.4	2.3
2.3	2.0
2.7	2.6
2.7	2.3
1.9	2.2

Does treatment with nifedipine affect the diameter of the coronary arteries in dogs who have received cocaine?

4-4 Rework Probs. 3-1 and 3-5 using the t test. What is the relationship between the value of t computed here and the value of F computed for these data in Chap. 3?

4-5 Problem 3-2 presented the data that White and Froeb collected on the lung function of nonsmokers working in smoke-free environments, nonsmokers working in smoky environments, and smokers of various intensity. Analysis of variance revealed that these data were inconsistent with the hypothesis that the lung function was the same in all these groups. Isolate the various subgroups with similar lung function. What does this result mean in terms of the original question they posed: Does chronic exposure to other people's smoke affect the health of healthy adult nonsmokers?

4-6 Directly test the limited hypothesis that exposure to other people's smoke affects the health of healthy nonsmokers by comparing each group of involuntary smokers and active smokers with the nonsmokers working in a clean environment as the control group. Use the data from Prob. 3-2 and Dunnett's test.

4-7 Problem 3-3 led to the conclusion that HDL concentration is not the same in inactive men, joggers, and marathon runners. Use Holm *t* tests to compare each of these groups pairwise.

4-8 Suppose that we were just interested in comparisons of the joggers and the marathon men with the inactive adults (as the control group). Use the data in Prob. 3-3 and make these comparisons with Holm *t* tests.

4-9 Use the data from Prob. 3-4 to determine which interventions have protective effects on the heart during a prolonged ischemic attack. Can a pharmacological agent offer the same benefit as a brief ischemic preconditioning?

4-10 Use the Bonferroni *t* test to isolate which strains of mice discussed in Prob. 3-7 differ in testicular response to estrogen treatment.

4-11 Repeat Prob. 4-10 using the SNK and Holm tests. Compare the results with those of Prob. 4-10 and explain any differences.

4-12 In Prob. 3-6 you determined there was a difference in burnout among nursing staffs of different patient care units. Isolate these differences and discuss them.

4-13 In a test of significance, the *P* value of the test statistic is .063. Are the data statistically significant at

a. both the $\alpha = .05$ and $\alpha = .01$ levels?

b. the $\alpha = .05$ level but not at the $\alpha = .01$ level?

c. the $\alpha = .01$ level but not at the $\alpha = .05$ level?

d. neither the $\alpha = .05$ nor the $\alpha = .01$ levels?

Chapter 5

How to Analyze Rates and Proportions

The statistical procedures developed in Chapters 2 to 4 are appropriate for analyzing the results of experiments in which the variable of interest takes on a continuous range of values, such as blood pressure, urine production, or length of hospital stay. These, and similar variables, are measured on an *interval scale* because they are measured on a scale with constant intervals, e.g., millimeters of mercury, milliliters, or days. Much of the information physicians, nurses, and medical scientists use cannot be measured on interval scales. For example, an individual may be male or female, dead or alive, or Caucasian, African American, Hispanic, or Asian. These variables are measured on a *nominal scale,* in which there is no arithmetic relationship between the different classifications. We now develop the statistical tools necessary to describe and analyze such information.*

*There is a third class of variables in which responses can be *ordered* without an arithmetic relationship between the different possible states. Ordinal scales often appear in clinical practice; Chaps. 8 and 10 develop statistical procedures to analyze variables measured on ordinal scales.

It is easy to describe things measured on a nominal scale: simply count the number of patients or experimental subjects with each condition and (perhaps) compute the corresponding percentages.

Let us continue our discussion of the use of halothane versus morphine in open-heart surgery.* We have already seen that these two anesthetic agents produce differences in blood pressure that are unlikely to be due to random sampling effects. This finding is interesting, but the important clinical question is: Was there any difference in mortality? Of the patients anesthetized with halothane, 8 of 61 (13.1 percent) died compared with 10 of the 67 anesthetized with morphine (14.9 percent). This study showed that halothane was associated with a 1.8 percent lower mortality rate *in the 128 patients who were studied.* Is this difference due to a real clinical effect or simply to random variation?

To answer this and other questions about nominal data, we must first invent a way to estimate the precision with which percentages based on limited samples approximate the true rates that would be observed if we could examine the entire population, in this case, *all* people who will be anesthetized for open-heart surgery. We will use these estimates to construct statistical procedures to test hypotheses.

BACK TO MARS

Before we can quantify the certainty of our descriptions of a population on the basis of a limited sample, we need to know how to describe the population itself. Since we have already visited Mars and met all 200 Martians (in Chapter 2), we will continue to use them to develop ways to describe populations. In addition to measuring the Martians' heights, we noted that 50 of them were left-footed and the remaining 150 were right-footed. Figure 5–1 shows the entire population of Mars divided according to footedness. The first way in which we can describe this population is by giving the *proportion p* of Martians who are in each class. In this case $p_{\text{left}} = 50/200 = 0.25$ and $p_{\text{right}} = 150/250 = 0.75$. Since there are only two possible classes, notice that

*When this study was discussed in Chap. 4, we assumed the same number of patients in each treatment group to simplify the computation. In this chapter we use the actual number of patients in the study.

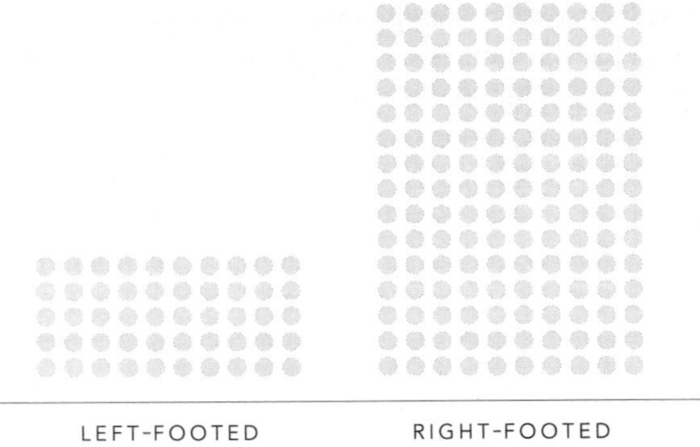

Figure 5–1 Of the 200 Martians 50 are left-footed, and the remaining 150 are right-footed. Therefore, if we select one Martian at random from this population, there is a $p_{\text{left}} = 50/200 = 0.25 = 25$ percent chance it will be left-footed.

$p_{\text{right}} = 1 - p_{\text{left}}$. Thus, whenever there are only two possible classes and they are mutually exclusive, we can completely describe the division in the population with the single parameter p, the proportion of members with one of the attributes. The proportion of the population with the other attribute is *always* $1 - p$.

Note that p also is the *probability* of drawing a left-footed Martian if one selects one member of the population at random.

Thus p plays a role exactly analogous to that played by the population mean μ in Chapter 2. To see why, suppose we associate the value $X = 1$ with each left-footed Martian and a value of $X = 0$ with each right-footed Martian. The mean value of X for the population is

$$\mu = \frac{\Sigma X}{N} = \frac{1 + 1 + \cdots + 1 + 0 + 0 + \cdots + 0}{200}$$
$$= \frac{50(1) + 150(0)}{200} = \frac{50}{200} = 0.25$$

which is p_{left}.

This idea can be generalized quite easily using a few equations. Suppose M members of a population of N individuals have some attribute and the remaining $N - M$ members of the population do not. Associate a value of $X = 1$ with the population members having the attribute and a value of $X = 0$ with the others. The mean of the resulting collection of numbers is

$$\mu = \frac{\Sigma X}{N} = \frac{M(1) + (N - M)(0)}{N} = \frac{M}{N} = p$$

the proportion of the population having the attribute.

Since we can compute a mean in this manner, why not compute a standard deviation in order to describe variability in the population? Even though there are only two possibilities, $X = 1$, and $X = 0$, the amount of variability will differ, depending on the value of p. Figure 5–2 shows three more populations of 200 individuals each. In Figure 5–2*A* only 10 of the individuals are left-footed; it exhibits less variability than the population shown in Fig. 5–1. Figure 5–2*B* shows the extreme case in which half the members of the population fall into each of the two classes; the variability is greatest. Figure 5–2*C* shows the other extreme; all the members fall into one of the two classes, and there is no variability at all.

To quantify this subjective impression, we compute the standard deviation of the 1s and 0s associated with each member of the population when we computed the mean. By definition, the population standard deviation is

$$\sigma = \sqrt{\frac{\Sigma(X - \mu)^2}{N}}$$

$X = 1$ for M members of the population and 0 for the remaining $N - M$ members, and $\mu = p$; therefore

$$\sigma = \sqrt{\frac{(1-p)^2+(1-p)^2+\cdots+(1-p)^2+(0-p)^2+(0-p)^2+\cdots+(0-p)^2}{N}}$$

$$= \sqrt{\frac{M(1 - p)^2 + (N - M)p^2}{N}} = \sqrt{\frac{M}{N}(1 - p)^2 + \left(1 - \frac{M}{N}\right)p^2}$$

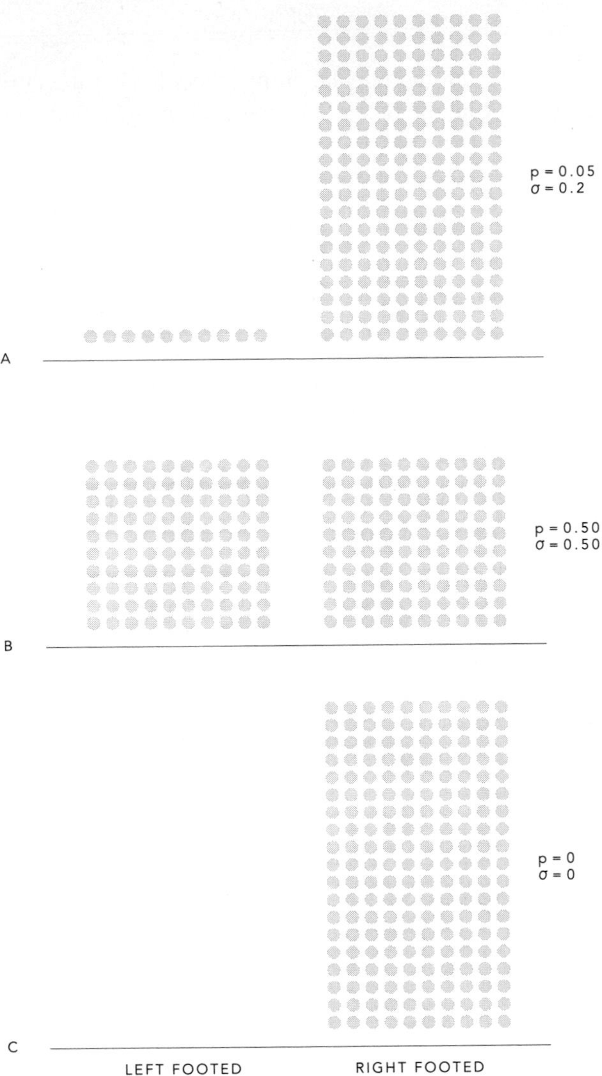

Figure 5–2 This figure illustrates three different populations, each containing 200 members but with different proportions of left-footed members. The standard deviation, $\sigma = \sqrt{p(1-p)}$ quantifies the variability in the population. ***(A)*** When most of the members fall in one class, σ is a small value, 0.2, indicating relatively little variability. ***(B)*** In contrast, if half the members fall into each class, σ reaches its maximum value of .5, indicating the maximum possible variability. ***(C)*** At the other extreme, if all members fall into the same class, there is no variability at all and $\sigma = 0$.

But since $M/N = p$ is the proportion of population members with the attribute,

$$\sigma = \sqrt{p(1-p)^2 + (1-p)p^2} = \sqrt{[p(1-p) + p^2](1-p)}$$

which simplifies to

$$\sigma = \sqrt{p(1-p)}$$

This equation for the population standard deviation produces quantitative results that agree with the qualitative impressions we developed from Figs. 5–1 and 5–2. As Figure 5–3 shows, $\sigma = 0$ when $p = 0$ or $p = 1$, that is, when all members of the population either do or do not have the attribute, and σ is maximized when $p = .5$, that is, when any given member of the population is as likely to have the attribute as not.

Since σ depends only on p, it really does not contain any additional information (in contrast to the mean and standard deviation of a normally distributed variable, where μ and σ provide two independent pieces of information). It will be most useful in computing a standard

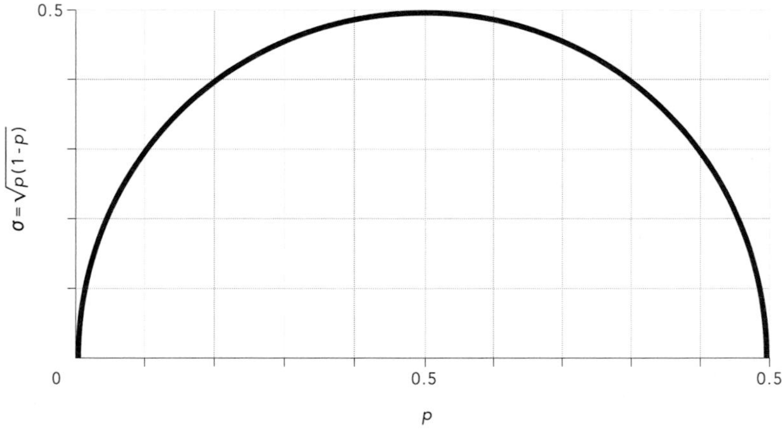

Figure 5–3 The relationship between the standard deviation of a population divided into two categories varies with p, the proportion of members in one of the categories. There is no variation if all members are in one category or the other (so $\sigma = 0$ when $p = 0$ or 1) and maximum variability when a given member is equally likely to fall in one class or the other ($\sigma = 0.5$ when $p = 0.5$).

error associated with estimates of p based on samples drawn at random from populations like those shown in Figs. 5–1 or 5–2.

ESTIMATING PROPORTIONS FROM SAMPLES

Of course, if we could observe all members of a population, there would not be any statistical question. In fact, all we ever see is a limited, hopefully representative, sample drawn from that population. How accurately does the proportion of members of a sample with an attribute reflect the proportion of individuals in the population with that attribute? To answer this question, we do a sampling experiment, just as we did in Chapter 2 when we asked how well the sample mean estimated the population mean.

Suppose we select 10 Martians at random from the entire population of 200 Martians. Figure 5–4 (top) shows which Martians were drawn; Fig. 5–4 (bottom) shows all the information the investigators who drew the sample would have. Half the Martians in the sample are left-footed

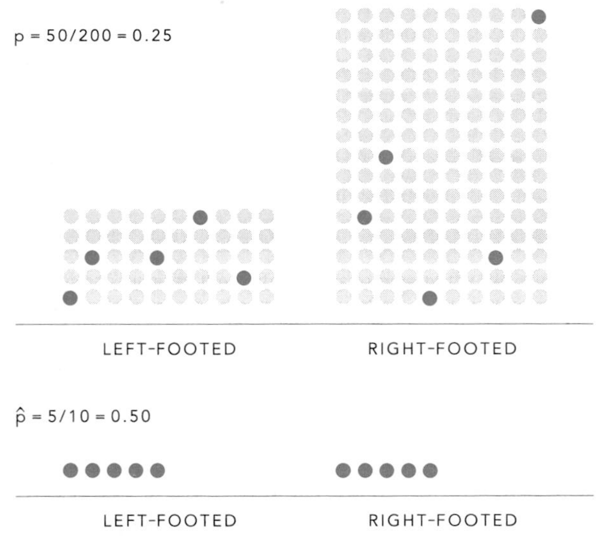

Figure 5–4 The top panel shows one random sample of 10 Martians selected from the population in Fig. 5–1; the bottom panel shows what the investigator would see. Since this sample included 5 left-footed Martians and 5 right-footed Martians, the investigator would estimate the proportion of left-footed Martians to be $\hat{p}_{\text{left}} = 5/10 = .5$, where the circumflex denotes an estimate.

and half are right-footed. Given only this information, one would probably report that the proportion of left-footed Martians is 0.5, or 50 percent.

Of course, there is nothing special about this sample, and one of the four other random samples shown in Figure. 5–5 could just as well have been drawn, in which case the investigator would have reported that the proportion of left-footed Martians were 30, 30, 10, or 20 percent, depending on which random sample happened to be drawn. In each case we have computed an estimate of the population proportion p based on a sample. Denote this estimate $\hat{p}$. Like the sample mean, the possible values of $\hat{p}$ depend on both the nature of the

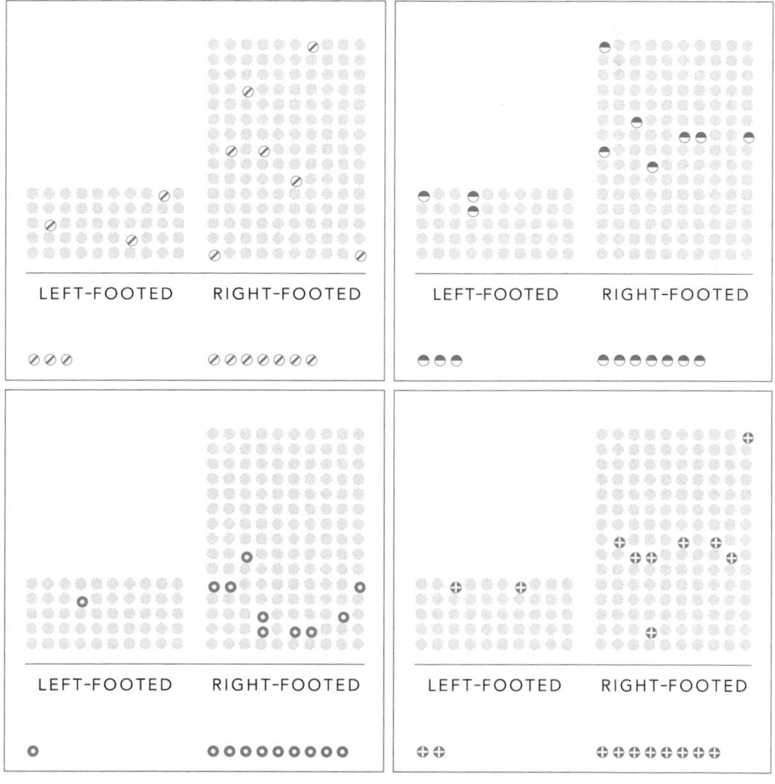

Figure 5–5 Four more random samples of 10 Martians each, together with the sample as it would appear to the investigator. Depending which sample happened to be drawn, the investigator would estimate the proportion of left-footed Martians to be 30, 30, 10, or 20 percent.

underlying population and the specific sample that is drawn. Figure 5–6 shows the five values of $\hat{p}$ computed from the specific samples in Figs. 5–4 and 5–5 together with the results of drawing another 20 random samples of 10 Martians each. Now we change our focus from the population of Martians to the population of all values of $\hat{p}$ computed from random samples of 10 Martians each. There are more than 10^{16} such samples with their corresponding estimates $\hat{p}$ of the value of p for the population of Martians.

The mean estimate of $\hat{p}$ for the 25 samples of 10 Martians each shown in Fig. 5–6 is 30 percent, which is remarkably close to the true proportion of left-footed Martians in the population (25 percent or 0.25). There is some variation in the estimates. To quantify the variability in the possible values of $\hat{p}$, we compute the *standard deviation* of values of $\hat{p}$ computed from random samples of 10 Martians each. In this case, it is about 14 percent or 0.14. This number describes the variability in the population of all possible values of the proportion of left-footed Martians computed from random samples of 10 Martians each.

Does this sound familiar? It should. It is just like the standard error of the mean. Therefore, we define the *standard error of the estimate of a proportion* to be the standard deviation of the population of all possible

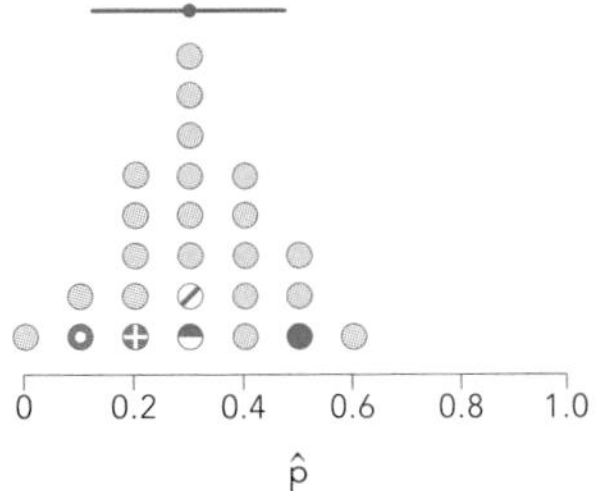

Figure 5–6 There will be a distribution of estimates of the proportion of left-footed Martians $\hat{p}_{\text{left}}$ depending on which random sample the investigator happens to draw. This figure shows the 5 specific random samples drawn in Figs. 5–4 and 5–5 together with 20 more random samples of 10 Martians each. The mean of the 25 estimates of p and the standard deviation of these estimates are also shown. The standard deviation of this distribution is the standard error of the estimate of the proportion $\sigma_{\hat{p}}$; it quantifies the precision with which $\hat{p}$ estimates p.

values of the proportion computed from samples of a given size. Just as with the standard error of the mean

$$\sigma_{\hat{p}} = \frac{\sigma}{\sqrt{n}}$$

in which $\sigma_{\hat{p}}$ is the standard error of the proportion, σ is the standard deviation of the population from which the sample was drawn, and n is the sample size. Since $\sigma = \sqrt{p(1 - p)}$,

$$\sigma_{\hat{p}} = \sqrt{\frac{p(1 - p)}{n}}$$

We estimate the standard error from a sample by replacing the true value of p in this equation with our estimate $\hat{p}$ obtained from the random sample. Thus,

$$s_{\hat{p}} = \sqrt{\frac{\hat{p}\,(1 - \hat{p})}{n}}$$

The standard error is a very useful way to describe the uncertainty in the estimate of the proportion of a population with a given attribute because the central-limit theorem (Chapter 2) also leads to the conclusion that the distribution of $\hat{p}$ is approximately normal, with mean p and standard deviation $\sigma_{\hat{p}}$ for large enough sample sizes. On the other hand, this approximation fails for values of p near 0 or 1 or when the sample size n is small. When can you use the normal distribution? Statisticians have shown that it is adequate when $n\hat{p}$ and $n(1 - \hat{p})$ both exceed about 5.* Recall that about 95 percent of all members of a normally distributed population fall within 2 standard deviations of the mean. When the distribution of $\hat{p}$ approximates the normal distribution, we can assert, with about 95 percent confidence, that the true

*When the sample size is too small to use the normal approximation, you need to solve the problem exactly using the binomial distribution. For a discussion of the binomial distribution, see J. H. Zar, *Biostatistical Analysis,* 4th ed, Prentice-Hall, Upper Saddle River, N.J., 1999, chap. 22 "The Binomial Distribution."

proportion of population members with the attribute of interest p lies within $2s_{\hat{p}}$ of $\hat{p}$.

These results provide a framework within which to consider the question we posed earlier in the chapter regarding the mortality rates associated with halothane and morphine anesthesia; 13.1 percent of 61 patients anesthetized with halothane and 14.9 percent of 67 patients anesthetized with morphine died following open-heart surgery. The standard errors of the estimates of these percentages are

$$s_{\hat{p}_{\text{hlo}}} = \sqrt{\frac{.131(1 - .131)}{61}} = .043 = 4.3\%$$

for halothane and

$$s_{\hat{p}_{\text{mor}}} = \sqrt{\frac{.149(1 - .149)}{67}} = .044 = 4.4\%$$

for morphine. Given that there was only a 1.8 percent difference in the observed mortality rate, it does not seem likely that the difference in observed mortality rate is due to anything beyond random sampling.

Before moving on, we should pause to list explicitly the assumptions that underlie this approach. We have been analyzing what statisticians call *independent Bernoulli trials,* in which

- *Each individual trial has two mutually exclusive outcomes.*
- *The probability* p *of a given outcome remains constant.*
- *All the trials are independent.*

In terms of a population, we can phrase these assumptions as follows:

- *Each member of the population belongs to one of two classes.*
- *The proportion of members of the population in one of the classes* p *remains constant.*
- *Each member of the sample is selected independently of all other members.*

HYPOTHESIS TESTS FOR PROPORTIONS

In Chapter 4 the sample mean and standard error of the mean provided the basis for constructing the *t* test to quantify how compatible observations were with the null hypothesis. We defined the *t* statistic as

$$t = \frac{\text{difference of sample means}}{\text{standard error of difference of sample means}}$$

The role of $\hat{p}$ is analogous to that of the sample mean in Chapters 2 and 4, and we have also derived an expression for the standard error of $\hat{p}$. We now use the observed proportion of individuals with a given attribute and its standard error to construct a test statistic analogous to *t* to test the hypothesis that the two samples were drawn from populations containing the same proportion of individuals with a given attribute.

The test statistic analogous to *t* is

$$z = \frac{\text{difference of sample proportions}}{\text{standard error of difference of sample proportions}}$$

Let $\hat{p}_1$ and $\hat{p}_2$ be the observed proportions of individuals with the attribute of interest in the two samples. The standard error is the standard deviation of the population of all possible values of $\hat{p}$ associated with samples of a given size, and since variances of differences add, the standard error of the difference in proportions is

$$s_{\hat{p}_1 - \hat{p}_2} = \sqrt{s_{\hat{p}_1}^2 + s_{\hat{p}_2}^2}$$

Therefore

$$z = \frac{\hat{p}_1 - \hat{p}_2}{s_{\hat{p}_1 - \hat{p}_2}} = \frac{\hat{p}_1 - \hat{p}_2}{\sqrt{s_{\hat{p}_1}^2 + s_{\hat{p}_1}^2}}$$

If n_1 and n_2 are the sizes of the two samples,

$$s_{\hat{p}_1} = \sqrt{\frac{\hat{p}_1(1 - \hat{p}_1)}{n_1}} \quad \text{and} \quad s_{\hat{p}_2} = \sqrt{\frac{\hat{p}_2(1 - \hat{p}_2)}{n_2}}$$

then

$$z = \frac{\hat{p}_1 - \hat{p}_2}{\sqrt{[\hat{p}_1(1 - \hat{p}_1)/n_1] + [\hat{p}_2(1 - \hat{p}_2)/n_2]}}$$

is our test statistic.

z replaces t because this ratio is approximately normally distributed for large enough sample sizes,* and it is customary to denote a normally distributed variable with the letter z.

Just as it was possible to improve the sensitivity of the t test by pooling the observations in the two sample groups to estimate the population variance, it is possible to increase the sensitivity of the z test for proportions by pooling the information from the two samples to obtain a single estimate of the population standard deviation s. Specifically, if the hypothesis that the two samples were drawn from the same population is true, $\hat{p}_1 = m_1/n_1$ and $\hat{p}_2 = m_2/n_2$, in which m_1 and m_2 are the number of individuals in each sample with the attribute of interest, are both estimates of the same population proportion p. In this case, we would consider all the individuals drawn as a single sample of size $n_1 + n_2$ containing a total of $m_1 + m_2$ individuals with the attribute and use this single pooled sample to estimate $\hat{p}$:

$$\hat{p} = \frac{m_1 + m_2}{n_1 + n_2} = \frac{n\hat{p}_1 + n_2\hat{p}_2}{n_1 + n_2}$$

in which case

$$s = \sqrt{\hat{p}(1 - \hat{p})}$$

and we can estimate

$$s_{\hat{p}_1 - \hat{p}_2} = \sqrt{\frac{s^2}{n_1} + \frac{s^2}{n_2}} = \sqrt{\hat{p}(1 - \hat{p})\left(\frac{1}{n_1} + \frac{1}{n_2}\right)}$$

*The criterion for a large sample is the same as in the last section, namely that $n\hat{p}$ and $n(1 - \hat{p})$ both exceed about 5 for both samples. When this is not the case, one should use the *Fisher exact test* discussed later in this chapter.

Therefore, our test statistic, based on a pooled estimate of the uncertainty in the population proportion, is

$$z = \frac{\hat{p}_1 - \hat{p}_2}{\sqrt{\hat{p}(1 - \hat{p})(1/n_1 + 1/n_2)}}$$

Like the t statistic, z will have a range of possible values depending on which random samples happen to be drawn to compute $\hat{p}_1$ and $\hat{p}_2$, even if both samples were drawn from the same population. If z is sufficiently "big," we will conclude that the data are inconsistent with this hypothesis and assert that there is a difference in the proportions. This argument is exactly analogous to that used to define the critical values of the t for rejecting the hypothesis of no difference. The only change is that in this case we use the standard normal distribution (Fig. 2–5) to define the cutoff values. In fact, the standard normal distribution and the t distribution with an infinite number of degrees of freedom are identical, so we can get the critical values for 5 or 1 percent confidence levels from the last line Table 4–1. This table shows that there is less than a 5 percent chance of z being beyond -1.96 or $+1.96$ and less than a 1 percent chance of z being beyond -2.58 or $+2.58$ when, in fact, the two samples were drawn from the same population.

The Yates Correction for Continuity

The standard normal distribution only approximates the actual distribution of the z test statistic in a way that yields P values that are always smaller than they should be. Thus, the results are biased toward concluding that the treatment had an effect when the evidence does not support such a conclusion. The mathematical reason for this problem has to do with the fact that the z test statistic can only take on discrete values, whereas the theoretical standard normal distribution is continuous. To obtain values of the z test statistic, which are more compatible with the theoretical standard normal distribution, statisticians have introduced the *Yates correction* (or *continuity correction*), in which the expression for z is modified to become

$$z = \frac{|\hat{p}_1 - \hat{p}_2| - \frac{1}{2}(1/n_1 + 1/n_2)}{\sqrt{\hat{p}(1 - \hat{p})(1/n_1 + 1/n_2)}}$$

This adjustment slightly reduces the value of z associated with the data and compensates for the mathematical problem just described.

Mortality Associated with Anesthesia for Open-Heart Surgery with Halothane or Morphine

We can now formally test the hypothesis that halothane and morphine are associated with the same mortality rate when used as anesthetic agents in open-heart surgery. Recall that the logic of the experiment was that halothane depressed cardiac function whereas morphine did not, so in patients with cardiac problems it ought to be better to use morphine anesthesia. Indeed, Chapters 3 and 4 showed that halothane produces lower mean arterial blood pressures during the operation than morphine; so the supposed physiological effect is present.

Nevertheless, the important question is: Does either anesthetic agent lead to a detectable improvement in mortality associated with this operation in the period immediately following the operation? Since 8 of the 61 patients anesthetized with halothane (13.1 percent) and 10 of the 67 patients anesthetized with morphine (14.9 percent) died,

$$\hat{p} = \frac{8 + 10}{61 + 67} = 0.141$$

$n\hat{p}$ for the two samples is $0.141(61) = 8.6$ and $0.141(67) = 9.4$. Since both exceed 5, we can use the test described in the last section.* Our test statistic is therefore

$$z = \frac{|\hat{p}_{\text{hlo}} - \hat{p}_{\text{mor}}| - \frac{1}{2}(1/n_{\text{hlo}} + 1/n_{\text{mor}})}{\sqrt{\hat{p}(1 - \hat{p})(1/n_{\text{hlo}} + 1/n_{\text{mor}})}}$$

$$= \frac{|0.131 - 0.149| - \frac{1}{2}\left(\frac{1}{61} + \frac{1}{67}\right)}{\sqrt{(0.141)(1 - 0.141)\left(\frac{1}{61} + \frac{1}{67}\right)}} = 0.04$$

*$n(1 - \hat{p})$ also exceeds 5 in both cases. We did not need to check this because $\hat{p} < 0.5$, so $n\hat{p} < n(1 - \hat{p})$.

which is quite small. Specifically, it comes nowhere near 1.96, the z value that defines the most extreme 5 percent of all possible values of z when the two samples were drawn from the same population. Hence, we do not have evidence that there is any difference in the mortality associated with these two anesthetic agents, despite the fact that they do seem to have different physiological effects on the patient during surgery.

This study illustrates the importance of looking at *outcomes* in clinical trials. The human body has tremendous capacity to adapt not only to trauma but also to medical manipulation. Therefore, simply showing that some intervention (like a difference in anesthesia) changed a patient's physiological state (by producing different blood pressure) does not mean that in the long run it will make any difference in the clinical outcome. Focusing on these intermediate variables, often called *process variables,* rather than the more important outcome variables may lead you to think something made a clinical difference when it did not. For example, in this study there was the expected change in the process variable, blood pressure, but not the outcome variable, mortality. If we had stopped with the process variables, we might have concluded that morphine anesthesia was superior to halothane in patients with cardiac problems, even though the choice of anesthesia does not appear to have affected the most important variable, whether or not the patient survived.

Keep this distinction in mind when reading medical journals and listening to proponents argue for their tests, procedures, and therapies. It is much easier to show that something affects process variables than the more important outcome variables. In addition to being easier to produce a demonstrable change in process variables than outcome variables, process variables are generally easier to measure. Observing outcomes may require following the patients for some time and often present difficult subjective problems of measurement, especially when one tries to measure "quality of life" variables. Nevertheless, when assessing whether or not some new procedure deserves to be adopted in an era of limited medical resources, you should seek evidence that something affects the patient's outcome. The patient and the patient's family care about outcome, not process.

Prevention of Thrombosis in People Receiving Hemodialysis

People with chronic kidney disease can be kept alive by dialysis; their blood is passed through a machine that does the work of their kidneys and removes metabolic products and other chemicals from their blood. The dialysis machine must be connected to one of the patient's arteries and veins to allow the blood to pass through the machine. Since patients must be connected to the dialysis machine on a regular basis, it is necessary to create surgically a more or less permanent connection that can be used to attach the person's body to the machine. One way of doing this is to attach a small Teflon tube containing a coupling fitting, called a *shunt,* between an artery and vein in the wrist or arm. When the patient is to be connected to the dialysis machine, the tubing is connected to these fittings on the Teflon tube; otherwise, the two fittings are simply connected together so that the blood just flows directly from the small artery to the vein. For a variety of reasons, including the surgical technique used to place the shunt, disease of the artery or vein, local infection, or a reaction to the Teflon adapter, blood clots (thromboses) tend to form in these shunts. These clots have to be removed regularly to permit dialysis and can be severe enough to require tying off the shunt and creating a new one. The clots can spread down the artery or vein, making it necessary to pass a catheter into the artery or vein to remove the clot. In addition, these clots may break loose and lodge elsewhere in the body, where they may cause problems. Herschel Harter and colleagues* knew that aspirin tends to inhibit blood clotting and wondered whether thrombosis could be reduced in people who were receiving chronic dialysis by giving them a low dose of aspirin (160 mg, one-half a common aspirin tablet) every day to inhibit the blood's tendency to clot.

They completed a randomized clinical trial in which all people being dialyzed at their institution who agreed to participate in the study and who had no reason for not taking aspirin (like an allergy) were randomly assigned to a group that received either a placebo or aspirin. To avoid bias on either the investigators' or patients' parts, the

*H. R. Harter, J. W. Burch, P. W. Majerus, N. Stanford, J. A. Delmez, C. B. Anderson, and C. A. Weerts, "Prevention of Thrombosis in Patients in Hemodialysis by Low-Dose Aspirin," *N. Engl. J. Med.,* **301:**577–579, 1979.

study was *double-blind.* Neither the physician administering the drug nor the patient receiving it knew whether the tablet was placebo or aspirin. This procedure adjusts for the placebo effect in the patients and prevents the investigators from looking harder for clots in one group or the other. The double-blind randomized clinical trial is the best way to test a new therapy.

They continued the study until 24 patients developed thrombi, because they assumed that with a total of 24 patients with thrombi any differences between the placebo and aspirin-treated groups would be detectable. Once they reached this point, they broke the code on the bottles of the pills and analyzed their results: 19 people had received aspirin and 25 people had received placebo (Table 5–1). There did not seem to be any clinically important difference in these two groups in terms of age distribution, sex, time on dialysis at entry into the study, or other variables.

Of the 19 people receiving aspirin, 6 developed thrombi; of the 25 people receiving placebo 18 developed thrombi. Is this difference beyond what we would expect if aspirin had no effect and acted like a placebo, so the two groups of patients could be considered as having been drawn from the same population in which a constant proportion p of patients were destined to develop thrombi?

We first estimate $\hat{p}$ for the two groups:

$$\hat{p}_{\text{asp}} = \frac{6}{19} = 0.32$$

Table 5–1 Thrombus Formation in People Receiving Dialysis and Treated with Placebo or Aspirin

	Number of patients		
Sample group	Developed thrombi	Free of thrombi	Treated
Placebo	18	7	25
Aspirin	6	13	19
Total	24	20	44

Source: H. R. Harter, J. W. Burch, P. W. Majerus, N. Stanford, J. A. Delmez, C. B. Anderson, and C. A. Weerts "Prevention of Thrombosis in Patients on Hemodialysis by Low-Dose Aspirin," *N. Engl. J. Med.,* **301**:577–579, 1979. Reprinted by permission of the *New England Journal of Medicine.*

for the people who received aspirin and

$$\hat{p}_{\text{pla}} = \frac{18}{25} = 0.72$$

for the people who received placebo.

Next, we make sure that $n\hat{p}$ and $n(1 - \hat{p})$ are greater than about 5 for both groups, to be certain that the sample sizes are large enough for the normal distribution to reasonably approximate the distribution of our test statistic z if the hypothesis that aspirin had no effect is true. For the people who received aspirin

$$n_{\text{asp}}\hat{p}_{\text{asp}} = 6$$
$$n_{\text{asp}}(1 - \hat{p}_{\text{asp}}) = 13$$

and for the people who received placebo

$$n_{\text{pla}}\hat{p}_{\text{pla}} = 18$$
$$n_{\text{pla}}(1 - \hat{p}_{\text{pla}}) = 7$$

We can use the methods we have developed.

The proportion of all patients who developed thromboses was

$$\hat{p} = \frac{6 + 18}{19 + 25} = 0.55$$

and so

$$s_{\hat{p}_{\text{asp}} - \hat{p}_{\text{pla}}} = \sqrt{\hat{p}(1 - \hat{p})\left(\frac{1}{n_{\text{asp}}} + \frac{1}{n_{\text{pla}}}\right)}$$
$$= \sqrt{0.55(1 - 0.55)\left(\frac{1}{19} + \frac{1}{25}\right)} = 0.15$$

Finally, we compute z according to

$$z = \frac{|\hat{p}_{\text{asp}} - \hat{p}_{\text{pla}}| - \dfrac{1}{2}\left(\dfrac{1}{19} + \dfrac{1}{25}\right)}{s_{\hat{p}_{\text{asp}} - p_{\text{pla}}}}$$

$$= \frac{|0.32 - 0.72| - 0.05}{0.15} = 2.33$$

Table 4–1 indicates that z will exceed 2.3263 in magnitude less than 2 percent of the time if the two samples are drawn from the same population. Since the value of z associated with our experiment is more extreme than 2.3263, it is very unlikely that the two samples were drawn from a single population. Therefore, we conclude that they were not, with $P < .02$.* In other words, we will conclude that giving patients low doses of aspirin while they are receiving chronic kidney dialysis decreases the likelihood that they will develop thrombosis in the shunt used to connect them to the dialysis machine.

ANOTHER APPROACH TO TESTING NOMINAL DATA: ANALYSIS OF CONTINGENCY TABLES

The methods we just developed based on the z statistic are perfectly adequate for testing hypotheses when there are only two possible attributes or outcomes of interest. The z statistic plays a role analogous to the t test for data measured on an interval scale. There are many situations, however, where there are more than two samples to be compared or more than two possible outcomes. To do this, we need to develop a testing procedure, analogous to analysis of variance, that is more flexible than the z test just described. While the following approach may seem quite different from the one we just used to design the z test for proportions, it is essentially the same.

*The value of z associated with these data, 2.33, is so close to the critical value of 2.3263 associated with $P < .02$ that it would be prudent to report $P < .05$ (corresponding to a critical value of 1.960) because the mathematical models that are used to compute the table of critical values are only approximations of reality.

To keep things simple, we begin with the problem we just solved, assessing the efficacy of low-dose aspirin in preventing thrombosis. In the last section we analyzed the *proportion* of people in each of the two treatment groups (aspirin and placebo) who developed thromboses. Now we change our emphasis slightly and analyze the *number* of people in each group who developed thrombi. Since the procedure we will develop does not require assuming anything about the nature of parameters of the population from which the samples were drawn, it is called a *nonparametric* method.

Table 5–1 shows the results of placebo and aspirin in the experiment, with the number of people in each treatment group who did and did not develop thromboses. This table is called a 2 × 2 *contingency table*. Most of the patients in the study fell along the diagonal in this table, suggesting an association between the presence of thrombi and the absence of aspirin treatment. Table 5–2 shows what the experimental results might have looked like *if the aspirin had no effect on thrombus formation*. It also shows the total number of patients who received each treatment as well as the total number who did and did not develop thrombi. These numbers are obtained by summing the rows and columns, respectively, in the table; these sums are the same as Table 5–1. More patients developed thrombi under each treatment; the differences in absolute numbers of patients are due to the fact that more patients received the placebo than aspirin. In contrast to Table 5–1, there does not seem to be a pattern relating treatment to thrombus formation.

To understand better why most people have this subjective impression, let us examine where the numbers in Table 5–2 came from. Of the 44 people in the study 25, or 25/44 = 57 percent, received

Table 5–2 Expected Thrombus Formation If Aspirin Had No Effect

	Number of patients		
Sample group	Developed thrombi	Free of thrombi	Treated
Aspirin	10.36	8.64	19
Placebo	13.64	11.36	25
Total	24	20	44

placebo and 19, or 19/44 = 43 percent, received aspirin. Of the people in the study 24, or 25/44 = 55 percent, developed thrombi and 20, or 20/44 = 45 percent, did not. Now, let us hypothesize that the treatment did *not* affect the likelihood that someone would develop a thrombus. In this case, we would expect 55 percent of the 25 patients treated with placebo (13.64 patients) to develop thrombi and 55 percent of the 19 patients treated with aspirin (10.36 patients) to develop thrombi. The remaining patients should be free of thrombi. Note that we compute the expected frequencies to two decimal places (i.e., to the hundredth of a patient); this procedure is necessary to ensure accurate results in the computation of the χ^2 test below. Thus, Table 5–2 shows how we would *expect* the data to look if 25 patients were given placebo and 19 patients were given aspirin and 24 of them were destined to develop thrombi *regardless of how they were treated.* Compare Tables 5–1 and 5–2. Do they seem similar? Not really; the actual pattern of observations seems quite different from what we expected if the treatment had no effect.

The next step in designing a statistical procedure to test the hypothesis that the pattern of observations is due to random sampling rather than a treatment effect is to reduce this subjective impression to a single number, a test statistic, like *F, t,* or *z*, so that we can reject the hypothesis of no effect when this statistic is "big."

Before constructing this test statistic, however, let us return to another example, the relationship between type of anesthesia and mortality following open-heart surgery. Table 5–3 shows the results of our investigation, presented in the same format as Table 5–1. Table 5–4 presents what the table might look like if the type of anesthesia had no effect on mortality. Out of 128 people, 110, or 110/128 = 86 percent, lived. If the type of anesthesia had no effect on mortality rate, 86 percent of the 61 people anesthetized with halothane (52.42 people)

Table 5–3 Mortality Associated with Open-Heart Surgery

Anesthesia	Lived	Died	Total no. of cases
Halothane	53	8	61
Morphine	57	10	67
Total	110	18	128

Table 5–4 Expected Mortality with Open-Heart Surgery If Anesthesia Did Not Matter

Anesthesia	Lived	Died	Total no. of cases
Halothane	52.42	8.58	61
Morphine	57.58	9.42	67
Total	110	18	128

and 86 percent of the 67 people anesthetized with morphine (57.58 people) would be expected to live, the rest dying in each case. Compare Tables 5–3 and 5–4; there is little difference between the expected and observed frequencies in each cell in the table. The observations are compatible with the assumption that there is no relationship between type of anesthesia and mortality.

The Chi-Square Test Statistic

Now we are ready to design our test statistic. It should describe, with a single number, how much the observed frequencies in each cell in the table differ from the frequencies we would expect if there is no relationship between the treatments and the outcomes that define the rows and columns of the table. In addition, it should allow for the fact that if we expect a large number of people to fall in a given cell, a difference of one person between the expected and observed frequencies is less important than in cases where we expect only a few people to fall in the cell.

We define the test statistic χ^2 (the square of the Greek letter chi) as

$$\chi^2 = \text{sum of } \frac{(\text{observed} - \text{expected number of individuals in cell})^2}{\text{expected number of individuals in cell}}$$

The sum is calculated by adding the results for all cells in the contingency table. The equivalent mathematical statement is

$$\chi^2 = \sum \frac{(O - E)^2}{E}$$

in which O is the observed number of individuals (frequency) in a given cell, E is the expected number of individuals (frequency) in that cell, and the sum is over all the cells in the contingency table. Note that if the observed frequencies are similar to the expected frequencies, χ^2 will be a small number and if the observed and expected frequencies differ, χ^2 will be a big number.

We can now use the information in Tables 5–1 and 5–2 to compute the χ^2 statistic associated with the data on the use of low-dose aspirin to prevent thrombosis in people undergoing chronic dialysis. Table 5–1 gives the observed frequencies, and Table 5–2 gives the expected frequencies. Thus,

$$\chi^2 = \sum \frac{(O - E)^2}{E} = \frac{(18 - 13.64)^2}{13.64} + \frac{(7 - 11.36)^2}{11.36} + \frac{(6 - 10.36)^2}{10.36} + \frac{(13 - 8.64)^2}{8.64} = 7.10$$

To begin getting a feeling for whether or not 7.10 is "big," let us compute χ^2 for the data on mortality associated with halothane and morphine anesthesia given in Table 5–3. Table 5–4 gives the expected frequencies, so

$$\chi^2 = \frac{(53 - 52.42)^2}{52.42} + \frac{(8 - 8.58)^2}{8.58} + \frac{(57 - 57.58)^2}{57.58} + \frac{(10 - 9.42)^2}{9.42} = 0.09$$

which is pretty small, in agreement with our intuitive impression that the observed and expected frequencies are quite similar. (Of course, it is also in agreement with our earlier analysis of the same data using the z statistic in the last section.) In fact, it is possible to show that $\chi^2 = z^2$ when there are only two samples and two possible outcomes.

Like all test statistics, χ^2 can take on a range of values even when there is no relationship between the treatments and outcomes because of the effects of random sampling. Figure 5–7 shows the distribution of possible values for χ^2 computed from data in 2×2 contingency tables

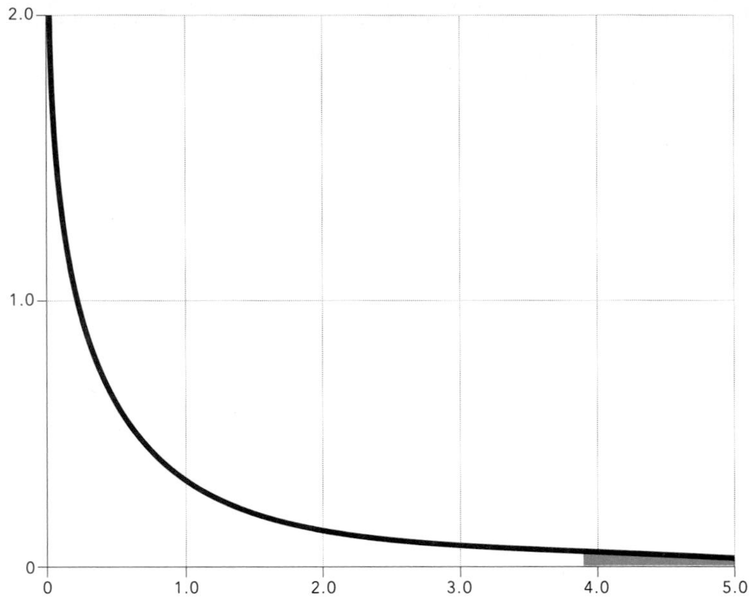

Figure 5–7 The chi-square distribution with 1 degree of freedom. The shaded area denotes the biggest 5 percent of possible values of the χ^2 test statistic when there is no relationship between the treatments and observations.

like those in Tables 5–1 or 5–3. It shows that when the hypothesis of no relationship between the rows and columns of the table is true, χ^2 would be expected to exceed 6.635 only 1 percent of the time. Because the observed value of χ^2, 7.10 exceeds this critical value of 6.635, we can conclude that the data in Table 5–1 are unlikely to occur when the hypothesis that aspirin and placebo have the same effect on thrombus formation is true. We report that aspirin is associated with lower rates of thrombus formation ($P < .01$).

In contrast, the data in Table 5–3 seem very compatible with the hypothesis that halothane and morphine produce the same mortality rates in patients being operated on for repair of heart valves.

Of course, neither of these cases *proves* that aspirin did or did not have an effect, or that halothane and morphine did or did not produce the same mortality rates. What they show is that in one case the pattern of the observations is unlikely to arise if the aspirin acts like a placebo, whereas on the other hand the pattern of observations are very likely to arise if halothane and morphine produce similar mortality rates. Like all the other procedures we have been using to test hypotheses, however, when we reject the hypothesis of no association at the 5 percent level, we are implicitly willing to accept the fact that, in the long run, about 1 reported effect in 20 will be due to random variation rather than a real treatment effect.

As with all theoretical distributions of test statistics used for testing hypotheses, there are assumptions built into the use of χ^2. For the resulting theoretical distribution to be reasonably accurate, *the expected number of individuals in all the cells must be at least 5.** (This is essentially the same as the restriction on the z test in the last section.)

Like most test statistics, the distribution of χ^2 depends on the number of treatments being compared. It also depends on the number of possible outcomes. This dependency is quantified in a *degrees of freedom* parameter ν equal to the number of rows in the table minus 1 times the number of columns in the table minus 1

$$\nu = (r - 1)(c - 1)$$

where r is the number of rows and c is the number of columns in the table. For the 2×2 tables we have been dealing with so far, $\nu = (2 - 1)(2 - 1) = 1$.

As with the z test statistic discussed earlier in this chapter, when analyzing 2×2 contingency tables ($\nu = 1$), the value of χ^2 computed using the formula above and the theoretical χ^2 distribution leads to P values that are smaller than they ought to be. Thus, the results are biased toward concluding that the treatment had an effect when the evidence does not support such a conclusion. The mathematical reason for this problem has to do with the fact that the theoretical χ^2 distribution is continuous whereas the set of all possible values that the χ^2 test statistics can take on is not. To obtain values of the test statistic that are more

*When the data do not meet this requirement, one should use the Fisher exact test.

compatible with the critical values computed from the theoretical χ^2 distribution when $\nu = 1$, apply the *Yates correction* (or *continuity correction*) to compute a corrected χ^2 test statistic according to

$$\chi^2 = \sum \frac{(|O - E| - \frac{1}{2})^2}{E}$$

This correction slightly reduces the value of χ^2 associated with the contingency table and compensates for the mathematical problem just described. The Yates correction is used only when $\nu = 1$, that is, for 2×2 tables.

To illustrate the use and effect of the continuity correction, let us recompute the value of χ^2 associated with the data on the use of low-dose aspirin to prevent thrombosis in people undergoing chronic dialysis. From the observed and expected frequencies in Tables 5–1 and 5–2, respectively

$$\chi^2 = \frac{(|18 - 13.64| - \frac{1}{2})^2}{13.64} + \frac{(|7 - 11.36| - \frac{1}{2})^2}{11.36} + \frac{(|6 - 10.36| - \frac{1}{2})^2}{10.36} + \frac{(|13 - 8.64| - \frac{1}{2})^2}{8.64} = 5.57$$

Note that this value of χ^2, 5.57, is smaller than the uncorrected value of χ^2, 7.10, we obtained before. The corrected value of χ^2 no longer exceeds the critical value of 6.635 associated with the greatest 1 percent of possible χ^2 values (i.e., for $P < .01$). After applying the continuity correction, χ^2 now only exceeds 5.024, the critical value that defines the greatest 2.5 percent of possible values (i.e., for $P < .025$).

CHI-SQUARE APPLICATIONS TO EXPERIMENTS WITH MORE THAN TWO TREATMENTS OR OUTCOMES

It is easy to generalize what we have just done to analyze the results of experiments with more than two treatments or outcomes. The z test we developed earlier in this chapter will not work for such experiments.

Recall that in Chapter 3 we demonstrated that women who jog regularly or engage in long-distance running have fewer menstrual periods

Table 5–5 Consult Physician for Menstrual Problem

Group	Yes	No	Total
Controls	14	40	54
Joggers	9	14	23
Runners	46	42	88
Total	69	96	165

Source: E. Dale, D. H. Gerlach, and A. L. Wilhite, "Menstrual Dysfunction in Distance Runners," *Obstet. Gynecol.*, **54:**47–53, 1979.

on the average than women who do not participate in this sport.* Does this physiological change lead women to consult their physician about menstrual problems? Table 5–5 shows the results of a survey of the same women discussed in conjunction with Fig. 3–9. Are these data consistent with the hypothesis that running does not increase the likelihood that a woman will consult her physician for a menstrual problem?

Of the 165 women in the study 69, or 69/165 = 42 percent, consulted their physicians for a menstrual problem, while the remaining 96, or 96/165 = 58 percent, did not. If the extent of running did not affect the likelihood that a woman would consult her physician, we would expect 42 percent of the 54 controls (22.58 women) to have visited their physicians, and 42 percent of the 23 joggers (9.62 women) to have consulted their physicians, and 42 percent of the 88 distance runners (36.80 women) to have consulted their physicians. Table 5–6 shows these expected frequencies, together with the expected frequencies of women who did not consult their physicians. Are the differences between the observed and expected frequencies "big?"

To answer this question, we compute the χ^2 statistic

$$\chi^2 = \frac{(14 - 22.58)^2}{22.58} + \frac{(40 - 31.42)^2}{31.42} + \frac{(9 - 9.62)^2}{9.62} + \frac{(14 - 13.38)^2}{13.38} + \frac{(46 - 36.80)^2}{36.80} + \frac{(42 - 51.20)^2}{51.20} = 9.63$$

*When this study was discussed in Chapter 3, we assumed the same number of patients in each treatment group to simplify the computation. In this chapter we use the actual number of patients in the study.

Table 5–6 Expected Frequencies of Physician Consultation If Running Did Not Matter

Group	Yes	No	Total
Controls	22.58	31.42	54
Joggers	9.62	13.38	23
Runners	36.80	51.20	88
Total	69	96	165

The contingency table in Table 5–5 has three rows and two columns, so the χ^2 statistic has

$$\nu = (r - 1)(c - 1) = (3 - 1)(2 - 1) = 2$$

degrees of freedom associated with it. Table 5–7 shows that χ^2 will exceed 9.21 less than 1 percent of the time when the difference between the observed and expected frequencies is due to random variation rather than an effect of the treatment (in this case, running). Thus, there is a relationship between running and the chances that a woman will consult her physician about a menstrual problem ($P < .01$). Note, however, that we do not yet know which group or groups of women account for this difference.

Let us now sum up how to use the χ^2 statistic.

- *Tabulate the data in a contingency table.*
- *Sum the number of individuals in each row and each column and figure the percentage of all individuals who fall in each row and column, independent of the column or row in which they fall.*
- *Use these percentages to compute the number of people that would be expected in each cell of the table if the treatment had no effect.*
- *Summarize the differences between these expected frequencies and the observed frequencies by computing χ^2. If the data form a 2 × 2 table, include the Yates correction.*
- *Compute the number of degrees of freedom associated with the contingency table and use Table 5–7 to see whether the observed value of χ^2 exceeds what would be expected from random variation.*

Recall that when the data fell into a 2 × 2 contingency table, all the expected frequencies had to exceed about 5 for the χ^2 test to be accurate. In larger tables, most statisticians recommend that the expected number of individuals in each cell never be less than 1 and that no more than 20 percent of them be less than 5. When this is not the case, the χ^2 test can be quite inaccurate. The problem can be remedied by collecting more data to increase the cell numbers or by reducing the number of categories to increase the numbers in each cell of the table.

Subdividing Contingency Tables

Our analysis of Table 5–6 revealed that there is probably a difference in the likelihood that the different groups of women will consult their physicians regarding a menstrual problem, but our analysis did not isolate *which* groups of women accounted for this effect. This situation is analogous to the multiple-comparison problem in analysis of variance. The analysis of variance will help decide whether *something* is different, but you need to go on to the multiple-comparison procedure to define *which group it was.* You can do the same thing with a contingency table.

Looking at the numbers in Table 5–5 suggests that joggers and runners are more likely to consult their physicians than women in the control group, but they seem similar to each other.

To test this latter hypothesis, we *subdivide* the contingency table to look only at the joggers and runners. Table 5–8 shows the data for the joggers and runners. The numbers in parentheses are the expected number of women in each cell. The observed and expected number of women in each cell appear quite similar; since it is a 2 × 2 contingency table, we compute χ^2 with the Yates correction

$$\chi^2 = \sum \frac{(|O - E| - \frac{1}{2})^2}{E}$$

$$= \frac{(|9 - 11.40| - \frac{1}{2})^2}{11.40} + \frac{(|14 - 11.60| - \frac{1}{2})^2}{11.60}$$

$$+ \frac{(|46 - 43.60| - \frac{1}{2})^2}{43.60} + \frac{(|42 - 44.40| - \frac{1}{2})^2}{44.40} = .79$$

Table 5–7 Critical Values for the χ^2 Distribution

ν	Probability of greater value P							
	.50	.25	.10	.05	.025	.01	.005	.001
1	.455	1.323	2.706	3.841	5.024	6.635	7.879	10.828
2	1.386	2.773	4.605	5.991	7.378	9.210	10.597	13.816
3	2.366	4.108	6.251	7.815	9.348	11.345	12.838	16.266
4	3.357	5.385	7.779	9.488	11.143	13.277	14.860	18.467
5	4.351	6.626	9.236	11.070	12.833	15.086	16.750	20.515
6	5.348	7.841	10.645	12.592	14.449	16.812	18.548	22.458
7	6.346	9.037	12.017	14.067	16.013	18.475	20.278	24.322
8	7.344	10.219	13.362	15.507	17.535	20.090	21.955	26.124
9	8.343	11.389	14.684	16.919	19.023	21.666	23.589	27.877
10	9.342	12.549	15.987	18.307	20.483	23.209	25.188	29.588
11	10.341	13.701	17.275	19.675	21.920	24.725	26.757	31.264
12	11.340	14.845	18.549	21.026	23.337	26.217	28.300	32.909
13	12.340	15.984	19.812	22.362	24.736	27.688	29.819	34.528
14	13.339	17.117	21.064	23.685	26.119	29.141	31.319	36.123
15	14.339	18.245	22.307	24.996	27.488	30.578	32.801	37.697
16	15.338	19.369	23.542	26.296	28.845	32.000	34.267	39.252
17	16.338	20.489	24.769	27.587	30.191	33.409	35.718	40.790
18	17.338	21.605	25.989	28.869	31.526	34.805	37.156	42.312
19	18.338	22.718	27.204	30.144	32.852	36.191	38.582	43.820
20	19.337	23.828	28.412	31.410	34.170	37.566	39.997	45.315
21	20.337	24.935	29.615	32.671	35.479	38.932	41.401	46.797
22	21.337	26.039	30.813	33.924	36.781	40.289	42.796	48.268
23	22.337	27.141	32.007	35.172	38.076	41.638	44.181	49.728
24	23.337	28.241	33.196	36.415	39.364	42.980	45.559	51.179
25	24.337	29.339	34.382	37.652	40.646	44.314	46.928	52.620
26	25.336	30.435	35.563	38.885	41.923	45.642	48.290	54.052
27	26.336	31.528	36.741	40.113	43.195	46.963	49.645	55.476
28	27.336	32.020	37.916	41.337	44.461	48.278	50.993	56.892
29	28.336	33.711	39.087	42.557	45.722	49.588	52.336	58.301
30	29.336	34.800	40.256	43.773	46.979	50.892	53.672	59.703
31	30.336	35.887	41.422	44.985	48.232	52.191	55.003	61.098
32	31.336	36.973	42.585	46.194	49.480	53.486	56.328	62.487
33	32.336	38.058	43.745	47.400	50.725	54.776	57.648	63.870
34	33.336	39.141	44.903	48.602	51.966	56.061	58.964	65.247
35	34.336	40.223	46.059	49.802	53.203	57.342	60.275	66.619
36	35.336	41.304	47.212	50.998	54.437	58.619	61.581	67.985
37	36.336	42.383	48.363	52.192	55.668	59.893	62.883	69.346

(continued)

	Probability of greater value P							
ν	.50	.25	.10	.05	.025	.01	.005	.001
38	37.335	43.462	49.513	53.384	56.896	61.162	64.181	70.703
39	38.335	44.539	50.660	54.572	58.120	62.428	65.476	72.055
40	39.335	45.616	51.805	55.758	59.342	63.691	66.766	73.402
41	40.335	46.692	52.949	56.942	60.561	64.950	68.053	74.745
42	41.335	47.766	54.090	58.124	61.777	66.206	69.336	76.084
43	42.335	48.840	55.230	59.304	62.990	67.459	70.616	77.419
44	43.335	49.913	56.369	60.481	64.201	68.710	71.893	78.750
45	44.335	50.985	57.505	61.656	65.410	69.957	73.166	80.077
46	45.335	52.056	58.641	62.830	66.617	71.201	74.437	81.400
47	46.335	53.127	59.774	64.001	67.821	72.443	75.704	82.720
48	47.335	54.196	60.907	65.171	69.023	73.683	76.969	84.037
49	48.335	55.265	62.038	66.339	70.222	74.919	78.231	85.351
50	49.335	56.334	63.167	67.505	71.420	76.154	79.490	86.661

Source: Adapted from J. H. Zar, *Biostatistical Analysis* (2nd ed). Prentice-Hall, Englewood Cliffs, N.J., 1984, pp. 479–482, table B. 1. Used by permission.

which is small enough for us to conclude that the joggers and runners are equally likely to visit their physicians. Since they are so similar, we combine the two groups and compare this combined group with the control group. Table 5–9 shows the resulting 2 × 2 contingency table, together with the expected frequencies in parentheses. χ^2 for this contingency table is 7.39, which exceeds 6.63, the critical value that defines the upper 1 percent of probable values of χ^2 when there is no relationship between the rows and columns in a 2 × 2 table.

Table 5–8 Physician Consultation among Women Joggers and Runners*

Group	Yes	No	Total
Joggers	9 (11.40)	14 (11.60)	23
Runners	46 (43.60)	42 (44.40)	88
Total	55	56	111

*Numbers in parentheses are expected frequencies if the amount of running does not affect physician consultation.

Table 5–9 Physician Consultation among Women Who Did and Did Not Run*

Group	Yes	No	Total
Controls	14 (22.58)	40 (31.42)	54
Joggers and runners	55 (46.42)	56 (64.58)	111
Total	69	96	165

*Numbers in parentheses are expected frequencies of physician consultation if a woman ran or did not affect the likelihood of her consulting a physician for a menstrual problem.

Note, however, that because we have done *two* tests on the same data, we must use a Bonferroni of Holm correction to adjust the *P* values to account for the fact that we are doing multiple tests. Since we did two tests, we multiply the nominal 1 percent *P* value obtained from Table 5–7 by 2 to obtain 2(1) = 2 percent.* Therefore, we conclude that the joggers and runners did not differ in their medical consultations from each other but did differ from the women in the control group ($P < .02$).

THE FISHER EXACT TEST

The χ^2 test can be used to analyze 2×2 contingency tables when each cell has an expected frequency of at least 5. In small studies, when the expected frequency is smaller than 5, *the Fisher exact test* is the appropriate procedure. This test turns the liability of small sample sizes into a benefit. When the sample sizes are small, it is possible to simply *list* all the possible arrangements of the observations, then compute the exact probabilities associated with each possible arrangement of the data. The total (two-tailed) probability of obtaining the observed data or more extreme patterns in the data is the *P* value associated with the hypothesis that the rows and columns in the data are independent.

*We could also use a Holm procedure to account for multiple comparisons.

Table 5–10 Notation for the Fisher Exact Test

			Row Totals
	O_{11}	O_{12}	R_1
	O_{21}	O_{22}	R_2
Column Totals	C_1	C_2	N

The Fisher exact test begins with the fact that the probability of observing any given pattern in the 2×2 contingency table with the observed row and column totals in Table 5–10 is

$$P = \frac{\dfrac{R_1!R_2!C_1!C_2!}{N!}}{O_{11}!O_{12}!O_{21}!O_{22}!}$$

where O_{11}, O_{12}, O_{21}, and O_{22} are the observed frequencies in the four cells of the contingency table, C_1 and C_2 are the sums of the two columns, R_1 and R_2 are the sums of the two rows, N is the total number of observations, and the exclamation mark "!" indicates the factorial operator.*

Unlike the χ^2 test statistic, there are one- and two-tailed versions of the Fisher exact test. Unfortunately, most descriptions of the Fisher exact test simply describe the one-tailed version and many computer programs compute the one-tailed version without clearly identifying it as such. Because many researchers do not recognize this issue, results (i.e., P values) may be reported for a single tail without the researchers realizing it. To determine whether or not investigators recognized whether they were using one- or two-tailed Fisher exact tests, W. Paul McKinney and colleagues† examined the use of the Fisher exact test in

*The definition $n!$ is $n! = (n)(n-1)(n-2) \times \times \times (2)(1)$; e.g., $5! = 5 \times 4 \times 3 \times 2 \times 1$.

†W. P. McKinney, M. J. Young, A. Harta, and M. B. Lee, "The Inexact Use of Fisher's Exact Test in Six Major Medical Journals," *JAMA*, **261**:3430–3433, 1989.

Table 5–11 Reporting of Use of Fisher Exact Test in the *New England Journal of Medicine* and *The Lancet*

	Test Identified?		
Group	Yes	No	Totals
New England Journal of Medicine	1	8	9
The Lancet	10	4	14
Totals	11	12	23

papers published in the medical literature to see whether or not the authors noted the type of Fisher exact test that was used. Table 5–11 shows the data for the two journals, *New England Journal of Medicine* and *The Lancet.* Because the numbers are small, χ^2 is not an appropriate test statistic. From the equation above, the probability of obtaining the pattern of observations in Table 5–11 for the given row and column totals is

$$P = \frac{\frac{9!14!11!12!}{23!}}{1!8!10!4!} = .00666$$

Thus, it is very unlikely that *this particular* table would be observed. To obtain the probability of observing a pattern in the data this extreme *or more extreme* in the direction of the table, reduce the smallest observation by 1, and recompute the other cells in the table to maintain the row and column totals constant.

In this case, there is one more extreme table, given in Table 5–12. This table has a probability of occurring of

$$P = \frac{\frac{9!14!11!12!}{23!}}{9!0!3!11!} = .00027$$

(Note that the numerator only depends on the row and column totals associated with the table, which does not change, and so only needs to be computed once.) Thus, the one-tailed Fisher exact test yields a

Table 5–12 More Extreme Pattern of Observations in Table 5–11, Using Smallest Observed Frequency (in This Case, 1)

	Test Identified?		
Group	Yes	No	Totals
New England Journal of Medicine	0	9	9
The Lancet	11	3	14
Totals	11	12	23

P value of $P = .00666 + .00027 = .00695$. This probability represents the probability of obtaining a pattern of observations as extreme or more extreme in one direction as the actual observations in Table 5–11.

To find the other tail, we list all the remaining possible patterns in the data that would give the same row and column totals. These possibilities, together with the associated probabilities, appear in Table 5–13. These tables are obtained by taking each of the remaining three elements in Table 5–11 one at a time and progressively making it smaller by one, then eliminating the duplicate tables. Two of these tables have probabilities at or below the probability of obtaining the original observations, .00666: the ones with probabilities of .00242 and .00007. These two tables constitute the "other" tail of the Fisher exact test. There is a total probability of being in this table of $.00242 + .00007 = .00249$.* Thus, the total probability of obtaining a pattern of observations as extreme or more extreme than that observed is $P = .00695 + .00249 = .00944$, and we conclude there is a significant difference in the correct presentation of the Fisher exact test in the *New England Journal of Medicine* and *The Lancet* ($P = .009$). Indeed, it is important when reading papers that use the Fisher exact test to make sure the authors know what they are doing and report the results appropriately.

*Note that the two tails have different probabilities; this is generally the case. The one exception is when either the two rows or two columns have the same sums, in which case the two-tail probability is simply twice the one-tail probability. Some books say that the two-tail value of P is always simply twice the one-tail value. This is not correct unless the row or column sums are equal.

Table 5–13 Other Patterns of Observations in Table 5–11 with the Same Row and Column Totals

			Totals				Totals
	2	7	9		6	3	9
	9	5	14		5	9	14
Totals	11	12	23	Totals	11	12	23
	$P = .05330$				$P = .12438$		

			Totals				Totals
	3	6	9		7	2	9
	8	6	14		4	10	14
Totals	11	12	23	Totals	11	12	23
	$P = .18657$				$P = .02665$		

			Totals				Totals
	4	5	9		8	1	9
	7	7	14		3	11	14
Totals	11	12	23	Totals	11	12	23
	$P = .31983$				$P = .00242$		

			Totals				Totals
	5	4	9		9	0	9
	6	8	14		2	12	14
Totals	11	12	23	Totals	11	12	23
	$P = .27985$				$P = .00007$		

Let us now sum up how to do the Fisher exact test.

- *Compute the probability associated with the observed data.*
- *Identify the cell in the contingency table with the smallest frequency.*
- *Reduce the smallest element in the table by 1, then compute the elements for the other three cells so that the row and column sums remain constant.*
- *Compute the probability associated with the new table.*

- *Repeat this process until the smallest element is zero.*
- *List the remaining tables by repeating this process for the other three elements.* List each pattern of observations only once.*
- *Compute the probabilities associated with each of these tables.*
- *Add all the probabilities together that are equal to or smaller than the probability associated with the observed data.*

This probability is the *two-tail* probability of observing a pattern in the data as extreme or more extreme than observed. Many computer programs show *P* values for the Fisher exact test, without clearly indicating whether they are one- or two-tail values. Make sure that you know which value is being reported before you use it in your work; the two-tailed *P* value is generally the one you want.

MEASURES OF ASSOCIATION BETWEEN TWO NOMINAL VARIABLES†

In addition to testing whether there are significant differences between two rates or proportions, people often want a measure of the strength of association between some event and different treatments or conditions, particularly in *clinical trials* and *epidemiological studies.* In a *prospective* clinical trial, such as the study of thrombus formation in people treated with aspirin or placebo discussed earlier in this chapter (Table 5–1), investigators randomly assign people to treatment (aspirin) or control (placebo), then follow them to see whether they develop a thrombus or not. In that example, 32 percent (6 out of 19) of the people receiving aspirin developed thrombi and 72 percent (18 out of 25) receiving placebo developed thrombi. These proportions are estimates of the probability of developing a thrombus associated with each of these treatments; these results indicate that the probability of

*Many of these computations can be avoided: see Appendix A.

†In an introductory course, this section can be skipped without loss of continuity.

developing a thrombus was cut by more than half by treatment with aspirin. We will now examine different ways to quantify this effect, *relative risk* and the *odds ratio.*[*]

Prospective Studies and Relative Risk

We quantify the size of the association between treatment and outcome with the *relative risk,* RR, which is defined as

$$\text{RR} = \frac{\text{Probability of event in } \textit{treatment} \text{ group}}{\text{Probability of event in } \textit{control} \text{ group}}$$

For the aspirin trial,

$$\text{RR} = \frac{\hat{p}_{asp}}{\hat{p}_{pla}} = \frac{0.32}{0.72} = 0.44$$

The fact that the relative risk is less than 1 indicates that aspirin reduces the risk of a thrombus. In clinical trials evaluating treatments against placebo (or standard treatment, when it would be unethical to administer a placebo), a relative risk less than 1 indicates that the treatment leads to better outcomes.

In an *epidemiological study,* the probability of an event among people *exposed* to some potential toxin or risk factor is compared to people who are *not exposed.* The calculations are the same as for clinical trials.[†]

[*]Another way to quantify this difference is to present the *absolute risk reduction,* which is simply the difference of the probability of an event (in this case, a thrombus) without and with the treatment, .72 − .32 = .40. Treatment with aspirin reduces the probability of a thrombus by .40. An alternative approach is to present the *number needed to treat,* which is the number of people that would have to be treated to avoid one event. The number needed to treat is simply 1 divided by the absolute risk reduction, in this case 1/.40 = 2.5. Thus, one would expect to avoid one thrombotic event for about every 2.5 people treated (or, if you prefer dealing with whole people, 2 events for every 5 people treated).

[†]In clinical trials and epidemiological studies one often wants to adjust for other so-called *confounding variables* that could be affecting the probability of an event. It is possible to account for such variables using multivariate techniques using *logistic regression* or the *Cox proportional hazards model.* For a discussion of these issues, see S. A. Glantz and B. K. Slinker, *Primer of Applied Regression and Analysis of Variance,* 2nd ed, New York, McGraw-Hill, 2000, chap. 12, "Regression with a Qualitative Dependent Variable."

Table 5–14 Arrangement of Data to Compute Relative Risk

	Number of people		
Sample group	Disease	No disease	Total
Treated (or exposed to risk factor)	a	b	a + b
Control (or not exposed to risk factor)	c	d	c + d
Total	a + c	b + d	

Relative risks greater than 1 indicate that exposure to the toxin *increases* the risk of disease. For example, being married to a smoker is associated with a relative risk of heart disease in nonsmokers of 1.3,* indicating that nonsmokers married to smokers are 1.3 times more likely to die from heart disease as nonsmokers married to nonsmokers (and so not breathing secondhand smoke at home).

Table 5–14 shows the general layout for a calculation of relative risk; it is simply a 2 × 2 contingency table. The probability of an event in the treatment group (also called the *experimental event rate*) is $a/(a + b)$ and the probability of an event in the treatment group (also called the *control event rate*) is $c/(c + d)$. Therefore, the formula for relative risk is

$$\text{RR} = \frac{a/(a + b)}{c/(c + d)}$$

Using the results of the aspirin trial in Table 5–1, we would compute

$$\text{RR} = \frac{6/(6 + 13)}{13/(18 + 7)} = \frac{0.32}{0.72} = 0.44$$

This formula is simply a restatement of the definition of relative risk presented above.

*S. A. Glantz and W. W. Parmley. "Passive Smoking and Heart Disease: Epidemiology, Physiology, and Biochemistry," *Circulation,* **83:**1–12, 1991. S. Glantz and W. Parmley. Passive Smoking and Heart Disease: Mechanisms and Risk, *JAMA,* **273:**1047–1053, 1995.

The most common null hypothesis that people wish to test related to relative risks is that the relative risk equals 1 (i.e., that the treatment or risk factor does not affect event rate). Although it is possible to test this hypothesis using the standard error of the relative risk, most people simply apply a χ^2 test to the contingency table used to compute the relative risk.*

To compute a relative risk, the data must be collected as part of a *prospective study* in which people are randomized to treatment or control or subjects in an epidemiological study† are followed forward in time after they are exposed (or not exposed) to the toxin or risk factor of interest. It is necessary to conduct the study prospectively to estimate the absolute event rates in people in the treatment (or exposed) and control groups.

Such prospective studies are often difficult and expensive to do, particularly if it takes several years for events to occur after treatment or exposure. It is, however, possible to conduct a similar analysis *retrospectively* based on so-called *case-control studies.*

Case-Control Studies and the Odds Ratio

Unlike prospective studies, case-control studies are done after the fact. In a case-control study, people who experienced the outcome of interest are identified and the number exposed to the risk factor of interest are counted. These people are the *cases.* You then identify people who did not experience the outcome of interest, but are similar to the cases in all other relevant ways and count the number that were exposed to the risk factor. These people are the *controls.* (Often investigators include more than one control per case in order to increase the sample size.) Table 5–15 shows the layout for data from a case-control study.

This information can be used to compute a statistic similar to the relative risk known as the *odds ratio.* The odds ratio, OR, is defined as

$$\text{OR} = \frac{\text{Odds of exposure in } \textit{cases}}{\text{Odds of exposure in } \textit{controls}}$$

*Traditionally direct hypothesis testing of relative risks is done by examining confidence intervals; see Chap. 7.

†Prospective epidemiological studies are also called *cohort studies.*

Table 5–15 Arrangement of Data to Compute Odds Ratio

	Number of People	
Sample group	Disease "cases"	No disease "controls"
Exposed to risk factor (or treatment)	a	b
Not exposed to risk factor (or treatment)	c	d
Total	a + c	b + d

The percentage of cases (people with the disease) exposed to the risk factor is $a/(a + c)$ and the percentage of cases not exposed to the risk factor is $c/(a + c)$. (Note that each of the denominators is appropriate for the numerator; this situation would not exist if one was using case-control data to compute a relative risk.) The odds of exposure in the cases is the ratio of these two percentages.

$$\text{Odds of exposure in } \textit{cases} = \frac{a/(a + c)}{c/(a + c)} = \frac{a}{c}$$

Likewise, the odds of exposure in the controls is

$$\text{Odds of exposure in } \textit{controls} = \frac{b/(b + d)}{d/(b + d)} = \frac{b}{d}$$

Finally, the odds ratio is

$$\text{OR} = \frac{a/c}{b/d} = \frac{ad}{bc}$$

Because the number of controls (and so b and d in Table 5–15) depends on how the investigator designs the study, you cannot use data from a case-control study to compute a relative risk. In a case-control study the investigator decides how many subjects with and without the disease will be studied. This is the opposite of the situation in prospective studies (clinical trials and epidemiological cohort studies), when the investigator decides how many subjects with and without the risk factor will be included in the study. The odds ratio may be used in both case-control and prospective studies, but *must* be used in case-control studies.

While the odds ratio is distinct from the relative risk, the odds ratio is a reasonable estimate of the relative risk when the number of people with the disease is small compared to the number of people without the disease.*

As with the relative risk, the most common null hypothesis that people wish to test related to relative risks is that the odds ratio equals 1 (i.e., that the treatment or risk factor does not affect the event rate). While it is possible to test this hypothesis using the standard error of the odds ratio, most people simply apply a χ^2 test to the contingency table used to compute the odds ratio.†

Passive Smoking and Breast Cancer

Breast cancer is the second leading cause of cancer death among women (behind lung cancer). Smoking causes lung cancer because of the cancer-causing chemicals in the smoke that enter the body and some of these chemicals appear in breast milk, indicating that they reach the breast. To examine whether exposure to secondhand tobacco smoke increased the risk of breast cancer in lifelong nonsmokers, Johnson and colleagues†† conducted a case-control study using cancer registries in Canada to identify premenopausal women with histologically confirmed invasive primary breast cancer. They contacted the women and interviewed them about their smoking habits and exposure to secondhand smoke at home and at work. They obtained a group of controls who did

*In this case, the number of people who have the disease, a and c, is much smaller than the number of people without the disease, b and d, so $a + b \cong b$ and $c + d \cong d$. As a result

$$\text{RR} = \frac{a/(a+b)}{c/(c+d)} \approx \frac{a/b}{c/d} = \frac{ad}{bc} = \text{OR}$$

†Direct hypothesis testing regarding odds ratios is usually done with confidence intervals; see Chapter 7.

††K. C. Johnson, J. Hu, Y. Mao, and the Canadian Cancer Registries Epidemiology Research Group, "Passive and Active Smoking and Breast Cancer Risk in Canada, 1994–1997," *Cancer Causes Control,* **11:**211–221, 2000.

Table 5–16 Passive Smoking and Breast Cancer

	Number of People	
Sample group	Cases (breast cancer)	Controls
Exposed to secondhand smoke	50	43
Not exposed to secondhand smoke	14	35
Total	64	78

not have breast cancer, matched by age group, from a mailing to women using lists obtained from the provincial health insurance authorities. Table 5–16 shows the resulting data.

The fraction of women with breast cancer (cases) who were exposed to secondhand smoke is $50/(50 + 14) = 0.781$ and the fraction of women with breast cancer not exposed to secondhand smoke is $14/(50 + 14) = 0.218$, so the odds of the women with breast cancer having been exposed to secondhand smoke is $0.781/0.218 = 3.58$. Similarly, the fraction of controls exposed to secondhand smoke is $43/(43 + 35) = 0.551$ and the fraction not exposed to secondhand smoke is $35/(43 + 35) = 0.449$, so the odds of the women without breast cancer having been exposed to secondhand smoke is $0.551/0.449 = 1.23$. Finally, the odds ratio of breast cancer associated with secondhand smoke exposure is

$$\text{OR} = \frac{\begin{array}{c}\text{Odds of secondhand smoke exposure}\\ \text{in women with breast cancer}\end{array}}{\begin{array}{c}\text{Odds of secondhand smoke}\\ \text{exposure in controls}\end{array}} = \frac{3.58}{1.23} = 2.91$$

Alternatively, we could use the direct formula for odds ratio and compute

$$\text{OR} = \frac{ad}{bc} = \frac{50 \cdot 35}{14 \cdot 43} = 2.91$$

Based on this study, we conclude that exposure to secondhand smoke increases the odds of having breast cancer by 2.91 times among this population. A χ^2 analysis of the data in Table 15–16 shows that this difference is statistically significant ($P = .007$).

We now have the tools to analyze data measured on a nominal scale. So far we have been focusing on how to demonstrate a difference and quantify the certainty with which we can assert this difference or effect with the *P* value. Now we turn to the other side of the coin: What does it mean if the test statistic is *not* big enough to reject the hypothesis of no difference?

PROBLEMS

5-1 Obtaining a blood sample of arterial blood permits measuring blood pH, oxygenation, and CO_2 elimination in order to see how well the lungs are functioning at oxygenating blood. The blood sample is often drawn from an artery in the wrist, which can be a painful procedure. Shawn Aaron and colleagues ("Topical tetracaine prior to arterial puncture: a randomized, placebo-controlled clinical trial," *Respir. Med.* **97:**1195–1199, 2003) compared the effectiveness of a topical anesthetic gel applied to the skin over the puncture point with a placebo cream. They observed adverse effects (redness, swelling, itching, or bruising) within 24 hours of administering the gel. Three of 36 people receiving the anesthetic gel and 8 of 40 receiving the placebo gel suffered an adverse reaction. Is there evidence of a difference in the rate of adverse effects between the anesthetic gel and the placebo gel?

5-2 Adolescent suicide is commonly associated with alcohol misuse. In a retrospective study involving Finnish adolescents who committed suicide, Sami Pirkola and colleagues ("Alcohol-Related Problems Among Adolescent Suicides in Finland," *Alcohol Alcohol.* **34:**320–328, 1999) compared situational factors and family background between victims who abused alcohol and those who did not. Alcohol use was determined by family interview several months following the suicide. Adolescents with alcohol problems, ranging from mild to severe, were classified together in a group called SDAM (Subthreshold or Diagnosable Alcohol Misuse) and compared to victims with no such reported alcohol problems. Some of Pirkola's findings appear below. Use these data to identify the characteristics of SDAM suicides. Are these factors specific enough to be of predictive value in a specific adolescent? Why or why not?

Factor	SDAM group ($n = 44$)	Not in SDAM group ($n = 62$)
Violent death (shooting, hanging, jumping, traffic)	32	51
Suicide under influence of alcohol	36	25
Blood alcohol concentration (BAC) ≥ 150 mg/dL	17	3
Suicide during weekend	28	26
Parental divorce	20	15
Parental violence	14	5
Parental alcohol abuse	17	12
Paternal alcohol abuse	15	9
Parental suicidal behavior	5	3
Institutional rearing	6	2

5-3 The 106 suicides analyzed in Prob. 5-2 were selected from 116 suicides that occurred between April 1987 and March 1988. Eight of the ten suicides not included in the study were due to lack of family interviews. Discuss the potential problems, if any, associated with these exclusions.

5-4 Major depression can be treated with medication, psychotherapy or a combination of the two. M. Keller and colleagues ("A Comparison of Nefazodone, the Cognitive Behavioral-Analysis System of Psychotherapy, and Their Combination for the Treatment of Chronic Depression," *N. Engl. J. Med.*, **342:**1462–1470, 2000) compared the efficacy of these approaches in outpatients diagnosed with a chronic major depressive disorder. Depression was diagnosed using the 24-item Hamilton Rating Scale for Depression, where a higher score indicates more severe depression. All subjects began the study with a score of at least 20. The investigators randomly assigned patients who met study criteria to the three groups—medication (nefazodone), psychotherapy, or both—for 12 weeks then measured remission, defined as having a follow-up score of 8 or less after 10 weeks of treatment. The responses of the people they studied fell into the following categories.

Treatment	Remission	No remission
Nefazodone	36	131
Psychotherapy	41	132
Nefazodone and psychotherapy	75	104

Is there any evidence that the different treatments produced different responses? If so, which one seems to work best? 5-5 Public health officials often investigate the source of widespread outbreaks of disease. Agnes O'Neil and coworkers ("A Waterborne Epidemic of Acute Infectious Non-Bacterial Gastroenteritis in Alberta, Canada." *Can. J. Public Health,* **76:**199–203, 1985) reported on an outbreak of gastroenteritis in a small Canadian town. They hypothesized that the source of contamination was the municipal water supply. They examined the association between amount of water consumed and the rate at which people got sick. What do these data suggest?

Water consumption, glasses per day	Number ill	Number not ill
Less than 1	39	121
1 to 4	265	258
5 or more	265	146

5-6 Authorship in biomedical publications establishes accountability, responsibility, and credit. The International Committee of Medical Journal Editors established authorship criteria in 1985, which boil down to playing an active role in the research and writing of the paper and being in a position to take responsibility for a paper's scientific content.* Misappropriation of authorship undermines the integrity of the authorship system. There are two ways that authorship is misappropriated: honorary authorship, when someone (typically a department or division chair or the person who obtained funding for the project) who did not actually participate in preparing the paper, is listed as an author, and ghost authorship, when someone who played an important role in writing the paper is not listed as an author. To investigate the prevalence of honorary and ghost authorship in medical journals, Annette Flanagin and her colleagues ("Prevalence of articles with honorary authors and ghost authors in peer-reviewed medical journals," *JAMA* **280:**222–224, 1998) sent questionnaires to a random sample of corresponding authors for papers published in three large circulation general medical journals (*Annals of Internal Medicine, Journal of the American Medical Association,* and *New England Journal of Medicine*) and three specialty journals (*American Journal of Cardiology, American Journal of Medicine,* and *American Journal of Obstetrics and Gynecology*). Here are their results:

*The full guidelines, which are accepted by most medical journals, are available at: International Committee of Medical Journal Editors. "Guidelines on Authorship," *BMJ.* **291:**722, 1985.

Journal	Total Number of Articles	Articles with Honorary Authors	Articles with Ghost Authors
American Journal of Cardiology	137	22	13
American Journal of Medicine	113	26	15
American Journal of Obstetrics and Gynecology	125	14	13
Annals of Internal Medicine	104	26	16
Journal of the American Medical Association	194	44	14
New England Journal of Medicine	136	24	22

Are there differences in the patterns of honorary authorship and ghost authorship among the different journals? Are there differences in patterns of honorary and ghost authorship between the specialty journals and large circulation generalist journals?

5-7 Dioxin is one of the most toxic synthetic environmental contaminants. An explosion at a herbicide plant in Sevaso, Italy in 1976 released large amounts of this long-lasting contaminant into the environment. Because exposure to dioxin during development is known to be dangerous, researchers have been carefully following the health status of exposed people and their children in Sevaso and surrounding areas. Peter Mocarelli and colleagues ("Paternal Concentrations of Dioxin and Sex Ratio of Offspring," *Lancet,* **355:**1858–1863, 2000) measured the serum concentration of dioxin in potentially exposed parents and analyzed the number of male and female babies born after 1976. They found that when both parents were exposed to greater that 15 parts per trillion (ppt) of dioxin the proportion of girl babies born was significantly increased compared to couples not exposed to this amount of dioxin. Mocarelli and colleagues also investigated whether there were differences in the proportion of female babies born if only one parent was exposed to greater than 15 ppt of dioxin and whether the sex of the parent (mother or father) made a difference. Based on numbers presented below, are there differences in the proportion of female babies born when only one parent is exposed to greater than 15 ppt of dioxin?

Parental exposure to dioxin	Female babies	Male babies
Father exposed; mother unexposed	105	81
Father unexposed; mother exposed	100	120

5-8 Fabio Lattanzi and coworkers ("Inhibition of Dipyridamole-Induced Ischemia by Antianginal Therapy in Humans: Correlation with Exercise Electrocardiography," *Circulation,* **83:**1256–1262, 1991) wished to compare the ability of electrocardiography (in which the electrical signals produced by the heart) and echocardiography (in which pictures of the heart are obtained with sound waves) to detect inadequate oxygen supply (ischemia) to the hearts of people with heart disease. To obtain the electrocardiographic test (EET), they had the people exercise to increase their heart rate until they developed chest pain or had abnormalities on their electrocardiogram indicating ischemia. To obtain the echocardiographic test (DET), they watched the heartbeat after increasing heart rate with the drug dipyridamole. They compared people receiving therapy for their heart disease in separate experiments. The results they obtained were:

	On therapy	
	Positive DET test	Negative DET test
Positive EET Test	38	2
Negative EET Test	14	3

	Off therapy	
	Positive DET test	Negative DET test
Positive EET Test	21	6
Negative EET Test	16	14

Was there a different response between the two tests in either group of patients?

5-9 Narrowing of the carotid arteries, which carry blood through the neck to the head, can reduce flow to the brain and starve the brain of oxygen, a condition called cerebral ischemia. To study whether medical or surgical treatment of the problem produced better results, W. Fields and his colleagues ("Joint Study of Extracranial Arterial Occlusion, V: Progress Report of Prognosis Following Surgery or Nonsurgical Treatment for Transient Ischemic Attacks and Cervical Carotid Artery Lesions," *JAMA,* **211:**1993–2003, 1970, copyright 1970–1973. American Medical Association) compared the outcomes among patients available for follow-up who received surgical and medical therapy and found:

	Recurrent ischemia, stroke, or death, no. of patients	
Therapy	Yes	No
Surgical	43	36
Medical	53	19

Is there sufficient evidence to conclude that one treatment is better than the other? David Sackett and Michael Gent ("Controversy in Counting and Attributing Events in Clinical Trials," *N. Engl. J. Med.,* **301:**1410–1412, 1979, used by permission) took note of two important points with regard to the study just described: (1) "available for follow-up" patients had to be discharged alive and free of stroke after their hospitalization; (2) this procedure excluded 15 surgically treated patients (5 who died and 10 who had strokes during or shortly after their operations) but only 1 medically treated patient. Including these 16 patients in the data from the previous problem yields the following result.

	Recurrent ischemia, stroke, or death, no. of patients	
Therapy	Yes	No
Surgical	58	36
Medical	54	19

Does including these patients change the conclusions of the trial? If so, should the trial be analyzed excluding them or including them? Why?

5-10 The chance of contracting disease X is 10 percent, regardless of whether or not a given individual has disease A or disease B. Assume that you can diagnose all three diseases with perfect accuracy and that in the entire population 1000 people have disease A and 1000 have disease B. People with X, A, and B have different chances of being hospitalized. Specifically, 50 percent of the people with A, 20 percent of the people with B, and 40 percent of the people with X are hospitalized. Then:

- Out of the 1000 people with A, 10 percent (100 people) also have X; 50 percent (50 people) are hospitalized because they have A. Of the remaining 50 (who also have X), 40 percent (20 people) are hospitalized because of X. Therefore, 70 people will be hospitalized with both A and X.
- Out of the 900 people with A but not X, 50 percent are hospitalized for disease A (450 people).
- Out of the 1000 with B, 10 percent (100 people) also have X; 20 percent (20 people) are hospitalized because of B, and of the 80, 40 percent (32 patients) are hospitalized because they have X. Thus, 52 people with B and X are in the hospital.
- Of the 900 with B but not X, 20 percent (180 people) are hospitalized because they have disease B.

A hospital-based investigator will encounter these patients in the hospital and observe the following relationship:

	Disease X	No disease X
Disease A	70	450
Disease B	52	180

Is there a statistically significant difference in the chances that an individual has X depending on whether or not he has A or B in the sample of patients the hospital-based investigator will encounter? Would the investigator reach the same conclusion if she could observe the entire population? If not, explain why. (This example is from D. Mainland, "The Risk of Fallacious Conclusions from Autopsy Data on the Incidence of Diseases with Applications to Heart Disease," *Am. Heart J.*, **45**:644–654, 1953.)

5-11 Cigarette smoking is associated with increased incidence of many types of cancers. Jian-Min Yuan and colleagues ("Tobacco Use in Relation to Renal Cell Carcinoma." *Cancer Epidemiol. Biomarkers*

Prev. **7:**429–433, 1998) wanted to investigate whether cigarette smoking was also associated with increased risk of renal cell cancer. They recruited patients with renal cell cancer from the Los Angeles County Cancer Surveillance Program to serve as cases in a retrospective case-control study. Control subjects without renal cell cancer were matched on sex, age (within 5 years), race, and neighborhood of residence to each case subject. After recruiting a total of 2314 subjects for the study, Yuan and colleagues visited subjects in their homes and interviewed them about their smoking habits, both past and present. What effect does smoking cigarettes have on the risk of developing renal cell cancer?

	Number of people	
	Renal cell cancer	No cancer
Ever smoked cigarettes	800	713
Never smoked cigarettes	357	444

5-12 Yuan and colleagues also collected information from subjects who had quit smoking. Is there any evidence that stopping smoking reduces risk of developing renal cell cancer compared to current smokers?

	Number of people	
	Renal cell cancer	No cancer
More than 20 years since quitting	169	177
Current smokers	337	262

5-13 Many postmenopausal women are faced with the decision of whether they want to take hormone replacement therapy or not. Benefits of hormone replacement include decreased risk of cardiovascular disease and osteoporosis. However, hormone replacement therapy has also been associated with increased risk of breast cancer and endometrial cancer. Francine Grodstein and colleagues ("Postmenopausal Hormone Therapy and Mortality." *N. Engl. J. Med.,* **336:** 1769–1775, 1997) investigated the relationship between hormone replacement therapy and overall mortality in a large group of postmenopausal women. The women used in this study were selected from a sample of registered nurses participating in the Nurses' Health Study. This prospective study has been tracking the health status of a large group of registered nurses since 1976, updating information every 2 years. Women became eligible for Grodstein's study when they became menopausal and were included as long as they did not report a history of cardiovascular disease or cancer on the original 1976 questionnaire. Is there any evidence that the risk of death differs in women who were identified as currently using hormone replacement therapy?

	Number of people	
	Deceased	Alive
Currently using hormone replacement therapy	574	8483
Never used hormone replacement therapy	2051	17,520

5-14 Is there an increase in risk of death in women who reported past hormone replacement therapy use compared to women who never used it?

	Number of people	
	Deceased	Alive
Past use of hormone replacement therapy	1012	8621
Never used hormone replacement therapy	2051	17,520

Chapter 6

What Does "Not Significant" Really Mean?

Thus far, we have used statistical methods to reach conclusions by seeing how compatible the observations were with the null hypothesis that the treatment had no effect. When the data were unlikely to occur if this null hypothesis was true, we rejected it and concluded that the treatment had an effect. We used a test statistic (F, t, q, q', z, or χ^2) to quantify the difference between the actual observations and those we would expect if the null hypothesis of no effect were true. We concluded that the treatment had an effect if the value of this test statistic was bigger than 95 percent of the values that would occur if the treatment had no effect. When this is so, it is common for medical investigators to report a *statistically significant* effect. On the other hand, when the test statistic is not big enough to reject the hypothesis of no treatment effect, investigators often report *no statistically significant difference* and then discuss their results as if they had proved that the treatment had no effect. *All they really did was fail to demonstrate that it did have an effect.* The distinction between positively demonstrating that a treatment had no effect and failing to demonstrate that it did have an effect is subtle but very important, especially in the light of the small numbers of subjects included in most clinical studies.*

As already mentioned in our discussion of the *t* test, the ability to detect a treatment effect with a given level of confidence depends on the size of the treatment effect, the variability within the population, and the size of the samples used in the study. Just as bigger samples make it more likely that you will be able to detect an effect, smaller sample sizes make it harder. In practical terms, this fact means that studies of therapies that involve only a few subjects and fail to reject the null hypothesis of no treatment effect may arrive at this result because the statistical procedures lacked the *power* to detect the effect because of a too small sample size, even though the treatment did have an effect. Conversely, considerations of the power of a test permit you to compute the sample size needed to detect a treatment effect of given size that you believe is present.

AN EFFECTIVE DIURETIC

Now, we make a radical departure from everything that has preceded: we assume that the treatment *does* have an effect.

Figure 6–1 shows the same population of people we studied in Fig. 4–4 except that this time the drug given to increase daily urine production works. It increases the average urine production for members of this population from 1200 to 1400 mL/day. Figure 6–1A shows the distribution of daily urine production for all 200 members of the population in the control (placebo) group, and Fig. 6–1B shows the distribution of urine production for all 200 members of the population in the diuretic group.

More precisely, the population of people taking the placebo consist of a normally distributed population with mean μ_{pla} = 1200 mL/day, and the population of people taking the drug consist of a normally

*This problem is particularly encountered in small clinical studies in which there are no "failures" in the treatment group. This situation often leads to overly optimistic assessments of therapeutic efficacy. See J. A. Hanley and A. Lippman-Hand, "If Nothing Goes Wrong, Is Everything All Right? Interpreting Zero Numerators," *JAMA* **249:**1743–1745, 1983.

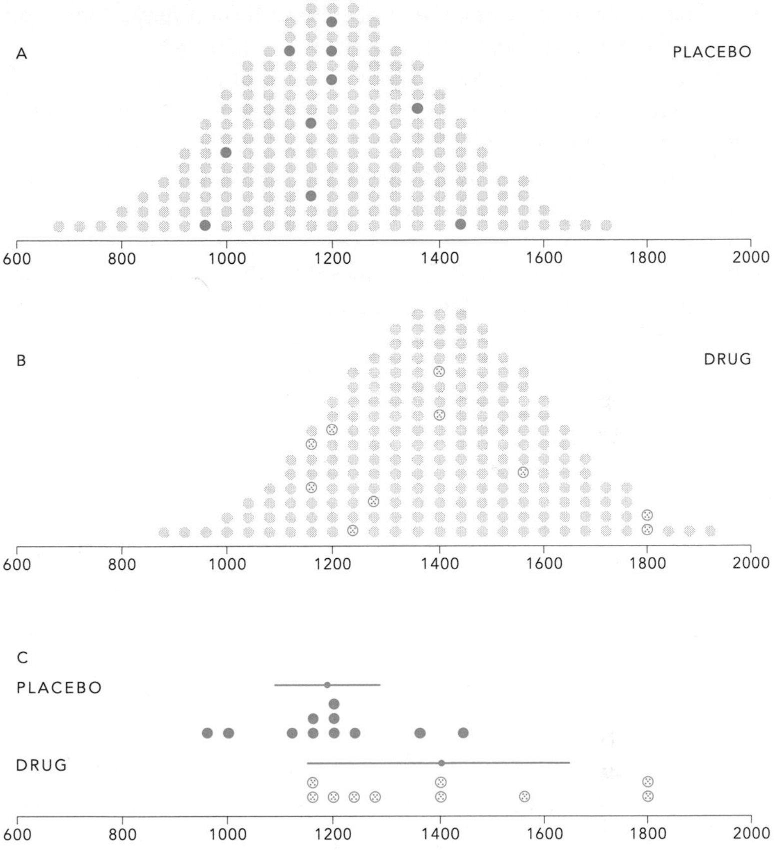

Figure 6–1 Daily urine production in a population of 200 people while they are taking a placebo and while they are taking an effective diuretic that increases urine production by 200 mL/day on the average. Panels ***A*** and ***B*** show the specific individuals selected at random for study. Panel ***C*** shows the results as they would appear to the investigator. $t = 2.447$ for these observations. Since the critical value of t for $P < .05$ with $2(10 - 1) = 18$ degrees of freedom is 2.101, the investigator would probably report that the diuretic was effective.

distributed population with a mean of $\mu_{dr} = 1400$ mL/day. Both populations have the same standard deviation, $\sigma = 200$ mL/day.

Of course, an investigator cannot observe all members of the population, so he or she selects two groups of 10 people at random, gives one group the diuretic and the other a placebo, and measures their daily urine production. Figure 6–1*C* shows what the investigator would see. The people receiving a placebo produce an average of 1180 mL/day, and those receiving the drug produce an average of 1400 mL/day. The standard deviations of these two samples are 144 and 245 mL/day, respectively. The pooled estimate of the population variance is

$$s^2 = \tfrac{1}{2}\,(s^2_{dr} + s^2_{pla}) = \tfrac{1}{2}\,(245^2 + 144^2) = 40{,}381 = 201^2$$

The value of t associated with these observations is

$$t = \frac{\bar{X}_{dr} - \bar{X}_{pla}}{\sqrt{(s^2/n_{dr}) + (s^2/n_{pla})}} = \frac{1400 - 1180}{\sqrt{(201^2/10) + (201^2/10)}} = 2.447$$

which exceeds 2.101, the value that defines the most extreme 5 percent of possible values of the t statistic when the two samples are drawn from the same population. (There are $\nu = n_{dr} + n_{pla} - 2 = 10 + 10 - 2 = 18$ degrees of freedom.) The investigator would conclude that the observations are not consistent with the assumption that two samples came from the same population and report that the drug increased urine production. And he or she would be right.

Of course, there is nothing special about the two random samples of people selected for the experiment. Figure 6–2 shows two more groups of people selected at random to test the drug, together with the results as they would appear to the investigator. In this case, the mean urine production is 1216 mL/day for the people given the placebo and 1368 mL/day for the people taking the drug. The standard deviations of urine production in the two samples are 97 and 263 mL/day, respectively, so the pooled estimate of the variance is $1/2\ (97^2 + 263^2) = 198^2$. The value of t associated with these observations is

$$t = \frac{1368 - 1216}{\sqrt{(198^2/10) + (198^2/10)}} = 1.71$$

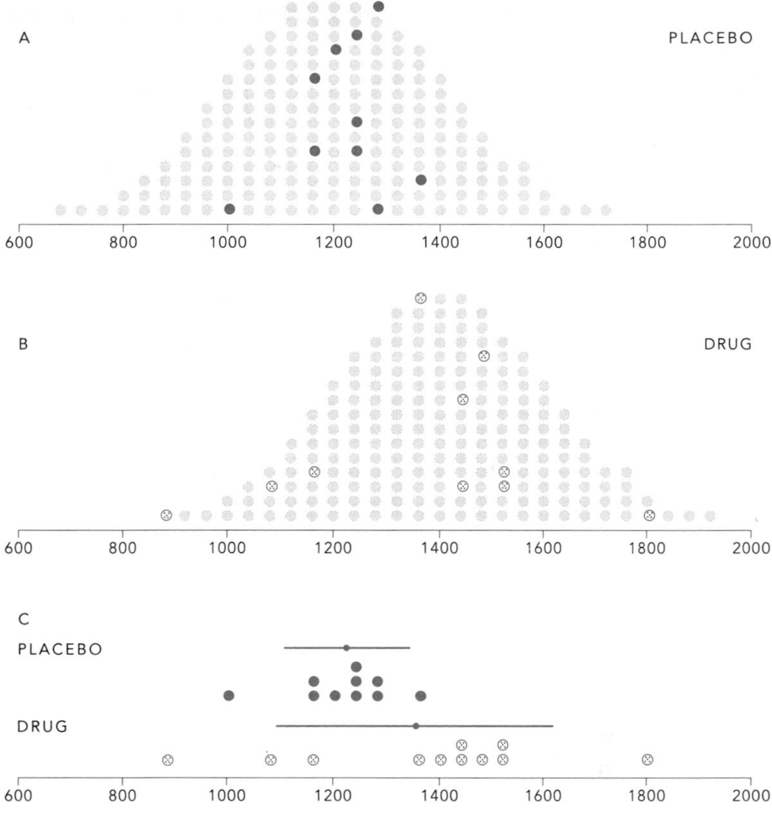

Figure 6–2 There is nothing special about the two random samples shown in Fig. 6–1. This illustration shows another random sample of two groups of 10 people each selected at random to test the diuretic and the results as they would appear to the investigator. The value of t associated with these observations is only 1.71, not great enough to reject the hypothesis of no drug effect with $P < 0.05$, that is, $\alpha = 0.05$. If the investigator reported the drug had no effect, he/she would be wrong.

which is less than 2.101. Had the investigator selected these two groups of people for testing, he or she would not have obtained a value of t large enough to reject the hypothesis that the drug had no effect, and probably report "no significant difference." If the investigator went on to conclude that the drug had no effect, he or she would be wrong.

Notice that this is a different type of error from that discussed in Chapters 3 to 5. In the earlier chapters we were concerned with *rejecting* the hypothesis of no effect when it was true. Now we are concerned with *not rejecting it when it is not true.*

What are the chances of making this second kind of error?

Just as we could repeat this experiment more than 10^{27} times when the drug had no effect to obtain the distribution of possible values of t (compare the discussion of Fig. 4–5), we can do the same thing when the drug does have an effect. Figure 6–3 shows the results of 200 such experiments; 111 out of the resulting values of t fall at or above 2.101, the value we used to define a "big" t. Put another way, if we wish to keep the P value at or below 5 percent, there is a 111/200 = 56 percent chance of concluding that the diuretic increases urine output when average urine output actually increases by 200 mL/day. We say the *power* of the test is .56.

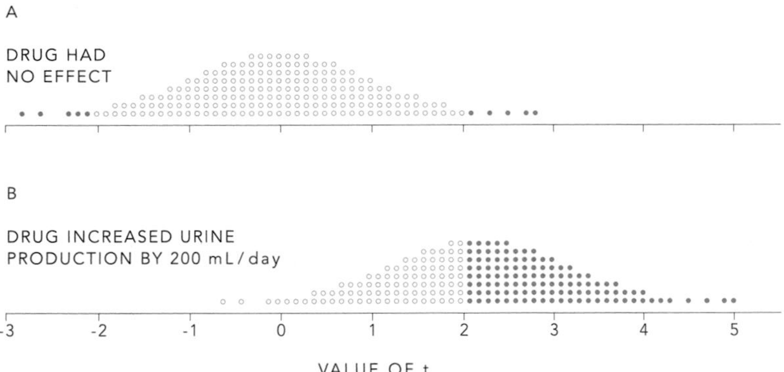

Figure 6–3 **(*A*)** The distribution of values of the t statistic computed from 200 experiments that consisted of drawing two samples of size 10 each from a single population; this is the distribution we would expect if the diuretic had no effect on urine production is centered on zero. (Compare with Fig. 4–5*A*.) **(*B*)** The distribution of t values from 200 experiments in which the drug increased average urine production by 200 mL/day. $t = 2.1$ defines the most extreme 5 percent of the possible values of t when the drug has no effect; 111 of the 200 values of t we would expect to observe from our data fall above this point when the drug increases urine production by 200 mL/day. Therefore, there is a 56 percent chance that we will conclude that the drug actually increases urine production from our experiment.

The power quantifies the chance of detecting a real difference of a given size.

Alternatively, we could concentrate on the 89 of the 200 experiments that produced t values below 2.101, in which case we would fail to reject the hypothesis that the treatment had no effect and be wrong. Thus, there is a 89/200 = 44 percent = .44 chance of continuing to accept the hypothesis of no effect when the drug really increased urine production by 200 mL/day on the average.

TWO TYPES OF ERRORS

Now we have isolated the two different ways the random-sampling process can lead to erroneous conclusions. These two types of errors are analogous to the false-positive and false-negative results one obtains from diagnostic tests. Before this chapter we concentrated on controlling the likelihood of making a false-positive error, that is, concluding that a treatment has an effect when it really does not. In keeping with tradition, we have generally sought to keep the chances of making such an error below 5 percent; of course, we could arbitrarily select any cutoff value we wanted at which to declare the test statistic "big." Statisticians denote the maximum acceptable risk of this error by α, the Greek letter alpha. If we reject the hypothesis of no effect whenever $P < .05$, $\alpha = 0.05$, or 5 percent. If we actually obtain data that lead us to reject the null hypothesis of no effect when the null hypothesis of no effect is true, statisticians say that we have made a *Type I error.* All this logic is relatively straightforward because we have specified how much we believe the treatment affects the variable of interest, that is, not at all.

What about the other side of the coin, the chances of making a false-negative conclusion and not reporting an effect when one exists? Statisticians denote the chance of erroneously accepting the hypothesis of no effect by β, the Greek letter beta. The chance of detecting a true-positive, that is, reporting a statistically significant difference when the treatment really produces an effect, is $1 - \beta$. The *power* of the test that we discussed earlier is equal to $1 - \beta$. For example, if a test has power equal to .56, there is a 56 percent chance of actually reporting a statistically significant effect when one is really present. Table 6–1 summarizes these definitions.

Table 6–1 Types of Erroneous Conclusions in Statistical Hypothesis Testing

	Actual situation	
Conclude from observations	Treatment has an effect	Treatment has no effect
Treatment has an effect	True positive Correct conclusion $1 - \beta$	False-positive Type I error α
Treatment has no effect	False-negative Type II error β	True negative Correct conclusion $1 - \alpha$

WHAT DETERMINES A TEST'S POWER?

So far we have developed procedures for estimating and controlling the Type I, or α, error; now we turn our attention to keeping the Type II, or β, error as small as possible. In other words, we want the power to be as high as possible. In theory, this problem is not very different from the one we already solved with one important exception. Since the treatment has an effect, *the size of this effect influences how easy it is to detect.* Large effects are easier to detect than small ones. To estimate the power of a test, you need to specify how small an effect is worth detecting.

Just as with false-positives and false-negatives in diagnostic testing, the Type I and Type II errors are intertwined. As you require stronger evidence before reporting that a treatment has an effect, i.e., make α smaller, you also increase the chance of missing a true effect, i.e., make β bigger or power smaller. The only way to reduce both α and β simultaneously is to increase the sample size, because with a larger sample you can be more confident in your decision, whatever it is.

In other words, the power of a given statistical test depends on three interacting factors:

- *The risk of error you will tolerate when rejecting the hypothesis of no treatment effect.*
- *The size of the difference you wish to detect relative to the amount of variability in the populations.*
- *The sample size.*

To keep things simple, we will examine each of these factors separately.

The Size of the Type I Error α

Figure 6–3 showed the complementary nature of the maximum size of the Type I error α and the power of the test. The acceptable risk of erroneously rejecting the hypothesis of no effect, α, determines the critical value of the test statistic above which you will report that the treatment had an effect, $P < \alpha$. (We have usually taken $\alpha = 0.05$.) This critical value is defined from the distribution of the test statistic for all possible experiments with a specific sample size *given that the treatment had no effect.* The power is the proportion of possible values of the test statistic that fall above this cutoff value *given that the treatment had a specified effect* (here a 200 mL/day increase in urine production). Changing α, or the P value required to reject the hypothesis of no difference, moves this cutoff point, affecting the power of the test.

Figure 6–4 illustrates this point further. Figure 6–4*A* essentially reproduces Fig. 6–3 except that it depicts the distribution of t values for all 10^{27} possible experiments involving two groups of 10 people as a continuous distribution. The top part, copied from Fig. 4–5*D*, shows the distribution of possible t values (with $\nu = 10 + 10 - 2 = 18$ degrees of freedom) that would occur if the drug did not affect urine production. Suppose we require $P < .05$ before we are willing to assert that the observations were unlikely to have arisen from random sampling rather than the effect of the drug. According to the table of critical values of the t distribution (see Table 4–1), for $\nu = 18$ degrees of freedom, 2.101 is the (two-tail) critical value that defines the most extreme 5 percent of possible values of the t test statistic if the null hypothesis of no effect of the diuretic on urine production is true. In other words, when we make $\alpha = 0.05$, in which case -2.101 and $+2.101$ delimit the most extreme 5 percent of all possible t values we would expect to observe if the diuretic did not affect urine production.

We know, however, that the drug actually increased average urine production by $\mu_{dr} - \mu_{pla} = 200$ mL/day. Therefore, the actual distribution of possible values of t associated with our experiment will not be given by the distribution at the top of Fig. 6–4 (which assumes that the null hypothesis that $\mu_{dr} - \mu_{pla} = 0$ is true and so is centered on 0).

To determine where the actual distribution of values of the t test statistic will be centered, recall, from Chapter 4, that the t test statistic

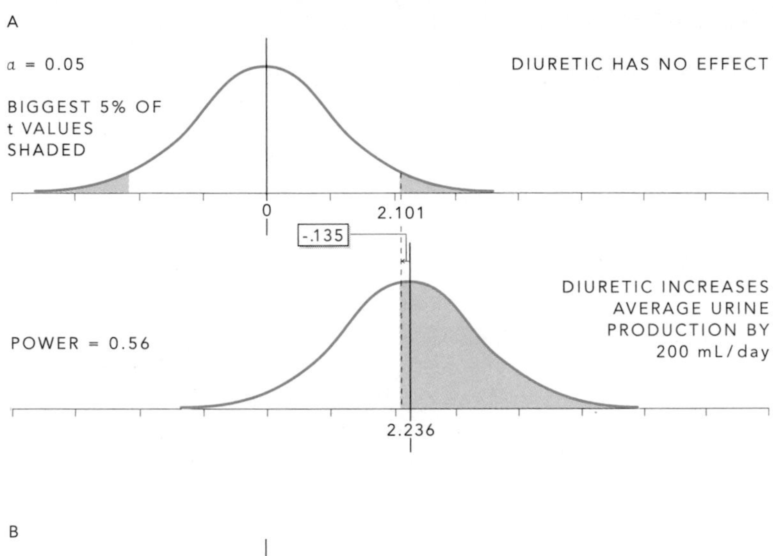

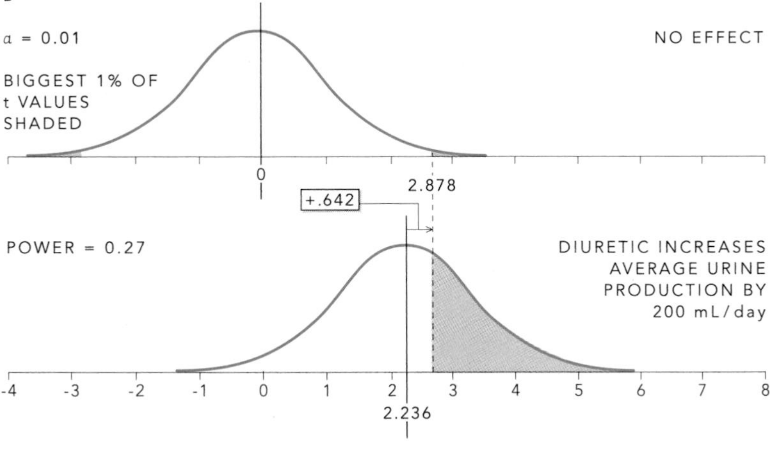

Figure 6–4 ***(A)*** The top panel shows the distribution of the *t* test statistic that would occur if the null hypothesis was true and the diuretic did not affect urine production. The distribution is centered on 0 (because the diuretic has no effect on urine production), and, from Table 4–1, $t = +2.101$ (and -2.101) define the (two-tail) 5 percent most extreme values of the *t* test statistic that would be expected to occur by chance if the drug had no effect. The second panel shows the actual distribution of the *t* test statistic that occurs when the diuretic increases urine output by 200 mL/day; the distribution of *t* values is shifted to the right, so the

to compare two means, is

$$t = \frac{\overline{X}_{dr} - \overline{X}_{pla}}{\sqrt{(s^2/n_{\text{dr}}) + (s^2/n_{\text{pla}})}}$$

$\overline{X}_{\text{dr}} - \overline{X}_{\text{pla}}$ computed from the observations is an estimate of the actual difference in mean urine production between the populations of people taking the drug and taking the placebo, $\mu_{\text{dr}} - \mu_{\text{pla}} = 200$ mL/day. The observed standard deviation, s, is an estimate of the standard deviation of the underlying populations, σ, which, from Fig. 6–1, is 200 mL/day. Therefore, we would expect the actual distribution of the *t* test statistic to be centered on

$$t' = \frac{\mu_{\text{dr}} - \mu_{\text{pla}}}{\sqrt{(\sigma^2/n_{\text{dr}}) + (\sigma^2/n_{\text{pla}})}}$$

n_{dr} and n_{pla} both are 10, so the actual distribution of the *t* test statistic will be centered on

$$t' = \frac{200}{\sqrt{(200^2/10) + (200^2/10)}} = 2.236$$

The lower distribution in Fig. 6–4*A* shows this actual distribution of possible *t* values associated with our experiment: the *t* distribution is moved to the right to be centered on 2.236 (rather than 0, as it was under the null hypothesis). Fifty-six percent of these possible values of *t*, that is, 56 percent of the area under the curve, fall above the 2.101 cutoff, so we say the power of the test is .56.

---

distribution is now centered on 2.236. The critical value of 2.101 is −.135 below 2.236, the center of this shifted distribution. From Table 6–2, .56 of the possible *t* values fall in the one-tail above −.135, so we conclude that the power of a *t* test to detect a 200 mL/day increase in urine production is 56 percent. (The power would also include the portion of the *t* distribution in the lower tail below −2.101, but because this area is so small, we will ignore it.) ***(B)*** If we require more evidence before rejecting the null hypothesis of no difference by reducing α to 0.01, the critical value of *t* that must be exceeded to reject the null hypothesis increases to 2.878 (and −2.878). Since the effect of the diuretic is unchanged, the actual distribution of *t* remains centered on 2.236; the critical value of 2.878 is .642 above 2.236, the center of the actual *t* distribution. From Table 6–2, .27 of the possible *t* values fall in the tail above .642, so the power of the test drops to 27 percent.

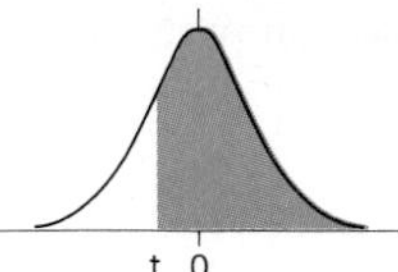

Table 6–2 Critical Values of *t* (One-Tailed)

	Probability of Larger Value (Upper Tail)									
	.995	.99	.98	.975	.95	.90	.85	.80	.70	.60
	Probability of Smaller Value (Lower Tail)									
ν	.005	.01	.02	.025	.05	.10	.15	.20	.30	.40
2	−9.925	−6.965	−4.849	−4.303	−2.920	−1.886	−1.386	−1.061	−0.617	−0.289
4	−4.604	−3.747	−2.999	−2.776	−2.132	−1.533	−1.190	−0.941	−0.569	−0.271
6	−3.707	−3.143	−2.612	−2.447	−1.943	−1.440	−1.134	−0.906	−0.553	−0.265
8	−3.355	−2.896	−2.449	−2.306	−1.860	−1.397	−1.108	−0.889	−0.546	−0.262
10	−3.169	−2.764	−2.359	−2.228	−1.812	−1.372	−1.093	−0.879	−0.542	−0.260
12	−3.055	−2.681	−2.303	−2.179	−1.782	−1.356	−1.083	−0.873	−0.539	−0.259
14	−2.977	−2.624	−2.264	−2.145	−1.761	−1.345	−1.076	−0.868	−0.537	−0.258
16	−2.921	−2.583	−2.235	−2.120	−1.746	−1.337	−1.071	−0.865	−0.535	−0.258
18	−2.878	−2.552	−2.214	−2.101	−1.734	−1.330	−1.067	−0.862	−0.534	−0.257
20	−2.845	−2.528	−2.197	−2.086	−1.725	−1.325	−1.064	−0.860	−0.533	−0.257
25	−2.787	−2.485	−2.167	−2.060	−1.708	−1.316	−1.058	−0.856	−0.531	−0.256
30	−2.750	−2.457	−2.147	−2.042	−1.697	−1.310	−1.055	−0.854	−0.530	−0.256
35	−2.724	−2.438	−2.133	−2.030	−1.690	−1.306	−1.052	−0.852	−0.529	−0.255
40	−2.704	−2.423	−2.123	−2.021	−1.684	−1.303	−1.050	−0.851	−0.529	−0.255
60	−2.660	−2.390	−2.099	−2.000	−1.671	−1.296	−1.045	−0.848	−0.527	−0.254
120	−2.617	−2.358	−2.076	−1.980	−1.658	−1.289	−1.041	−0.845	−0.526	−0.254
∞	−2.576	−2.326	−2.054	−1.960	−1.645	−1.282	−1.036	−0.842	−0.524	−0.253
normal	−2.576	−2.326	−2.054	−1.960	−1.645	−1.282	−1.036	−0.842	−0.524	−0.253

In other words, if the drug increases average urine production by 200 mL/day in this population and we do an experiment using two samples of 10 people each to test the drug, there is a 55 percent chance that we will conclude that the drug is effective ($P < .05$). To understand how we obtain this estimate of the power, we need to consult another table of critical values of the t distribution, one that gives the *one-tail* probability of being in the upper tail of the distribution as a function of the value of t (Table 6–2). The information in this table is essentially the same as in Table 4–1, with the difference that it presents critical values for one tail only, so the P values associated with each value of t in this table are half

Probability of Larger Value (Upper Tail)										
.50	.40	.30	.20	.15	.10	.05	.025	.02	.01	.005
Probability of Smaller Value (Lower Tail)										
.50	.60	.70	.80	.85	.90	.95	.975	.98	.99	.995
0	0.289	0.617	1.061	1.386	1.886	2.920	4.303	4.849	6.965	9.925
0	0.271	0.569	0.941	1.190	1.533	2.132	2.776	2.999	3.747	4.604
0	0.265	0.553	0.906	1.134	1.440	1.943	2.447	2.612	3.143	3.707
0	0.262	0.546	0.889	1.108	1.397	1.860	2.306	2.449	2.896	3.355
0	0.260	0.542	0.879	1.093	1.372	1.812	2.228	2.359	2.764	3.169
0	0.259	0.539	0.873	1.083	1.356	1.782	2.179	2.303	2.681	3.055
0	0.258	0.537	0.868	1.076	1.345	1.761	2.145	2.264	2.624	2.977
0	0.258	0.535	0.865	1.071	1.337	1.746	2.120	2.235	2.583	2.921
0	0.257	0.534	0.862	1.067	1.330	1.734	2.101	2.214	2.552	2.878
0	0.257	0.533	0.860	1.064	1.325	1.725	2.086	2.197	2.528	2.845
0	0.256	0.531	0.856	1.058	1.316	1.708	2.060	2.167	2.485	2.787
0	0.256	0.530	0.854	1.055	1.310	1.697	2.042	2.147	2.457	2.750
0	0.255	0.529	0.852	1.052	1.306	1.690	2.030	2.133	2.438	2.724
0	0.255	0.529	0.851	1.050	1.303	1.684	2.021	2.123	2.423	2.704
0	0.254	0.527	0.848	1.045	1.296	1.671	2.000	2.099	2.390	2.660
0	0.254	0.526	0.845	1.041	1.289	1.658	1.980	2.076	2.358	2.617
0	0.253	0.524	0.842	1.036	1.282	1.645	1.960	2.054	2.326	2.576
0	0.253	0.524	0.842	1.036	1.282	1.645	1.960	2.054	2.326	2.576

the corresponding values in Table 4–2. For example, the critical value of $t = +2.101$, the two-tail critical value associated with $P = .05$ for $\nu = 18$ degrees of freedom in Table 4–2, corresponds to a one (upper) tail probability of .025 in Table 6–2. This situation arises because in a two-tail test of the null hypothesis of *no difference,* half the risk of a false-positive conclusion resides in the upper tail of the distribution of possible values of t and the other half resides in the lower end of the distribution, below -2.101 in this case. Note, from Table 6–2, that the probability of being in the lower tail of the distribution of possible values of t (with $\nu = 18$) at or below -2.101 is .025. The .025 probability of being *at or below*

−2.101 plus the .025 probability of being *at or above +2.101* add up to the .05 two-tailed probability we found in Table 4–1.

As noted above, the actual distribution of values of the t test statistic given that there is actually a 200 mL/day increase in urine production with the diuretic is centered on 2.236, rather than 0, as it would be if the null hypothesis was true. The critical value of 2.101 that leads us to reject the null hypothesis (from the top distribution in Fig. 6–4*A*) is below the center of the actual distribution of the t test statistic by $2.101 - 2.236 = -.135$. We can use Table 6–2 to determine the probability of being in the upper tail of this t distribution* (with $\nu = 18$ degrees of freedom) is .56 (between .60, which corresponds to −.257 and .50, which corresponds to .000), yielding the power of 56 percent.

Conversely, we can say that β, the probability that we will make a false-negative, or Type II, error and accept the null hypothesis of no effect when it is not true is $1 - .56 = .44 = 44$ percent. Alternatively, we can use Table 6–2 to note that the probability of being in the lower tail of the t distribution (at or below −.135) is .44.

Now look at Fig. 6–4*B*. The two distributions of t values are identical to those in Fig. 6–4*A*. (After all, the drug's true effect is still the same.) This time, however, we will insist on stronger evidence before concluding that the drug actually increased urine production. We will require that the test statistic fall in the most extreme 1 percent of possible values before concluding that the data are inconsistent with the null hypothesis that the drug has no effect. Thus, $\alpha = 0.01$ and t must be below −2.878 or above +2.878 to fall in the most extreme 1 percent of values. The top part of panel *B* shows this cutoff point. The actual distribution of the t test statistic is still centered on 2.236, so the 2.878 critical value is now above the center of this distribution by $2.878 - 2.236 = .642$. From Table 6–2, we find that only .27 or 27 percent of the actual distribution of t falls above 2.878 in Fig. 6–4*B*, so the power of the test has fallen to .27. In other words, there is less than an even chance that we will report that the drug is effective even though it actually is.

By requiring stronger evidence that there be a treatment effect before reporting it we have decreased the chances of erroneously reporting an

*Technically, we should also consider the portion of the actual t distribution in the lower tail of Fig. 6–4*A* below −2.101, but this portion is extremely small and, so, we will ignore it.

effect (a Type I error), but we have increased the chances of failing to detect a difference when one actually exists (a Type II error) because we decreased the power of the test. This trade-off always exists.

The Size of the Treatment Effect

We just demonstrated that the power of a test decreases as we reduce the acceptable risk of making a Type I error, α. The entire discussion was based on the fact that the drug increased average urine production by 200 mL/day, from 1200 to 1400 mL/day. Had this change been different, the actual distribution of t values connected with the experiment also would have been different. In other words, the power of a test depends on the size of the difference to be detected.

Let us consider three specific examples. Figure 6–5*A* shows the t distribution (the distribution of possible values of the t statistic) for a sample size of 10 if the diuretic had no effect and the two treatment groups could be considered two random samples drawn from the same population. The most extreme 5 percent of the values are shaded, just as in Fig. 6–4. Figure 6–5*B* shows the distribution of t values we would expect if the drug increased urine production an average of 200 mL/day over the placebo; 56 percent of the possible values are beyond -2.101 or $+2.101$, so the power of the test is .56. (So far we are just recapitulating the results in Fig. 6–4). Now, suppose that the drug only increased urine production by 100 mL/day. In this case, as Fig. 6–5*C* shows, the actual distribution of the t test statistic will no longer be centered on 0, but on

$$t' = \frac{100}{\sqrt{(200^2/10) + (200^2/10)}} = 1.118$$

Thus, we need to determine the fraction of the actual possible values of the t distribution that fall above $2.101 - 1.118 = .983$. The sample size is the same as before (n = 10 in each group), so there are still $\nu = 10 + 10 - 2 = 18$ degrees of freedom. From Table 6–2 we find that .17 of the possible values fall above .983, so the power of the test to detect a 100 mL/day change in urine production is only .17 (or 17 percent). In other words, there is less than a 1 in 5 chance that doing a study of two groups of 10 people would detect a change in urine production of 100 mL/day if we required that $P < .05$ before reporting an effect.

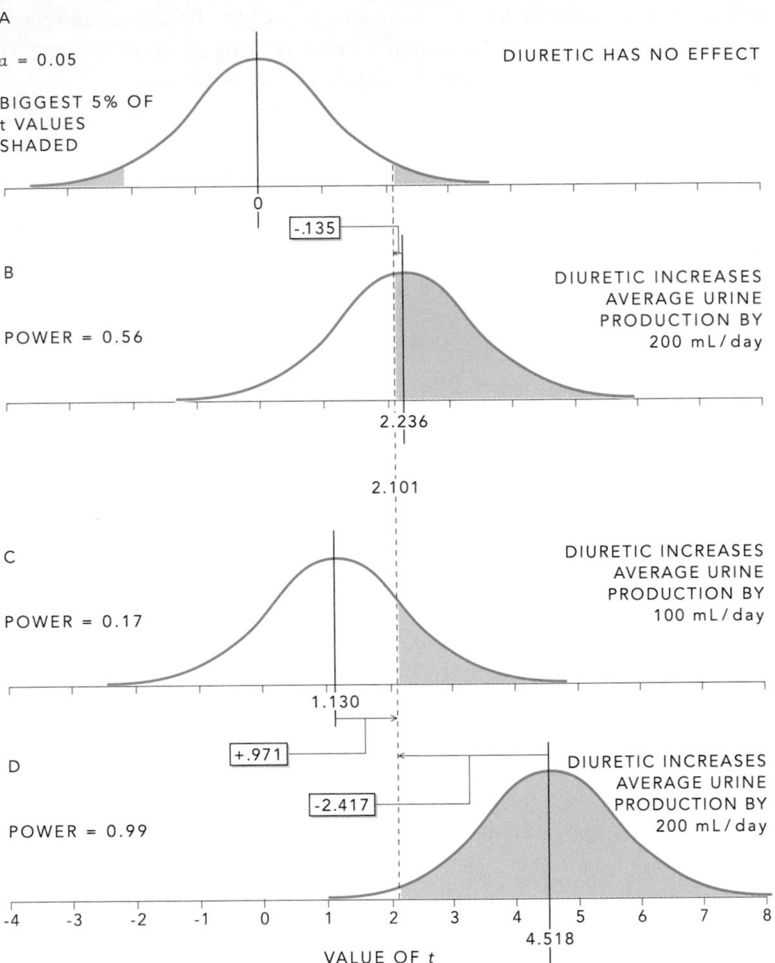

Figure 6–5 The larger the size of the treatment effect, the further the actual distribution of the *t* test statistic will shift away from zero, and the more of the actual distribution of *t* values will exceed the critical value of 2.101 that determines the most extreme (two-tail) 5 percent of the values of *t* that will occur if the null hypothesis of no effect is true. As a result, the greater the effect of the diuretic, the greater the power to detect the fact that the diuretic increases urine production.

Finally, Fig. 6–5*D* shows the distribution of *t* values that would occur if the drug increased urine production by an average of 400 mL/day. Because of this larger effect, the actual distribution of the *t* test statistic will be centered on

$$t' = \frac{400}{\sqrt{(200^2/10) + (200^2/10)}} = 4.472$$

The power of the test to detect this difference will be the fraction of the *t* distribution larger than $2.101 - 4.472 = -2.371$. From Table 6–2, with $\nu = 18$ degrees of freedom, .985 of all possible *t* values fall above 2.101, so the power of the test is 99 percent. The chance is quite good that our experiment will lead to the conclusion that the diuretic affects urine production (with $P < .05$).

Figure 6–5 illustrates the general rule: *It is easier to detect big differences than small ones.*

We could repeat this process for all possible sizes of the treatment effect, from no effect at all up to very large effects, then plot the power of the test as it varies with the change in urine production actually produced by the drug. Figure 6–6 shows a plot of the results, called a *power function,* of the test. It quantifies how much easier it is to detect a change (when we require a value of *t* corresponding to $P < .05$ and two samples of 10 people each) in urine production as the actual drug effect gets larger and larger. This plot shows that if the drug increases urine production by 200 mL/day, there is a 55 percent chance that we will detect this change with the experiment designed as we have it; if urine production increases by 350 mL/day, the chance of our detecting this effect improves to 95 percent.

The Population Variability

The power of a test increases as the size of the treatment effect increases, but the variability in the population under study also affects the likelihood with which we can detect a treatment effect of a given size.

Recall that the actual distribution of the *t* test statistic is centered on

$$t' = \frac{\mu_{dr} - \mu_{pla}}{\sqrt{(\sigma^2/n_{dr}) + (\sigma^2/n_{pla})}}$$

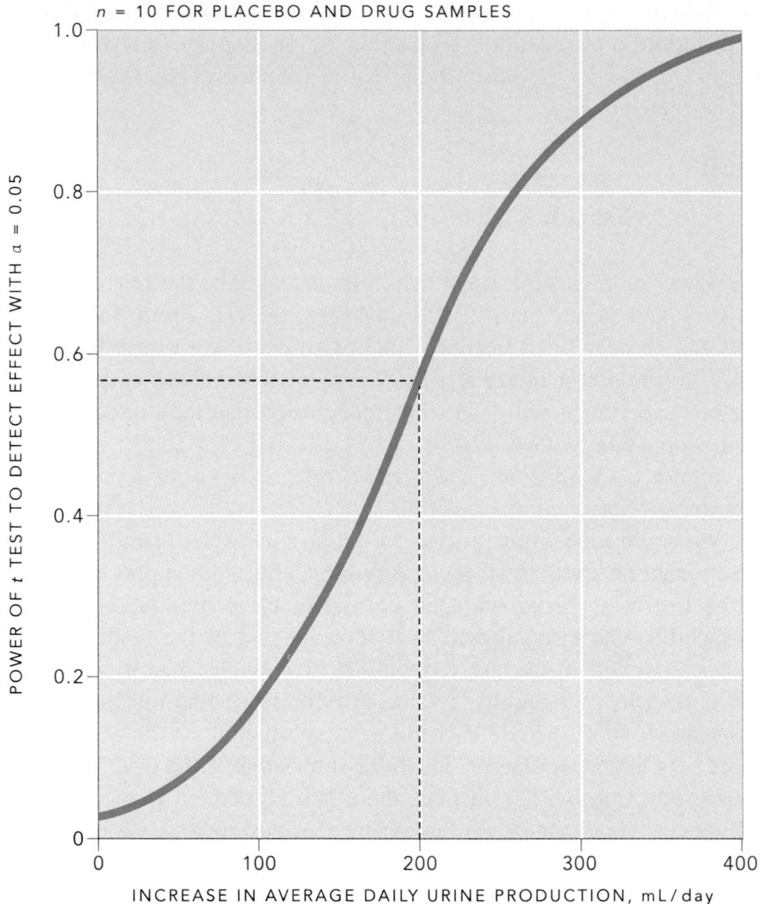

Figure 6–6 The power of a *t* test to detect a change in urine production based on experiments with two groups of people, each containing 10 individuals. The dashed line indicates how to read the graph. A *t* test has a power of .56 for detecting a 200 mL per day change in urine production.

in which $\mu_{dr} - \mu_{pla}$ is the actual size of the treatment effect, σ is the standard deviation of the two (different) underlying populations, and n_{dr} and n_{pla} are the sizes of the two samples. In the interest of simplicity, we assume that the two samples are the same size; that is $n_{dr} = n_{pla} = n$. Denote the change in the population mean due to the treatment with the

Greek letter delta, δ; then $\mu_{dr} - \mu_{pla} = \delta$, and the center of the actual t distribution will be

$$t' = \frac{\delta}{\sqrt{(\sigma^2/n) + (\sigma^2/n)}} = \frac{\delta}{\sigma}\sqrt{\frac{n}{2}}$$

Therefore, t', how far from being centered on 0 the center of the actual distribution of the t test statistic moves, depends on the change in the mean response (δ) normalized by the population standard deviation (σ).

For example, the standard deviation in urine production in the population we are studying is 200 mL/day (from Fig. 6–1). In this context, an increase in urine production of 200 or 400 mL/day can be seen to be 1 or 2 standard deviations, a fairly substantial change. These same absolute changes in urine production would be even more striking if the population standard deviation were only 50 mL/day, in which case a 200 mL/day absolute change would be 4 standard deviations. On the other hand, these changes in urine production would be hard to detect—indeed one wonders if you would want to detect them—if the population standard deviation were 500 mL/day. In this case, 200 mL/day would be only 0.4 standard deviation of the population.

As the variability in the population σ decreases, the power of the test to detect a fixed absolute treatment effect δ increases and vice versa. In fact, we can combine the influence of these two factors by considering the dimensionless ratio $\phi = \delta/\sigma$, known as the *noncentrality parameter,* rather than each one separately.

Bigger Samples Mean More Powerful Tests

So far we have seen two things: (1) The power of a test to correctly reject the hypothesis that a treatment has no effect decreases as the confidence with which you wish to reject that hypothesis increases; (2) the power increases as the size of the treatment effect, measured with respect to the population standard deviation, increases. In most cases, investigators cannot control either of these factors and for a given sample size are stuck with whatever the power of the test is. However, the situation is not totally beyond their control. They can increase the power of the test without sacrificing the confidence with which they reject the hypothesis of no treatment effect (α) by *increasing the sample size.*

Increasing the sample size generally increases the power, for two reasons. First, as the sample size grows, the number of degrees of freedom increases, and the value of the test statistic that defines the "biggest" 100α percent of possible values under the assumption of no treatment effect generally decreases. Second, as the equation for t' above shows, the value of t (and many other test statistics) increases as sample size n increases. As a result, the distribution of t values that occur when the treatment has an effect of a given size δ/σ is located at higher t values as sample size increases.

For example, Figure 6–7*A* shows the same information as Fig. 6–4*A*, with the sample size equal to 10 in each of the two groups. Figure 6–7*B* shows the distribution of possible t values if the hypothesis of no effect were true as well as the distribution of t values that would appear if the drug still increased urine production by 200 mL/day but now based on an experiment with 20 people in each group. Even though the size of the treatment effect (δ = 200 mL/day) and the standard deviations of the underlying populations (σ = 200 mL/day) are the same as before, the actual distribution of the t test statistic moves further to the right to

$$t' = \frac{200}{\sqrt{(200^2/20) + (200^2/20)}} = 3.162$$

because the sample size of each group increased from $n = 10$ to $n = 20$.

In addition, because there are now 20 people in each group, the experiment has $\nu = 2(20 - 1) = 38$ degrees of freedom. From Table 4–1, the critical value of t defining the most extreme (two-tail) 5 percent of possible t values under the null hypothesis of no effect falls to 2.024. To obtain the power of this test to reject the null hypothesis, we find the proportion of the t distribution at or above $2.204 - 3.162 = -.958$ with $\nu = 38$ degrees of freedom. From Table 6–2, we find that the power of this study to detect an effect has increased to .83, up substantially from the value of .56 associated with a sample size of 10 in each treatment group.

We could repeat this analysis over and over again to compute the power of this test to detect a 200 mL/day increase in urine production for a variety of sample sizes. Figure 6–8 shows the results of such

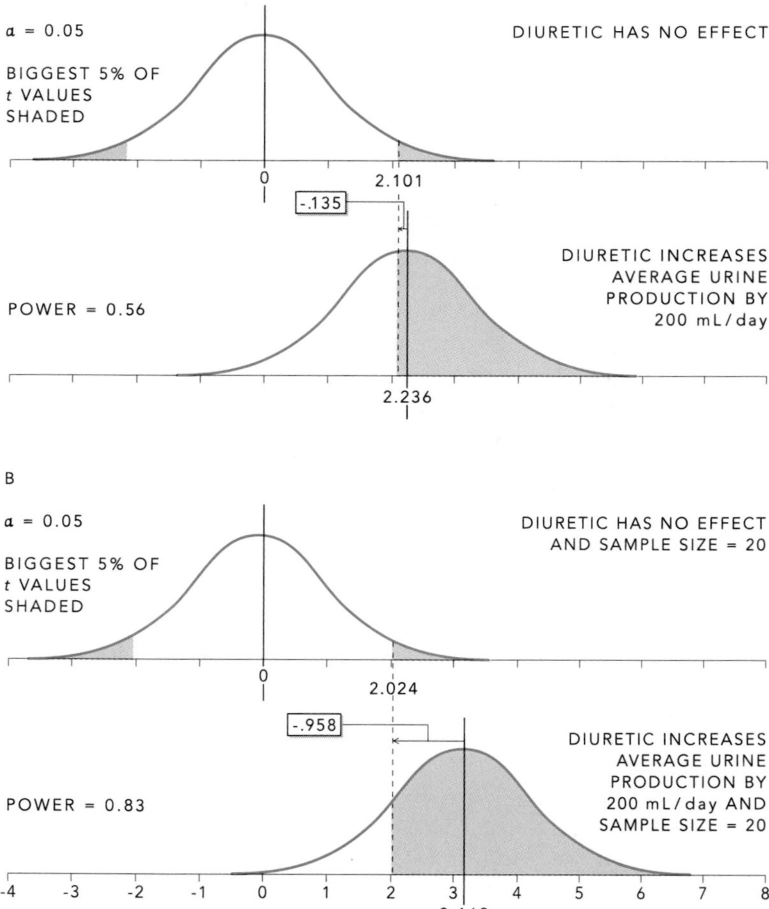

Figure 6–7 As the sample size increases, the power of the test increases for two reasons: (1) the critical value of t for a given confidence level in concluding that the treatment had an effect decreases, and (2) the values of the t statistic associated with the experiment increase.

computations. As the sample size increases, so does the test's power. In fact, estimating the sample size required to detect an effect large enough to be clinically significant is probably the major practical use to which power computations are put. Such computations are especially

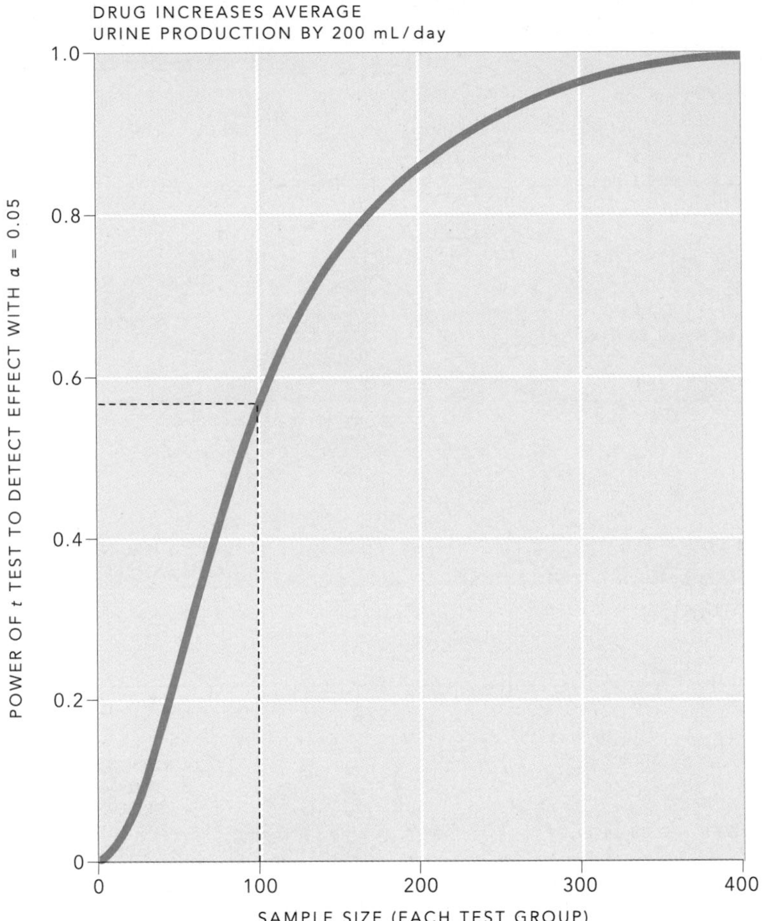

Figure 6–8 The effect of sample size on the power of a t test to detect a 200 mL per day increase in urine production with $\alpha = 0.05$ and a population standard deviation in urine production of 200 mL per day. The dashed line illustrates how to read the graph. A sample size of 10 yields a power of .56 for a t test to detect a 200 mL/day change in urine production.

important in planning randomized clinical trials to estimate how many patients will have to be recruited and how many centers will have to be involved to accumulate enough patients to obtain a large enough sample to complete a meaningful analysis.

What Determines Power? A Summary

Figure 6–9 shows a general power curve for the t test, allowing for a variety of sample sizes and differences of interest. All these curves assume that we will reject the null hypothesis of no treatment effect whenever we compute a value of t from the data that corresponds to $P < .05$ (so $\alpha = 0.05$). If we were more or less stringent in our requirement concerning the size of t necessary to report a difference, we would obtain a family of curves different from those in Fig. 6–9.

There is one curve for each value of the sample size n in Fig. 6–9. This value of n represents the size of *each* of the two sample groups being compared with the t test. Most power charts (and tables) present the results assuming that each of the experimental groups is of the same size because, for a given total sample size, power is greatest when there are equal numbers of subjects in each treatment group. Thus, when using power analysis to estimate the sample size for an experiment, the result actually yields the size of each of the sample groups. Power analysis also can be used to estimate the power of a test that yielded a negative finding; in the case of unequal sample sizes, use the size of the smaller sample in the power analysis with the charts in this book.* This procedure will give you a conservative (low) estimate for the power of the test.

To illustrate the use of Fig. 6–9, again consider the effects of diuretic presented in Fig. 6–1. We wish to compute the power of a t test (with a 5 percent risk of a Type I error, $\alpha = 0.05$) to detect a mean change in urine production of 200 mL/day when the population has a standard deviation of 200 mL/day. Hence

$$\phi = \frac{\delta}{\sigma} = \frac{200 \text{ mL/day}}{200 \text{ mL/day}} = 1$$

Since the sample size is $n = 10$ (in both the placebo and drug groups), we use the "$n = 10$" line in Fig. 6–9 to find that this test will have a power of .56.

All the examples in this chapter so far deal with estimating the power of an experiment that is analyzed with a t test. It is also possible

*There are computer programs that yield exact power calculations when sample sizes are not equal.

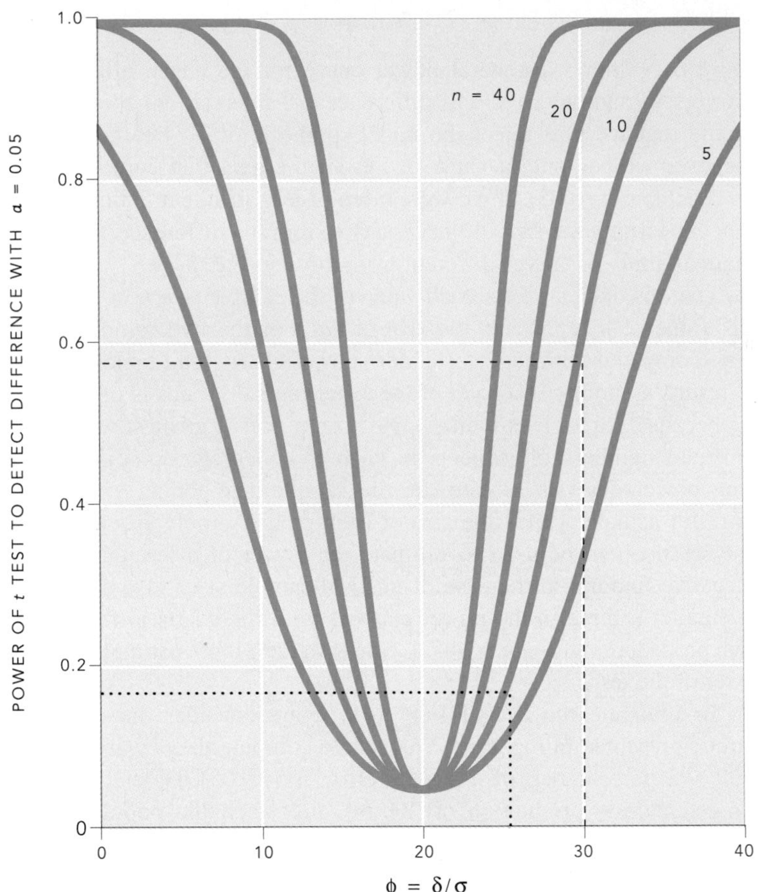

Figure 6–9 The power function for a *t* test for comparing two experimental groups, each of size *n*, with $\alpha = 0.05$. δ is the size of the change we wish to detect, σ is the population standard deviation. If we had taken $\alpha = 0.01$ or any other value, we would have obtained a different set of curves. The dashed line indicates how to read the power of a test to detect a $\delta = 200$ mL/day change in urine production with a $\sigma = 200$ mL/day standard deviation in the underlying population with a sample size of $n = 10$ in each test group; the power of this test is .56. The dotted line indicates how to find the power of an experiment designed to study the effects of anesthesia on the cardiovascular system in which $\phi = \delta/\sigma = .55$ with a sample size of 9; the power of this test is only .16.

to compute the power for all the other statistical procedures described in this book. Although the details of the computations are different, the same variables are important and play the same general roles in the computation.

Another Look at Halothane versus Morphine for Open-Heart Surgery

Table 4–2 presented data on the effects of anesthesia on the cardiovascular system. When we analyzed these data with a t test, we did not conclude that halothane and morphine anesthesia produced significantly different values of cardiac index, which is defined as the rate at which the heart pumps blood (the cardiac output) divided by body surface area. This conclusion, however, was based on relatively small samples ($n = 9$ for the halothane group and $n = 16$ for the morphine group), and there was a 15 percent change in mean cardiac index (from 2.08 L/m^2 for halothane to 1.75 L/m^2 for morphine) between these two anesthetic regimes. While a 15 percent change in cardiac index may not be clinically important, a 25 percent change could be. The question then becomes: What is the power of this experiment to detect a 25 percent change in cardiac index?

We have already decided that a 25 percent change in cardiac index, 0.52 L/m^2 (25 percent of 2.08 L/m^2), is the size of the treatment effect worth detecting. From the data in Table 4–2, the pooled estimate of the variance in the underlying population is $s^2_{wit} = 0.88(L/m^2)^2$; take the square root of this number to obtain the estimate of the population standard deviation of 0.94 L/m^2. Hence

$$\phi = \frac{\delta}{\sigma} = \frac{.52\ L/m^2}{.94\ L/m^2} = 0.553$$

Since the two sample groups have different sizes, we estimate the power of the test based on the size of the smaller group, 9. From Fig. 6–9, the power is only .16! Thus it is very unlikely that this experiment would be able to detect a 25 percent change in cardiac index.

We summarize our discussion of the power of hypothesis-testing procedures with these five statements:

- *The power of a test tells the likelihood that the hypothesis of no treatment effect will be rejected when the treatment has an effect.*
- *The more stringent our requirement for reporting that the treatment produced an effect (i.e., the smaller the chances of erroneously reporting that the treatment was effective), the lower the power of the test.*
- *The smaller the size of the treatment effect (with respect to the population standard deviation), the harder it is to detect.*
- *The larger the sample size, the greater the power of the test.*
- *The exact procedure to compute the power of a test depends on the test itself.*

POWER AND SAMPLE SIZE FOR ANALYSIS OF VARIANCE*

The issues underlying power and sample size calculations in analysis of variance are no different than for the t test. The only difference is the way in which the size of the minimum detectable treatment effect is quantified and the mathematical relationship relating this magnitude and the risk of erroneously concluding a treatment effect. The measure of the treatment effect to be detected is more complicated than in a t test because it must be expressed as more than a simple difference of two groups (because there are generally more than two groups in an analysis of variance). The size of the treatment effect is again quantified by the *noncentrality parameter,* ϕ, although it is defined differently than for a t test. To estimate the power of an analysis of variance, you specify the number of treatment groups, sample size, risk of a false-positive (α) you are willing to accept, and size of the treatment effect you wish to detect (ϕ), then look the power up in charts for analysis of variance, just as we used Figure 6–9 for t tests.

The first step is to define the size of the treatment effect with the noncentrality parameter. We specify the minimum difference between any two treatment groups we wish to detect, δ, just as when computing the power of the t test. In this case, we define

*In an introductory course, this section can be skipped without interfering with the remaining material in the book.

$$\phi = \frac{\delta}{\sigma}\sqrt{\frac{n}{2k}}$$

where σ is the standard deviation within the underlying population, k is the number of treatment groups, and n is the sample size of each treatment group.* (Note the similarity with the definition of $\phi = \delta/\sigma$ for the t test.) Once ϕ is determined, obtain the power by looking in a power chart such as Figure 6–10 with the appropriate number of numerator degrees of freedom, $\nu_n = k - 1$ and denominator degrees of freedom $\nu_d = k(n - 1)$. (A more complete set of power charts for analysis of variance appears in Appendix B.)

These same charts can be used to estimate the sample size necessary to detect a given effect with a specified power. The situation is a little more complicated than it was in the t test because the sample size, n, appears in the noncentrality parameter, ϕ, and the denominator degrees of freedom, ν_d. As a result, you must apply successive guesses to find n. You first guess n, compute the power, then adjust the guess until the computed power is close to the desired value. The example below illustrates this process.

*We present the analysis for equal sample sizes in all treatment groups and the case where all the means but one are equal and the other differs by δ. This arrangement produces the maximum power for a given total sample size. An alternative definition of ϕ involves specifying the means for the different treatment groups that you expect to detect, μ, for each of the k groups. In this case

$$\phi = \sqrt{\frac{n\Sigma(\mu_i - \mu)^2}{k\sigma^2}}$$

where

$$\mu = \frac{\Sigma\mu_i}{k}$$

is the grand population mean. The definition of ϕ in terms of the minimum detectable difference is generally easier to use because it requires fewer assumptions.

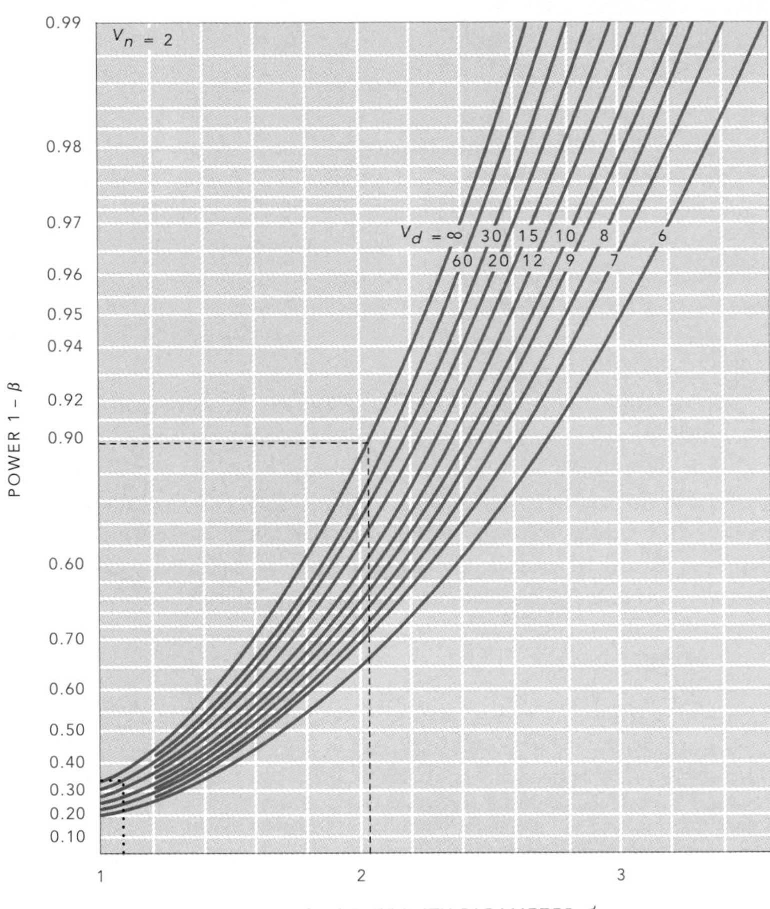

Figure 6–10 The power function for analysis of variance for $\nu_n = 2$ and $\alpha = 0.05$. Appendix B contains a complete set of power charts for a variety of values of ν_n and $\alpha = 0.05$ and .01. *(Adapted from E. S. Pearson and H. O. Hartley, "Charts for the Power Function for Analysis of Variance Tests, Derived from the Non-Central F Distribution,"* Biometrika, ***38:****112–130, 1951.)*

Power, Menstruation, and Running

To illustrate power and sample size computations for analysis of variance, let us return to the study of the effect of running on menstruation we discussed in conjunction with Figure 3–9. The essential question is whether women who jog or are serious runners have menstrual patterns different from sedentary women. Suppose we wish to detect a change of $\delta = 1$ menses per year when there is an underlying variation of $\sigma = 2$ menses per year among $k = 3$ groups of women (controls, joggers, and long-distance runners), and $n = 26$ women in each group with 95 percent confidence ($\alpha = 0.05$). (This is about the magnitude of the effect observed in the example in Chapter 3.) To find the power of this test, we first compute the noncentrality parameter

$$\phi = \frac{1}{2}\sqrt{\frac{26}{2 \cdot 3}} = 1.04$$

There are $\nu_n = k - 1 = 3 - 1 = 2$ numerator and $\nu_d = k(n - 1) = 3(26 - 1) = 75$ denominator degrees of freedom. From Fig. 6–10, the power is only about .32!

As with most power computations, this result is sobering. Suppose that we wanted to increase the power of the test to .80; how big will the samples have to be? We already know that 26 women per group is too small. Examining Fig. 6–10 suggests that we need to get ϕ up to about 2. Since the sample size, n, appears under a square root in the definition of ϕ, let us increase n by about a factor of 4 to 100 women per group. Now,

$$\phi = \frac{1}{2}\sqrt{\frac{100}{2 \cdot 3}} = 2.04$$

and $\nu_d = k(n - 1) = 3(100 - 1) = 297$. From Fig. 6–10, the power is .90. Given the uncertainties in the estimates of σ before actually conducting the experiment, this is probably close enough to stop working. The problem is that getting large samples is often difficult (and expensive). To get closer to the desired power of .80, let us try a smaller sample size, say 75. Now,

$$\phi = \frac{1}{2}\sqrt{\frac{75}{2 \cdot 3}} = 1.77$$

and $\nu_d = 3(75 - 1) = 222$. From Fig. 6–10, the power is .80. Therefore, to have an 80 percent chance of detecting a change of 1 menses per year among three groups of women when the standard deviation of the underlying population is 2 menses per year with 95 percent confidence, we need 77 women in each group.

POWER AND SAMPLE SIZE FOR COMPARING TWO PROPORTIONS*

The development of formulas for power and sample size when comparing two proportions is similar to the procedure that we used for the t test, except that we will be basing the computations on the normal distribution. We wish to find the power of a z test to detect a difference between two proportions, p_1 and p_2 with sample sizes n_1 and n_2. Recall, from Chapter 5, that the z test statistic used to compare two observed proportions, is

$$z = \frac{\hat{p}_1 - \hat{p}_2}{s_{p_1 - p_2}}$$

Under the null hypothesis of no difference, this test statistic follows the standard normal distribution (with mean 0 and standard deviation 1) given in the last row of Table 6–2. We denote the two-tailed critical value of z that we require to reject the null hypothesis of no difference with Type I error α, $z_{\alpha(2)}$. For example, if we follow the convention of accepting a 5 percent risk of a false-positive (i.e., reject the null hypothesis of no difference when $P < .05$), from Table 4–1, $z_{\alpha(2)} = 1.960$ (Figure 6–11*A*).

If there is actually a difference in the two proportions, p_1 and p_2, then the actual distribution of the z test statistic will be centered on

$$z' = \frac{p_1 - p_2}{s_{p_1 - p_2}}$$

where

$$s_{p_1 - p_2} = \sqrt{\frac{p_1(1 - p_1)}{n_1} + \frac{p_2(1 - p_2)}{n_2}}$$

*In introductory courses, this material can be skipped without loss of continuity.

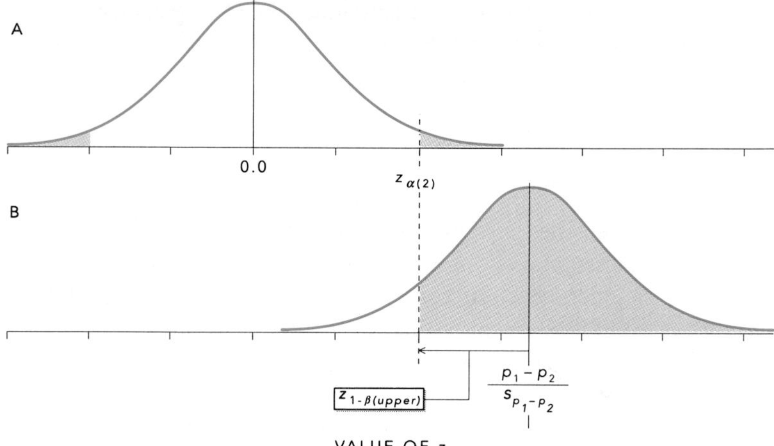

Figure 6–11 ***(A)*** $z_{\alpha(2)}$ is the two-tail critical value of the z test statistic that defines the α percent most extreme values of the z test statistic that we would expect to observe in an experiment comparing two proportions if the null hypothesis of no differences in the underlying populations was true. ***(B)*** If there is a difference in the proportions with the characteristic of interest in the two populations, the distribution of possible values of the z test statistic will no longer be centered on 0, but rather a value that depends on how big the actual differences in proportions between the two populations, $p_1 - p_2$, is. The fraction of this actual distribution of the z test statistic that fall above $z_{\alpha(2)}$ is the power of the test. (Compare this figure with Fig. 6–4.)

Note that we do not base our estimate of the standard deviation on sample estimates, since p_1 and p_2 are specified as part of the problem. As we did with the t test, we determine the power to detect the difference $p_1 - p_2$ as the proportion of the actual distribution of the z test statistic (Fig. 6–11*B*) that falls above $z_{\alpha(2)}$. Hence, the power of the test to detect the specified difference is the proportion of the normal distribution above

$$z_{1-\beta(\text{upper})} = z_{\alpha(2)} - z' = z_{\alpha(2)} - \frac{p_1 - p_2}{s_{p_1 - p_2}}$$

where $z_{1-\beta(\text{upper})}$ is the value of z that defines the (1 − β) percentage of the normal distribution (from Table 6–2).*

Mortality Associated with Anesthesia for Open-Heart Surgery

When we studied the mortality associated with halothane (13.1 percent of 61 patients) and morphine (14.9 percent of 67 patients) anesthesia in open-heart surgery in Chapter 5, we did not find a significant difference. What is the power of this study to detect a 30 percent difference in mortality, from 14 to 10 percent with 95 percent confidence?

In this case, $p_1 = .14$ and $p_2 = .10$; $n_1 = 61$ and $n_2 = 67$, so

$$s_{p_1 - p_2} = \sqrt{\frac{.14(1 - .14)}{61} + \frac{.10(1 - .10)}{67}} = .0576$$

The two-tail 95 percent critical value of the normal distribution, $z_{.05(2)}$ is, from Table 6–2, 1.960, so the power of the test is the fraction of the normal distribution above

$$z_{1-\beta(\text{upper})} = 1.960 - \frac{.14 - .10}{.0576} = 1.960 - .694 = 1.265$$

From Table 6–2, the power of the test is only 11 percent, so you should be careful about negative conclusions in such a study!

*Technically, we should also include the part of the distribution in Fig. 6–11*A* that falls below the lower z_α tail of the distribution in Fig. 6–11*B*, but this tail of the distribution rarely contributes anything of consequence. Note that these calculations do not include the Yates correction. It is possible to include the Yates correction by replacing $(p_1 - p_2)$ with $|p_1 - p_2| - (1/n_1 + 1/n_2)$. Doing so makes the arithmetic more difficult, but does not represent a theoretical change. Including the Yates correction lowers the power or increases the sample size.

Sample Size for Comparing Two Proportions

To obtain the sample size to compare two proportions, simply take $z_{1-\beta(\text{upper})}$ as given and solve the resulting equations for n, the size of each group. Assuming that the two groups are the same size, this process yields

$$n = \frac{A\left[1 + \sqrt{1 + \dfrac{4\delta}{A}}\right]^2}{4\delta^2}$$

where

$$A = \left[z_{\alpha(2)}\sqrt{2p(1-p)} + z_{1-\beta(\text{upper})}\sqrt{p_1(1-p_1) + p_2(1-p_2)}\right]^2$$

$$p = \frac{p_1 + p_2}{2}$$

$$\delta = |p_1 - p_2|$$

POWER AND SAMPLE SIZE FOR RELATIVE RISK AND ODDS RATIO

The formulas developed above can be used to estimate power and sample sizes for relative risks and odds ratios. Instead of specifying both proportions, you simply specify one proportion, the desired relative risk or odds ratio, and compute the other proportion. Let p_1 be the probability of disease in the unexposed members of the population and p_2 be the probability of disease in the exposed members of the population.

The relative risk is the ratio of the probability of disease in those exposed to the toxin of interest over those not exposed,

$$RR = \frac{p_{\text{exposed}}}{p_{\text{unexposed}}} = \frac{p_2}{p_1}$$

so use the formulas above with

$$p_2 = RR \cdot p_1$$

Likewise, the odds ratio is

$$OR = \frac{p_{\text{exposed}}/(1 - p_{\text{exposed}})}{p_{\text{unexposed}}/(1 - p_{\text{unexposed}})} = \frac{p_2/(1 - p_2)}{p_1/(1 - p_1)}$$

so

$$p_2 = \frac{OR \cdot p_1}{1 + p_1(OR - 1)}$$

POWER AND SAMPLE SIZE FOR CONTINGENCY TABLES*

Figure 6–10 (and the corresponding charts in Appendix B) can also be used to compute the power and sample size for contingency tables. As with other power computations, the first step is to define the pattern you wish to be able to detect. This effect is specified by selecting the proportions of row and column observations that appear in each cell of the contingency table.

Table 6–3 shows the notation for the computation for a 3 × 2 contingency table: p_{11} is the proportion of all observations expected in the upper left cell of the table, p_{12} the proportion in the upper right corner, and so on. All the proportions must add up to 1. The r row and c column sums are denoted with R's and C's with subscripts corresponding to the rows and columns. The noncentrality parameter for such a contingency table is defined as

$$\phi = \sqrt{\frac{N}{(r - 1)(c - 1) + 1} \sum \frac{(p_{ij} - R_i C_j)^2}{R_i C_j}}$$

where r is the number of rows, c is the number of columns, and N is the total number of observations. This value of ϕ is used with Fig. 6–10 with $\nu_n = (r - 1)(c - 1)$ and $\nu_d = \beta$ degrees of freedom.

*In introductory courses, this section can be skipped without loss of continuity.

Table 6–3 Notation for Computing Power for Contingency Tables

p_{11}	p_{12}	R_1
p_{21}	p_{22}	R_2
p_{31}	p_{32}	R_3
C_1	C_2	1.00

To compute the sample size necessary to achieve a given power, simply reverse this process. Determine the necessary value of ϕ to achieve the desired power with $\nu_n = (r - 1)(c - 1)$ and $\nu_d = \infty$ from Fig. 6–10 (or the power charts in Appendix B). We obtain the sample size by solving the equation above for N, to obtain

$$N = \frac{\phi^2[(r - 1)(c - 1) + 1]}{\sum \frac{(p_{ij} - R_iC_j)^2}{R_iC_j}}$$

Physicians, Perspiration, and Power

In addition to studying the effect of running on menstruation, Dale and colleagues also studied how likely women were to consult a physician depending on their running status. (This example was discussed in conjunction with Table 5–5.) Let us examine the power of a contingency table to detect the pattern of proportions shown in Table 6–4 with 95 percent confidence (α) from a sample of $N = 165$ women. Substituting into the equation above

$$\phi = \left[\frac{165}{(3 - 1)(2 - 1) + 1}\left[\frac{(.025 - .250 \cdot .350)^2}{.250 \cdot .350} + \frac{(.225 - .250 \cdot .650)^2}{.250 \cdot .650} + \frac{(.100 - .300 \cdot .350)^2}{.300 \cdot .350} + \frac{(.200 - .300 \cdot .650)^2}{.300 \cdot .650} + \frac{(.225 - .450 \cdot .350)^2}{.450 \cdot .350} + \frac{(.225 - .450 \cdot .650)^2}{.450 \cdot .650}\right]\right]^{1/2}$$

$$\phi = 2.50$$

Table 6–4 Pattern of Physician Consultation for Menstrual Problems to be Detected

Group	Yes	No	Total
Controls	.025	.225	.250
Joggers	.100	.200	.300
Runners	.225	.225	.450
Total	.350	.650	1.00

Consult Fig. 6–10 with $\phi = 2.50$, $\nu_n = (r - 1)(c - 1) = (3 - 1)(2 - 1) = 2$ and $\nu_d = \infty$ degrees of freedom to obtain a power of .98 to detect this pattern with 95 percent confidence.

PRACTICAL PROBLEMS IN USING POWER

If you know the size of the treatment effect, population standard deviation, α, and sample size, you can use graphs like Fig. 6–9 to estimate the power of a t test after the fact. Unfortunately, in practice, one does not know how large an effect a given treatment will have (finding that out is usually the reason for the study in the first place), so you must specify how large a change is *worth detecting* to compute the power of the test.

This requirement to go on record about how small a change is worth detecting may be one reason that very few people report the power of the tests they use. While such information is not especially important when investigators report that they detected a difference, it can be quite important when they report that they failed to detect one. If the power of the test to detect a clinically significant effect is small, say 25 percent, this report will mean something quite different than if the test was powerful enough to detect a clinically significant difference 85 percent of the time.

These difficulties are even more acute when using power computations to decide on the sample size for a study in advance. Completing this computation requires that investigators estimate not only the size of the effect they think is worth detecting and the confidence with which they hope to accept (β) or reject (α) the hypothesis that the treatment is effective but also the standard deviation of the population being studied. Sometimes existing information can be used to estimate these numbers; sometimes investigators do a pilot study to estimate them; sometimes they simply guess.

WHAT DIFFERENCE DOES IT MAKE?

In Chapter 4 we discussed the most common error in the use of statistical methods in the medical literature, inappropriate use of the t test. Repeated use of t tests increases the chances of reporting a "statistically significant" difference above the nominal levels one obtains from the t distribution. In the language of this chapter, it increases the Type I error. In practical terms, this increases the chances that an investigator will report some procedure or therapy capable of producing an effect beyond what one would expect from chance variation when the evidence does not actually support this conclusion.

This chapter examined the other side of the coin, the fact that perfectly correctly designed studies employing statistical methods correctly may fail to detect real, perhaps clinically important, differences simply because the sample sizes are too small to give the procedure enough power to detect the effect. This chapter shows how you can estimate the power of a given test after the results are reported in the literature and also how investigators can estimate the number of subjects they need to study to detect a specified difference with a given level of confidence (say, 95 percent; that is, $\alpha = 0.05$). Such computations are often quite distressing because they often reveal the need for a large number of experimental subjects, especially compared with the relatively few patients who typically form the basis for clinical studies.* Sometimes the investigators increase the size of the difference they say they wish to detect, decrease the power they find acceptable, or ignore the whole problem in an effort to reduce the necessary sample size. Most medical investigators never confront these problems because they have never heard of power.

In 1979, Jennie Freiman and colleagues† examined 71 randomized clinical trials published between 1960 and 1977 in journals, such as *The Lancet*, the *New England Journal of Medicine*, and the *Journal*

*R. A. Fletcher and S. W. Fletcher ("Clinical Research in General Medical Journals: A 30-Year Perspective," *N. Engl. J. Med.*, **301:**180–183, 1979) report the median number of subjects included in clinical studies published in the *Journal of the American Medical Association, The Lancet,* and the *New England Journal of Medicine* in 1946 to 1976 ranged from 16 to 36 people.

†J. A. Freiman, T. C. Chalmers, H. Smith, Jr., and R. R. Kuebler, "The Importance of Beta, the Type II Error and Sample Size in the Design and Interpretation of the Randomized Controlled Trial," *N. Engl. J. Med.*, **299:**690–694, 1978.

of the American Medical Association, reporting that the treatment studied did not produce a "statistically significant" ($P < .05$) improvement in clinical outcome. Only 20 percent of these studies included enough subjects to detect a 25 percent improvement in clinical outcome with a power of .50 or better. In other words, if the treatment produced a 25 percent reduction in mortality rate or other clinically important endpoint, there was less than a 50 : 50 chance that the clinical trial would be able to detect it with $P < .05$. Moreover, Freiman and colleagues found that *only one* of the 71 papers stated that α and β were considered at the start of the study; 18 recognized a trend in the results, whereas 14 commented on the need for a larger sample size.

Fifteen years later, in 1994, Mohler and colleagues* revisited this question by examining randomized controlled trials in these same journals published in 1975, 1980, 1985, and 1990. While the number of randomized controlled trials published in 1990 was more than twice the number published in 1975, the proportion reporting negative results remained reasonably constant, at about 27 percent of all the trials. Only 16 percent and 36 percent of the negative studies had an adequate power (.80) to detect a 25 percent or 50 percent change in outcome, respectively. Only one third of the studies with negative results reported information regarding how the sample sizes were computed. An evaluation of randomized controlled trials published in the surgical literature between 1988 and 1998 found that only 25 percent of the trials were large enough to detect a 50 percent difference in therapeutic effect with .80 power, and only 29 percent of the papers included a formal sample size calculation.†

Another study of papers published between 1999 and 2002 showed that half the studies were powered to detect a 50 percent difference in therapeutic effect.††

*D. Mohler, C. S. Dulberg, G. A. Wells, "Statistical Power, Sample Size, and Their Reporting in Randomized Clinical Trials," *JAMA* **272:**122–124, 1994.

†J. B. Dimick, M. Diener-West, P. A. Lipsett, "Negative Results of Randomized Clinical Trials Published in the Surgical Literature," *Arch. Surg.* **136:**796–800, 2001.

††M. A. Maggard, J. B. O'Connell, J. H. Liu, D. A. Etzioni, C. Y. Ko, "Sample Size Calculations in Surgery: Are They Done Correctly?" *Surgery,* **134:**275–279, 2003.

Things are improving, but slowly.

The fact remains, however, that publication of "negative" studies without adequate attention to having a large enough sample size to draw definitive conclusions remains a problem. Thus, in this area, like the rest of statistical applications in the medical literature, it is up to responsible readers to interpret what they read rather than take it at face value.

Other than throwing your hands up when a study with low power fails to detect a statistically significant effect, is there anything an investigator or clinician reading the literature can learn from the results? Yes. Instead of focusing on the accept–reject logic of statistical hypothesis testing,* one can try to estimate how strongly the observations *suggest* an effect by estimating the size of the hypothesized effect together with the uncertainty of this estimate.† We laid the groundwork for this procedure in Chapters 2, 4, and 5 when we discussed the standard error and the t distribution. The next chapter builds on this base to develop the idea of confidence limits.

*There is another approach that can be used in some clinical trials to avoid this accept–reject problem. In a *sequential trial* the data are analyzed after each new individual is added to the study and the decision made to (1) accept the hypothesis of no treatment effect, (2) reject the hypothesis, or (3) study another individual. Sequential tests generally allow one to achieve the same levels of α and β for a given size treatment effect with a smaller sample size than the methods discussed in this book. This smaller sample size is purchased at the cost of increased complexity of the statistical procedures. Sequential analyses are often performed by repeated use of the statistical procedures presented in this book, such as the t test. This procedure is incorrect because it produces overoptimistic P values, just as the repeated use of t tests (without the Bonferroni correction) produces erroneous results when one should do an analysis of variance. See W.J. Dixon and F.J. Massey, *Introduction to Statistical Analysis* (4 ed.), McGraw-Hill, New York, 1983, chapter 18, "Sequential Analysis," for an introduction to sequential analysis.

†One quick way to use a computerized statistical package to estimate if getting more cases would resolve a power problem is to simply copy the data twice and rerun the analysis on the doubled data set. If the results become less ambiguous, it suggests that obtaining more cases (on the assumption that the data will be similar to that which you have already obtained) will yield less ambiguous results. This procedure is, of course, not a substitute for a formal power analysis and would certainly not be reportable in a scientific paper, but it is an easy way to get an idea of whether gathering more data would be worthwhile.

PROBLEMS

6-1 Use the data in Table 4–2 to find the power of a *t* test to detect a 50 percent difference in cardiac index between halothane and morphine anesthesia.

6-2 How large a sample size would be necessary to have an 80 percent chance of detecting a 25 percent difference in cardiac index between halothane and morphine anesthesia?

6-3 Use the data in Table 4–2 to find the power of the experiments reported there to detect a 25 percent change in mean arterial blood pressure and total peripheral resistance.

6-4 In Prob. 3-5 (and again in Prob. 4-4), we decided that there was insufficient evidence to conclude that men and women who have had at least one vertebral fracture differ in vertebral bone density. What is the power of this test to detect average (with $\alpha = 0.05$) bone density in men 20 percent lower than the average bone density for women?

6-5 How large a sample would be necessary to be 90 percent confident that men have vertebral bone densities of at least 30 percent of the values for women when you wish to be 95 percent confident in any conclusion that vertebral bone densities differ between men and women?

6-6 Use the data in Prob. 3-2 to find the power of detecting a change in mean forced midexpiratory flow of 0.25 L/s with 95 percent confidence.

6-7 Use the data in Prob. 3-3 to find the power of detecting an increase in HDL of 5 mg/dL and 10 mg/dL with 95 percent confidence.

6-8 How large must each sample group be to have an 80 percent power to detect a change of 5 mg/dL with 95 percent confidence?

6-9 What is the power of the experiment in Prob. 5-4 to detect a situation in which nefazodone and psychotherapy each causes remission one-third of the time, and nefazodone and psychotherapy cause remission one-half of the time? Assume that the same number of people take each treatment as in Prob. 5-4. Use $\alpha = 0.05$.

6-10 How large would the sample size need to be in Prob. 6-9 to reach 80 percent power?

Chapter 7

Confidence Intervals

All the statistical procedures developed so far were designed to help decide whether or not a set of observations is compatible with some hypothesis. These procedures yielded P values to estimate the chance of reporting that a treatment has an effect when it really does not and the power to estimate the chance that the test would detect a treatment effect of some specified size. This decision-making paradigm does not characterize the size of the difference or illuminate results that may not be statistically significant (i.e., not associated with a value of P below .05) but does nevertheless suggest an effect. In addition, since P depends not only on the magnitude of the treatment effect but also the sample size, it is not unusual for experiments with large sample sizes to yield very small values of P (what investigators often call "highly significant" results) when the magnitude of the treatment effect is so small that it is clinically or scientifically unimportant. As Chapter 6 noted, it can be more informative to think not only in terms of the accept–reject approach of statistical hypothesis testing but also to estimate the size of the treatment effect together with some measure of the uncertainty in that estimate.

This approach is not new; we used it in Chapter 2 when we defined the standard error of the mean to quantify the certainty with which we could estimate the population mean from a sample. We observed that since the population of all sample means at least approximately follows a normal distribution, the true (and unobserved) population mean will lie within about 2 standard errors of the mean of the sample mean 95 percent of the time. We now develop the tools to make this statement more precise and generalize it to apply to other estimation problems, such as the size of the effect a treatment produces. The resulting estimates, called *confidence intervals,* can also be used to test hypotheses.* This approach yields exactly the same conclusions as the procedures we discussed earlier because it simply represents a different perspective on how to use concepts like the standard error, t, and normal distributions. Confidence intervals are also used to estimate the range of values that include a specified proportion of all members of a population, such as the "normal range" of values for a laboratory test.

THE SIZE OF THE TREATMENT EFFECT MEASURED AS THE DIFFERENCE OF TWO MEANS

In Chapter 4, we defined the t statistic to be

$$t = \frac{\text{difference of sample means}}{\text{standard error of difference of sample means}}$$

then computed its value for the data observed in an experiment. Next, we compared the result with the value t_α that defined the most extreme 100α percent of the possible values to t that would occur (in both tails) if the two samples were drawn from a single population. If the observed value of t exceeded t_α (given in Table 4–1), we reported a "statistically significant" difference, with $P < \alpha$. As Fig. 4–5 showed, the distribution of possible values of t has a mean of zero and is symmetric about zero when the two samples are drawn from the *same* population.

On the other hand, if the two samples are drawn from populations with *different* means, the distribution of values of t associated with

*Some statisticians believe that confidence intervals provide a better way to think about the results of experiments than traditional hypothesis testing. For a brief exposition from this perspective, see K. J. Rothman, "A Show of Confidence," *N. Engl. J. Med.*, **299:**1362–1363, 1978.

all possible experiments involving two samples of a given size is *not* centered on zero; it does not follow the t distribution. As Figs. 6–3 and 6–5 showed, the actual distribution of possible values of t has a nonzero mean that depends on the size of the treatment effect. It is possible to review the definition of t so that it will be distributed according to the t distribution in Fig. 4–5 *regardless of whether or not the treatment actually has an effect.* This modified definition of t is

$$t = \frac{\text{difference of sample means} - \text{true difference in population means}}{\text{standard error of difference of sample means}}$$

Notice that if the hypothesis of no treatment effect is correct, the difference in population means is zero and this definition of t reduces to the one we used before. The equivalent mathematical statement is

$$t = \frac{(\bar{X}_1 - \bar{X}_2) - (\mu_1 - \mu_2)}{s_{\bar{X}_1 - \bar{X}_2}}$$

In Chapter 4 we computed t from the observations, then compared it with the critical value for a "big" value of t with $\nu = n_1 + n_2 - 2$ degrees of freedom to obtain a P value. Now, however, we cannot follow this approach since we do not know all the terms on the right side of the equation. Specifically, *we do not know the true difference in mean values of the two populations* from which the samples were drawn, $\mu_1 - \mu_2$. We can, however, use this equation to estimate the size of the treatment effect, $\mu_1 - \mu_2$.

Instead of using the equation to determine t, we will select an appropriate value of t and use the equation to estimate $\mu_1 - \mu_2$. The only problem is that of selecting an appropriate value for t.

By definition, 100α percent of all possible values of t are more negative than $-t_\alpha$ or more positive than $+t_\alpha$. For example, only 5 percent of all possible t values will fall outside the interval between $-t_{.05}$ and $+t_{.05}$, where $t_{.05}$ is the critical value of t that defines the most extreme 5 percent of the t distribution (tabulated in Table 4–1). Therefore, $100(1 - \alpha)$

percent of all possible values of t fall between $-t_\alpha$ and $+t_\alpha$. For example, 95 percent of all possible values of t will fall between $-t_{.05}$ and $+t_{.05}$.

Every different pair of random samples we draw in our experiment will be associated with different values of $\overline{X}_1$, $\overline{X}_2$, and $s_{\overline{X}_1-\overline{X}_2}$ and $100(1 - \alpha)$ percent of all possible experiments involving samples of a given size will yield values of t that fall between $-t_\alpha$ and $+t_\alpha$. Therefore, for $100(1 - \alpha)$ percent of all possible experiments

$$-t_\alpha < \frac{(\overline{X}_1 - \overline{X}_2) - (\mu_1 - \mu_2)}{s_{\overline{X}_1-\overline{X}_2}} < +t_\alpha$$

Solve this equation for the true difference in sample means

$$(\overline{X}_1 - \overline{X}_2) - t_\alpha s_{\overline{X}_1-\overline{X}_2} < \mu_1 - \mu_2 < (\overline{X}_1 - \overline{X}_2) + t_\alpha s_{\overline{X}_1-\overline{X}_2}$$

In other words, the actual difference of the means of the two populations from which the samples were drawn will fall within t_α standard errors of the difference of the sample means of the observed difference in the sample means (t_α has $\nu = n_1 + n_2 - 2$ degrees of freedom, just as when we used the t distribution in hypothesis testing.) This range is called the $100(1 - \alpha)$ percent *confidence interval for the difference of the means.* For example, the 95 percent confidence interval for the true difference of the sample means is

$$(\overline{X}_1 - \overline{X}_2) - t_{.05}\, s_{\overline{X}_1-\overline{X}_2} < \mu_1 - \mu_2 < (\overline{X}_1 - \overline{X}_2) + t_{.05}\, s_{\overline{X}_1-\overline{X}_2}$$

This equation defines the range that will include the true difference in the means for 95 percent of all possible experiments that involve drawing samples from the two populations under study.

Since this procedure to compute the confidence interval for the difference of two means uses the t distribution, it is subject to the same limitations as the t test. In particular, the samples must be drawn from populations that follow a normal distribution at least approximately.*

*It is also possible to define confidence intervals for differences in means when there are multiple comparisons, using q and q' in place of t. For a detailed discussion of these computations, see J. H. Zar, *Biostatistical Analysis*, 4th ed., Prentice-Hall, Upper Saddle River, N.J., 1999.

THE EFFECTIVE DIURETIC

Figure 6–1 showed the distributions of daily urine production for a population of 200 individuals when they are taking a placebo or a drug that is an effective diuretic. The mean urine production of the entire population when all members are taking the placebo is $\mu_{\text{pla}} = 1200$ mL/day. The mean urine production for the population when all members are taking the drug is $\mu_{\text{dr}} = 1400$ mL/day. Therefore, the drug increases urine production by an average of $\mu_{\text{dr}} - \mu_{\text{pla}} = 1400 - 1200 = 200$ mL/day. An investigator, however, cannot observe every member of the population and must estimate the size of this effect from samples of people observed when they are taking the placebo or the drug. Figure 6–1 shows one pair of such samples, each of 10 individuals. The people who received the placebo had a mean urine output of 1180 mL/day, and the people receiving the drug had a mean urine output of 1400 mL/day. Thus, these two samples suggest that the drug increased urine production by $\bar{X}_{\text{dr}} - \bar{X}_{\text{pla}} = 1400 - 1180 = 220$ mL/day. The random variation associated with the sampling procedure led to a different estimate of the size of the treatment effect from that really present. Simply presenting this single estimate of 220 mL/day increase in urine output ignores the fact that there is some uncertainty in the estimates of the true mean urine output in the two populations, so there will be some uncertainty in the estimate of the true difference in urine output. We now use the confidence interval to present an alternative description of how large a change in urine output accompanies the drug. This interval describes the average change seen in the people included in the experiment and also reflects the uncertainty introduced by the random sampling process.

To estimate the standard error of the difference of the means $s_{\bar{X}_{\text{dr}} - \bar{X}_{\text{pla}}}$ we first compute a pooled estimate of the population variance. The standard deviations of observed urine production were 245 and 144 mL/day for people taking the drug and the placebo, respectively. Both samples included 10 people; therefore,

$$s^2 = \frac{1}{2}(s_{\text{dr}}^2 + s_{\text{pla}}^2) = \frac{1}{2}(245^2 + 144^2) = 201^2$$

and

$$s_{\bar{X}_{\text{dr}} - \bar{X}_{\text{pla}}} = \sqrt{\frac{s^2}{n_{\text{dr}}} + \frac{s^2}{n_{\text{pla}}}} = \sqrt{\frac{201^2}{10} + \frac{201^2}{10}} = 89.9 \text{ mL/day}$$

To compute the 95 percent confidence interval, we need the value of $t_{.05}$ from Table 4–1. Since each sample contains $n = 10$ individuals, we use the value of $t_{.05}$ corresponding to $\nu = 10 + 10 - 2 = 18$ degrees of freedom. From Table 4–1, $t_{.05} = 2.101$.

Now we are ready to compute the 95 percent confidence interval for the mean change in urine production that accompanies use of the drug

$$(\bar{X}_{dr} - \bar{X}_{pla}) - t_{.05}\, s_{\bar{X}_{dr}-\bar{X}_{pla}} < \mu_{dr} - \mu_{pla} < (\bar{X}_{dr} - \bar{X}_{pla}) + t_{.05}\, s_{\bar{X}_{dr}-\bar{X}_{pla}}$$

$$220 - 2.101(89.9) < \mu_{dr} - \mu_{pla} < 220 + 2.101(89.9)$$

$$31 \text{ mL/day} < \mu_{dr} - \mu_{pla} < 409 \text{ mL/day}$$

Thus, on the basis of this particular experiment, we can be 95 percent confident that the drug increases average urine production somewhere between 61 and 439 mL/day. The *range* of values from 61 to 439 *is* the 95 percent *confidence interval* corresponding to this experiment. As Figure 7–1*A* shows, this interval includes the actual change in mean urine production, $\mu_{dr} - \mu_{pla}$, 200 mL/day.

More Experiments

Of course, there is nothing special about the two samples of 10 people each selected in the study we just analyzed. Just as the values of the sample mean and standard deviation vary with the specific random

---

Figure 7–1 **(*A*)** The 95 percent confidence interval for the change in urine production produced by the drug using the random samples shown in Fig. 6–1. The interval contains the true change in urine production, 200 mL/day (indicated by the dashed line). Since the interval does not include zero (indicated by the solid line), we can conclude that the drug increases urine output ($P < .05$). **(*B*)** The 95 percent confidence interval for change in urine production computed for the random samples shown in Fig. 6–2. The interval includes the actual change in urine production (200 mL/day), but it also includes zero, so that it is not possible to reject the hypothesis of no drug effect (at the 5 percent level). **(*C*)** The 95 percent confidence intervals for 48 more sets of random samples, e.g., experiments, drawn from the two populations in Fig. 6–1*A*. All but 3 of the 50 intervals shown in this figure include the actual change in urine production; 5 percent of *all* possible 95 percent confidence intervals will not include the 200 mL/day. Of the 50 confidence intervals, 22 include zero, meaning that the data do not permit rejecting the hypothesis of no difference at the 5 percent level. In these cases, we would make a Type II error. Since 44 percent of *all* possible 95 percent confidence intervals include zero, the probability of detecting a change in urine production is $1 - \beta = .56$.

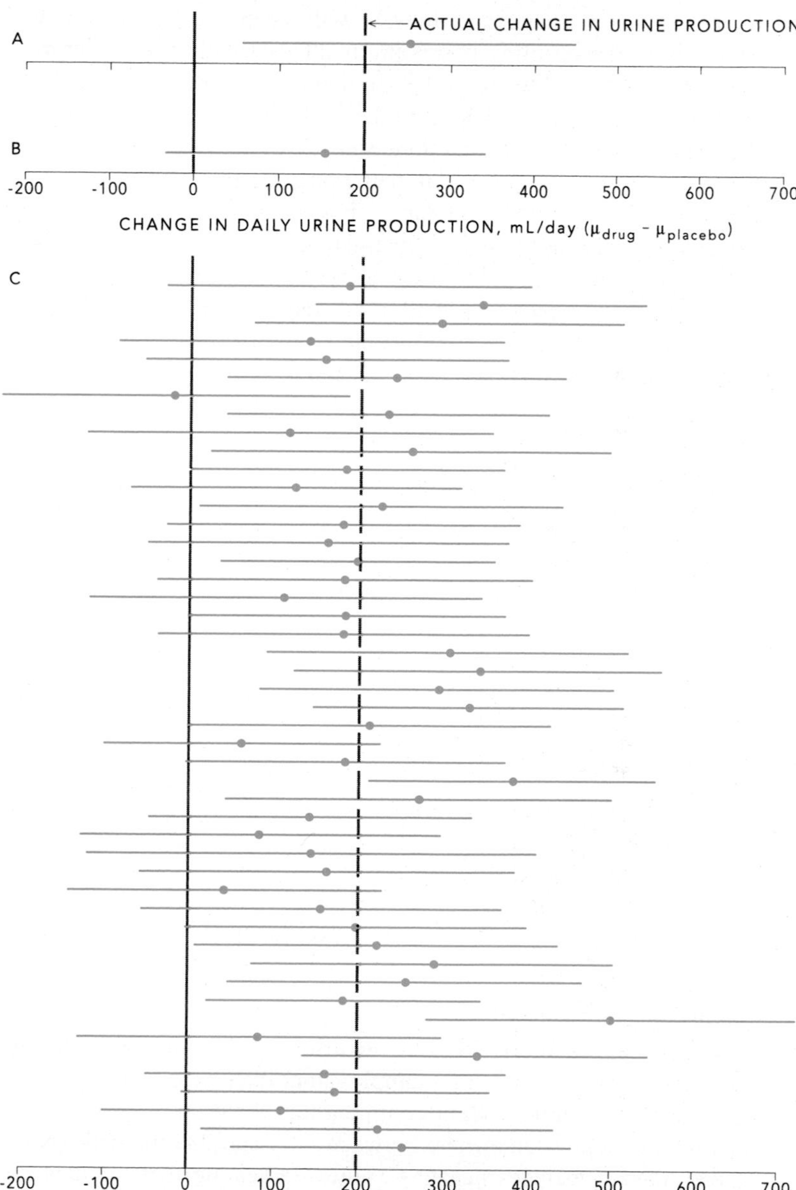
ACTUAL CHANGE IN URINE PRODUCTION
A
B
C
-200
-100
0
100
200
300
400
500
600
700
CHANGE IN DAILY URINE PRODUCTION, mL/day ($\mu_{drug} - \mu_{placebo}$)

sample of people we happen to draw, so will the confidence interval we compute from the resulting observations. (This should not be surprising, since the confidence interval is computed from the sample means and standard deviations.) The confidence interval we just computed corresponds to the specific random sample of individuals shown in Fig. 6–1. Had we selected a *different random sample* of people, say those in Fig. 6–2, we would have obtained a *different 95 percent confidence interval* for the size of the treatment effect.

The individuals selected at random for the experiment in Fig. 6–2 show a mean urine production of 1216 mL/day for the people taking the placebo and 1368 mL/day for the people taking the drug. The standard deviations of the two samples are 97 and 263 mL/day, respectively. In these two samples, the drug increased average urine production by $\bar{X}_{dr} - \bar{X}_{pla} = 1368 - 1216 = 152$ mL/day. The pooled estimate of the population variance is

$$s^2 = \frac{1}{2}(97^2 + 263^2) = 198^2$$

in which case,

$$s_{\bar{X}_{dr}-\bar{X}_{pla}} = \sqrt{\frac{198^2}{10} + \frac{198^2}{10}} = 89.9 \text{ mL/day}$$

So the 95 percent confidence interval for the mean change in urine production associated with the sample shown in Fig. 6–2 is

$$152 - 2.101(89.9) < \mu_{dr} - \mu_{pla} < 152 + 2.101(89.9)$$
$$-35 \text{ mL/day} < \mu_{dr} - \mu_{pla} < 339 \text{ mL/day}$$

This interval, while different from the first one we computed, also includes the actual mean increase in urine production, 200 mL/day (Fig. 7–1*B*). Had we drawn this sample rather than the one in Fig. 6–1, we would have been 95 percent confident that the drug increased average urine production somewhere between −35 and 339 mL/day. (Note that this interval includes negative values, indicating that the data do not permit us to exclude the possibility that the drug decreased as well as increased average urine production. This observation is the basis for using confidence intervals to test hypotheses later in this chapter.) In sum, *the specific 95 percent confidence interval we obtain depends on the specific random sample we happen to select for observation.*

So far, we have seen two such intervals that could arise from random sampling of the populations in Fig. 6–1; there are more than 10^{27} possible samples of 10 people each, so there are more than 10^{27} possible 95 percent confidence intervals. Figure 7–1*C* shows 48 more of them, computed by selecting two samples of 10 people each from the populations of placebo and drug takers. Of the 50 intervals shown in Fig. 7–1, all but 3 (about 5 percent) include the value of 200 mL/day, the actual change in average urine production associated with the drug.

WHAT DOES "CONFIDENCE" MEAN?

We are now ready to attach a precise meaning to the term *95 percent confident.* The specific 95 percent confidence interval associated with a given set of data will or will not actually include the true size of the treatment effect, but in the long run 95 percent of *all possible 95 percent confidence intervals* will include the true difference of mean values associated with the treatment. As such, it describes not only the size of the effect but quantifies the certainty with which one can estimate the size of the treatment effect.

The size of the interval depends on the level of confidence you want to have that it will actually include the true treatment effect. Since t_α increases as α decreases, requiring a greater and greater fraction of all possible confidence intervals to cover the true effect will make the intervals larger. To see this, let us compute the 90 percent, 95 percent, and 99 percent confidence intervals associated with the data in Fig. 6–1. To do so, we need only substitute the values of $t_{.10}$ and $t_{.01}$ corresponding to $\nu = 18$ from Table 4–1 for t_α in the formula derived above. (We have already solved the problem for $t_{.05}$.)

For the 90 percent confidence interval, $t_{.10} = 1.734$, so the interval associated with the samples in Fig. 6–1 is

$$250 - 1.734(89.9) < \mu_{dr} - \mu_{pla} < 250 + 1.734(89.9)$$

$$90 \text{ mL/day} < \mu_{dr} - \mu_{pla} < 410 \text{ mL/day}$$

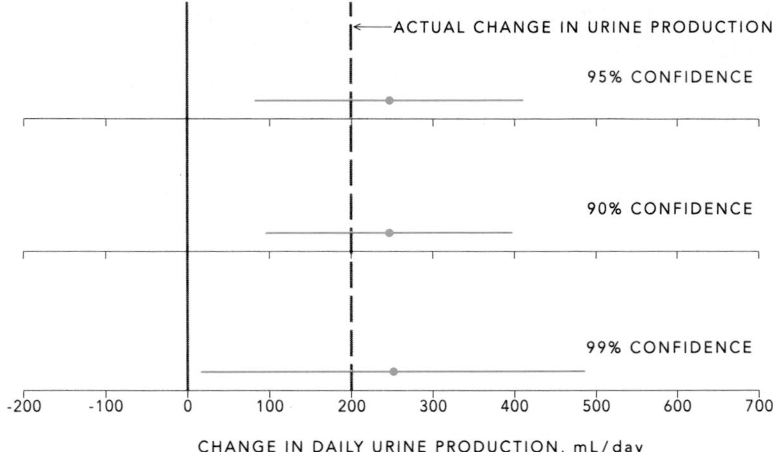

Figure 7–2 Increasing the level of confidence you wish to have that a confidence interval includes the true treatment effect makes the interval wider. All the confidence intervals in this figure were computed from the two random samples shown in Fig. 6–1. The 90 percent confidence interval is narrower than the 95 percent confidence interval, and the 99 percent confidence interval is wider. The actual change in urine production, 200 mL/day, is indicated with the dashed line.

which, as Figure 7–2 shows, is narrower than the 95 percent interval. Does this mean the data now magically yield a more precise estimate of the treatment effect? No. If you are willing to accept the risk that 10 percent of all possible confidence intervals will not include the true change in mean values, you can get by with a narrower interval.

On the other hand, if you want to specify an interval selected from a population of confidence intervals, 99 percent of which include the true change in population means, you compute the confidence interval with $t_{.01} = 2.552$. The 99 percent confidence interval associated with the samples in Fig. 6–1 is

$$250 - 2.552(89.9) < \mu_{\text{dr}} - \mu_{\text{pla}} < 250 + 2.552(89.9)$$

$$21\ \text{mL/day} < \mu_{\text{dr}} - \mu_{\text{pla}} < 479\ \text{mL/day}$$

This interval is wider than the other two in Fig. 7–2.

In sum, the confidence interval gives a range that is computed in the hope that it will include the parameter of interest (in this case, the difference of two population means). The confidence level associated with the interval (say 95, 90, or 99 percent) gives the percentage of all such possible intervals that will actually include the true value of the parameter. A *particular* interval will or will not include the true value of the parameter. Unfortunately, you can never know whether or not that interval does. All you can say is that the chances of selecting an interval that does not include the true value is small (say 5, 10, or 1 percent). The more confidence you wish to have that the interval will cover the true value, the wider the interval.

CONFIDENCE INTERVALS CAN BE USED TO TEST HYPOTHESES

As already noted, confidence intervals can provide another route to testing statistical hypotheses. This fact should not be surprising because we use all the same ingredients, the difference of the sample means, the standard error of the difference of sample means, and the value of t that corresponds to the biggest α fraction of the possible values defined by the t distribution with ν degrees of freedom.

Given a confidence interval, one cannot say where within the interval the true difference in population means lies. If the confidence interval contains zero, the evidence represented by the experimental observations is not sufficient to rule out the possibility that $\mu_1 - \mu_2 = 0$, that is, that $\mu_1 = \mu_2$, the hypothesis that the t test tests. Hence, we have the following rule:

> *If the 100(1 − a) percent confidence interval associated with a set of data includes zero, there is not sufficient evidence to reject the hypothesis of no effect with P < a. If the confidence interval does not include zero, there is sufficient evidence to reject the hypothesis of no effect with P < a.*

Apply this rule to the two examples just discussed. The 95 percent confidence interval in Fig. 7–1*A* does not include zero, so we can report that the drug produced a statistically significant change in urine production ($P < .05$), just as we did using the t test. The 95 percent confidence interval in Fig. 7–1*B* includes zero, so the random sample (shown in Fig. 6–2) used to compute it does not provide sufficient evidence to reject the hypothesis that the drug has no effect. This, too, is the same conclusion we reached before.

Of the fifty 95 percent confidence intervals shown in Fig. 7–1, twenty-two include zero. Hence 22/50 = 44 percent of these random samples do not permit reporting a difference with 95 percent confidence, i.e., with $P < .05$. If we looked at all possible 95 percent confidence intervals computed for these two populations with two samples of 10 people each, we would find that 44 percent of them include zero, meaning that we would fail to report a true difference, that is, would make a Type II error, 44 percent of the time. Hence, $\beta = .44$, and the power of the test is .56, which is what we found before (compare Fig. 6–4).

The confidence interval approach to hypothesis testing offers two potential advantages. In addition to permitting you to reject the hypothesis of no effect when the interval does not include zero, it also gives information about the size of the effect. Thus, if a result reaches statistical significance more because of a large sample size than because of a large treatment effect, the confidence interval will show it. In other words, it will make it easier to recognize effects that can be detected with confidence but are too small to be of clinical or scientific significance.

For example, suppose we wish to study the potential value of a proposed antihypertensive drug. We select two samples of 100 people each and administer a placebo to one group and the drug to the other. The treated group has a mean diastolic pressure of 81 mmHg and a standard deviation of 11 mmHg; the control (placebo) group has a mean blood pressure of 85 mmHg and a standard deviation of 9 mmHg. Are these data consistent with the hypothesis that the diastolic blood pressure among people taking the drug and placebo were actually no different? To answer this question, we use the data to complete a t test. The pooled-variance estimate is

$$s^2 = \frac{1}{2}(11^2 + 9^2) = 10^2 \text{ mmHg}^2$$

so

$$t = \frac{\overline{X}_{\text{dr}} - \overline{X}_{\text{pla}}}{s_{\overline{X}_{\text{dr}} - \overline{X}_{\text{pla}}}} = \frac{81 - 85}{\sqrt{(10^2/100) + (10^2/100)}} = -2.83$$

This value is more negative than -2.61, the critical value of t that defines the 1 percent most extreme of the t distribution with $\nu = 2(n-1) = 198$ degrees of freedom (from Table 4–1). Thus, we conclude that the drug lowers diastolic blood pressure ($P < .01$).

But is this result clinically significant? To gain a feeling for this, compute the 95 percent confidence interval for the mean difference in diastolic blood pressure for people taking placebo versus the drug. Since $t_{.05}$ for 198 degrees of freedom is (from Table 4–1) 1.973, the confidence interval is

$$-4 - 1.973(1.42) < \mu_{dr} - \mu_{pla} < -4 + 1.973(1.42)$$

$$-6.9 \text{ mmHg} < \mu_{dr} - \mu_{pla} < -1.2 \text{ mmHg}$$

In other words, we can be 95 percent confident that the drug lowers blood pressure between 1.2 and 6.9 mmHg. This is not a very large effect, especially when compared with standard deviations of the blood pressures observed within each of the samples, which are around 10 mmHg. Thus, while the drug does seem to lower blood pressure on the average, examining the confidence interval permitted us to see that the size of the effect is not very impressive. The small value of P was more a reflection of the sample size than the size of the effect on blood pressure.

This example also points up the importance of examining not only the P values reported in a study but also the *size* of the treatment effect compared with the variability within each of the treatment groups. Usually this comparison requires converting the standard errors of the mean reported in the paper to standard deviations by multiplying them by the square root of the sample size. This simple step often shows clinical studies to be of potential interest in illuminating physiological mechanisms but of little value in diagnosing or managing a specific patient because of person-to-person variability.

CONFIDENCE INTERVAL FOR THE POPULATION MEAN

The procedure we developed above can be used to compute a confidence interval for the mean of the population from which a sample was drawn. The resulting confidence interval is the origin of the rule, stated in Chapter 2, that the true (and unobserved) mean of the original population will lie within about 2 standard errors of the mean of the sample mean for 95 percent of all possible samples.

The confidence intervals we computed up to this point are based on the fact that

$$t = \frac{\text{difference of sample means} \; - \text{difference in population means}}{\text{standard error of difference of sample means}}$$

follows the t distribution. It is also possible to show that

$$t = \frac{\text{sample mean} - \text{population mean}}{\text{standard error of mean}}$$

follows the t distribution. The equivalent mathematical statement is

$$t = \frac{\overline{X} - \mu}{s_{\overline{X}}}$$

We can compute the $100(1 - \alpha)$ percent confidence interval for the population mean by obtaining the value of t_α corresponding to $\nu = n - 1$ degrees of freedom, in which n is the sample size. Substitute this value for t in the equation and solve for μ (just as we did for $\mu_1 - \mu_2$ earlier).

$$\overline{X} - t_\alpha s_{\overline{X}} < \mu < \overline{X} + t_\alpha s_{\overline{X}}$$

The interpretation of the confidence interval for the mean is analogous to the interpretation of the confidence interval for the difference of two means: every possible random sample of a given size can be used to compute a, say, 95 percent confidence interval for the population mean, and this same percentage (95 percent) of all such intervals will include the true population mean.

It is common to approximate the 95 percent confidence interval with the sample mean plus or minus twice the standard error of the mean because the values of $t_{.05}$ are approximately 2 for sample sizes above about 20 (see Table 4–1). This approximate rule of thumb does underestimate the size of the confidence interval for the mean, however, especially for the small sample sizes common in biomedical research.

THE SIZE OF THE TREATMENT EFFECT MEASURED AS THE DIFFERENCE OF TWO RATES OR PROPORTIONS

It is easy to generalize the procedures we just developed to permit us to compute confidence intervals for rates and proportions. In Chapter 5 we used the statistic

$$z = \frac{\text{difference of sample proportions}}{\text{standard error of difference of proportions}}$$

to test the hypothesis that the observed proportions of events in two samples were consistent with the hypothesis that the event occurred at the same rate in the two populations. It is possible to show that even when the two populations have different proportions of members with the attribute, the ratio

$$z = \frac{\begin{array}{c}\text{difference of sample proportions}\\ -\ \text{difference of population proportions}\end{array}}{\text{standard error of difference of sample proportions}}$$

is distributed approximately according to the normal distribution so long as the sample sizes are large enough.

If p_1 and p_2 are the actual proportions of members of each of the two populations with the attribute, and if the corresponding estimates computed from the samples are $\hat{p}_1$ and $\hat{p}_2$, respectively,

$$z = \frac{(\hat{p}_1 - \hat{p}_2) - (p_1 - p_2)}{s_{\hat{p}_1 - \hat{p}_2}}$$

We can use this equation to define the $100(1 - \alpha)$ percent confidence interval for the difference in proportions by substituting z_α for z in this equation and solving just as we did before. z_α is the value that defines the most extreme α proportion of the values in the normal distribution;* $z_\alpha = z_{.05} = 1.960$ is commonly used, since it is used to define the 95 percent confidence interval. Thus,

$$(\hat{p}_1 - p_2) - z_\alpha s_{\hat{p}_1 - \hat{p}_2} < p_1 - p_2 < (\hat{p}_1 - p_2) + z_\alpha s_{\hat{p}_1 - \hat{p}_2}$$

for 100(1 − α) percent of all possible samples.

Difference in Mortality Associated with Anesthesia for Open-Heart Surgery

In Chapter 5 we tested the hypothesis that the mortality rates associated with halothane and morphine anesthesia were no different. What is the 95 percent confidence interval for the difference in mortality rate for these two agents?

The mortality rates observed with these two anesthetic agents were 13.1 percent (8 of 61 people) and 14.9 percent (10 of 67 people). Therefore, the difference in observed mortality rates is $\hat{p}_{\text{hlo}} - \hat{p}_{\text{mor}} = 0.131 - 0.15 = -0.020$ and the standard error of the difference, based on a pooled estimate of the proportion of all patients who died is,

$$\hat{p} = \frac{8 + 10}{61 + 67} = .14$$

$$s_{\hat{p}_{\text{hlo}} - \hat{p}_{\text{mor}}} = \sqrt{\hat{p}\,(1 - \hat{p})\left(\frac{1}{n_{\text{hlo}}} + \frac{1}{n_{\text{mor}}}\right)}$$

$$= \sqrt{.14(1 - .14)\left(\frac{1}{61} + \frac{1}{67}\right)} = .062 = 6.2\%$$

*This value can be obtained from a t table, e.g., Table 4–1, by taking the value of t corresponding to an infinite number of degrees of freedom.

Therefore, the 95 percent confidence interval for the difference in mortality rates is

$$(\hat{p}_{\text{hlo}} - \hat{p}_{\text{mor}}) - z_{.05}\, s_{\hat{p}_{\text{hlo}}+\hat{p}_{\text{mor}}} < p_{\text{hlo}} - p_{\text{mor}} < (\hat{p}_{\text{hlo}} - \hat{p}_{\text{mor}}) + z_{.05}\, s_{\hat{p}_{\text{hlo}}+\hat{p}_{\text{mor}}}$$

$$-.020 - 1.960(.062) < p_{\text{hlo}} - p_{\text{mor}} < -.020 + 1.960(.062)$$

$$-.142 < p_{\text{hlo}} - p_{\text{mor}} < .102$$

We can be 95 percent confident that the true difference in mortality rate lies between a 14.2 percent better rate for morphine and a 10.2 percent better rate for halothane.* Since the confidence interval contains zero, there is not sufficient evidence to reject the hypothesis that the two anesthetic agents are associated with the same mortality rate. Furthermore, the confidence interval ranges about equally on both sides of zero, so there is not even a suggestion that one agent is superior to the other.

Difference in Thrombosis with Aspirin in People Receiving Hemodialysis

Chapter 5 also discussed the evidence that administering low-dose aspirin to people receiving regular kidney dialysis reduces the proportion of people who develop thrombosis. Of the people taking the placebo, 72 percent developed thrombosis, as did 32 percent of the people taking aspirin. Given only this information, we would report that aspirin reduced the proportion of patients who developed thrombosis by 40 percent. What is the 95 percent confidence interval for the improvement?

The standard error of the difference in the proportion of patients who developed thrombosis is .15 (from Chapter 5). So the 95 percent confidence interval for the true difference in proportion of patients who developed thrombosis is

$$.40 - 1.96(.15) < p_{\text{pla}} - p_{\text{asp}} < .40 + 1.96(.15)$$

$$.11 < p_{\text{pla}} - p_{\text{asp}} < .69$$

*To include the Yates correction, widen the upper and lower bounds of the confidence interval by $1/2(1/n_{\text{hlo}} + 1/n_{\text{mor}})$.

We can be 95 percent confident that aspirin reduces the rate of thrombosis somewhere between 11 and 69 percent compared with placebo.

How Negative Is a "Negative" Clinical Trial?

Chapter 6 discussed the study of 71 randomized clinical trials that did not demonstrate a statistically significant improvement in clinical outcome (mortality, complications, or the number of patients who showed no improvement, depending on the study). Most of these trials involved too few patients to have sufficient power to be confident that the failure to detect a treatment effect was not due to an inadequate sample size. To get a feeling for how compatible the data are with the hypothesis of no treatment effect, let us examine the 90 percent confidence intervals for the proportion of "successful" cases (the definition of success varied with the study) for all 71 trials. Figure 7–3 shows these confidence intervals.

All the confidence intervals include zero, so we cannot rule out the possibility that the treatments had no effect. Note, however, that some of the trials are also compatible with the possibility that the treatments produced sizable improvements in the success rate. Remember that while we can be 90 percent confident that the true change in proportion of successes lies in the interval, it could be anywhere. Does this prove that some of these treatments improved clinical outcome? No. The important point is that the confidence with which we can assert that there was no treatment effect is often the same as the confidence with which we can assert that the treatment produced a sizable improvement. While the size and location of the confidence interval cannot be used as part of a formal statistical argument to prove that the treatment had an effect, it certainly can help you look for trends in the data.

Meta-analysis

While the ideal solution to avoiding the problem we have been discussing would be to do large, well-powered studies that would yield estimates of the size of the effect that was studied along with a narrow confidence interval, the unfortunate fact remains that doing so is not always possible, either because of practical limitations

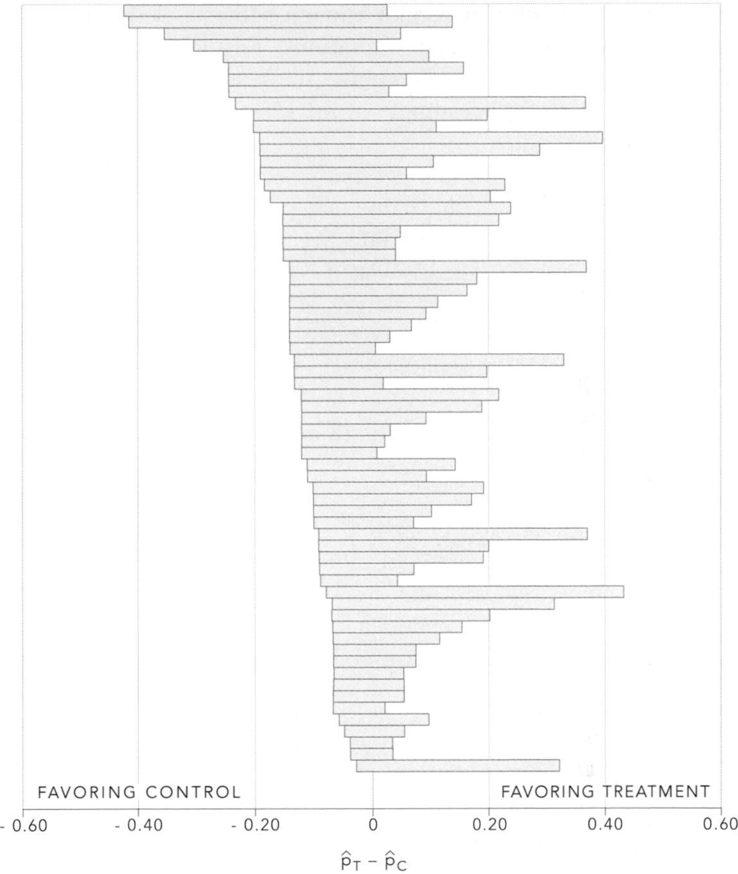

Figure 7–3 The 90 percent confidence intervals for 71 negative clinical trials. Since all the intervals contain zero, there is not sufficient evidence that the success rate is different for the treatment and control groups. Nevertheless, the data are also compatible with the treatment producing a substantial improvement in success rate in many of the trials. While this study was done in 1978, based on clinical trials conducted before then, the problem of drawing negative conclusions based on underpowered clinical trials persists in the 21st century. *(Data from Fig. 2 of J. A. Freiman, T. C. Chalmers, H. Smith, Jr., and R. R. Keubler, "The Importance of Beta, the Type II Error and Sample Size in the Design and Interpretation of the Randomized Control Trial: Survey of 71 'Negative' Trials,"* N. Engl. J. Med., ***299:****690–694, 1978.)*

(such as not being able to recruit enough subjects at the institution doing the study) or financial limitations. Fortunately, there is an approach that permits you to combine the results of several similar studies to obtain a single estimate of the effect that integrates all the available information.

This approach, known as *meta-analysis,* is essentially a procedure for pooling the results of the individual studies as if they were one much larger study.* Because the effective sample size is increased by combining all the studies, the associated confidence interval is narrower and the power of the combined analysis is increased. These two effects create a situation in which you can be more confident of both positive and negative conclusions than is possible when considering each individual study separately.

Figure 7–4 shows the results of 18 different studies of the relative risk of developing heart disease associated with being regularly exposed to secondhand tobacco smoke (defined as a nonsmoker living or working with a smoker) compared with people not exposed. Each line on the top part of Figure 7–4 represents the results of one of the studies. The points represent the observed risk in each study and the lines span the 95 percent confidence interval associated with each study. Not surprisingly, there is variability in the estimates of the effect sizes from study to study (because of the random sampling process inherent in making estimates from any sample). Several of the confidence intervals exclude a relative risk of 1.0, meaning that those studies found a statistically significant elevation in heart disease risk associated with secondhand smoke exposure. At the same time, several of the studies yielded confidence intervals including 1.0, meaning that you could not conclude that secondhand smoke increased the risk of heart disease based on those individual studies taken alone. Note also that many of the studies had wide confidence intervals associated with them, because of small sample sizes.

The estimate at the bottom of Figure 7–4 shows the results of combining all the individual studies with a meta-analysis. While

*The calculations involved in—and limitations of—meta-analysis are beyond the scope of this book. For a discussion of how to conduct a meta-analysis, see Diana B. Petitti, *Meta-analysis, Decision Analysis, and Cost-effectiveness Analysis: Methods for Quantitative Synthesis in Medicine,* 2nd ed. New York: Oxford University Press, 2000.

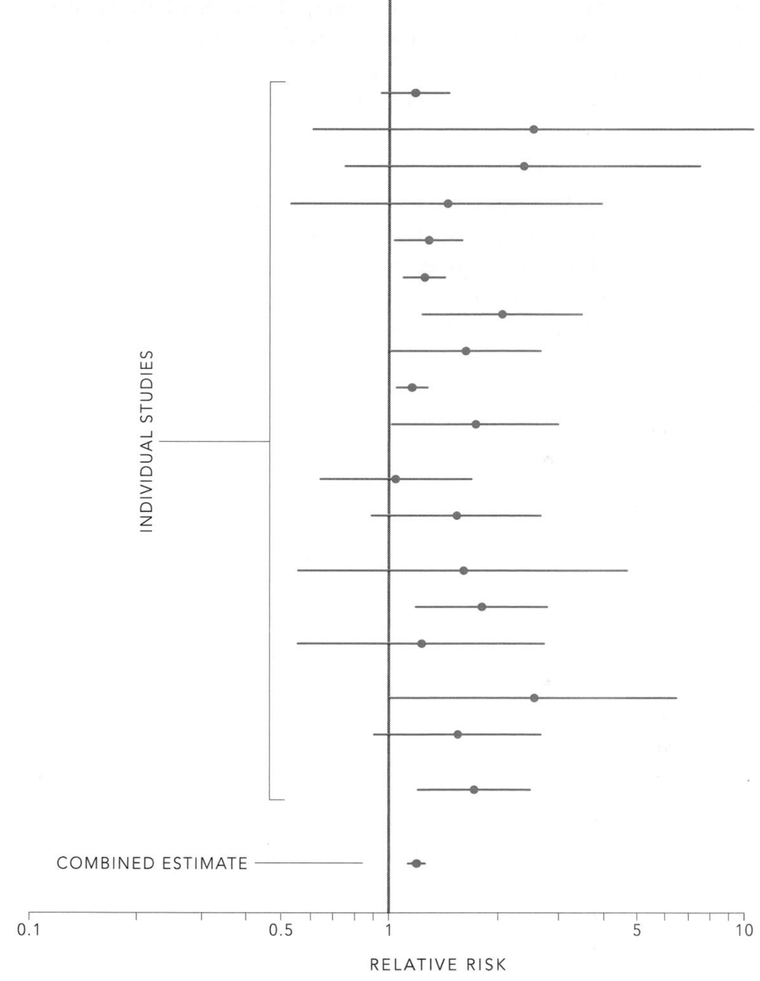

Figure 7–4 A meta-analysis of 18 studies of the relative risk of developing heart disease when exposed to secondhand smoke yields a single estimate of the risk with a much narrower confidence interval than any of the individual studies. This more precise estimate of the risk is obtained because the combined risk estimate uses information from all 18 studies, and so has a much larger effective sample size than the individual studies do. *(Adapted from J. He, S. Vupputuri, K. Allen, M. R. Prerost, J. Hughes, and P. K. Whelton, "Passive Smoking and the Risk of Coronary Heart Disease—A Meta-Analysis of Epidemiologic Studies,"* N. Engl. J. Med. ***340:****920–926, 1999. Used by permission.)*

only some of the 18 individual studies of the risk of heart disease associated with breathing secondhand smoke were large enough to reach conventional statistical significance (at the .05 level), the combined estimate of a relative risk of 1.25 and the narrow confidence interval (from 1.17 to 1.25) means that we can have a high level of confidence in concluding that there is an increased risk of heart disease in people regularly exposed to secondhand smoke. Because this estimate is based on all the data from all 18 studies, the effective sample size is substantially greater than any of the individual studies, which is the reason that the 95 percent confidence interval for the combined estimate of the effect size is so much narrower than for the individual studies.

While not perfect, meta-analysis has become an important tool for combining information from several related studies and dealing with the problem that individual studies lack adequate power to provide high confidence in drawing negative conclusions.

CONFIDENCE INTERVAL FOR RATES AND PROPORTIONS

It is possible to use the normal distribution to compute approximate confidence intervals for proportions from observations, so long as the sample size is large enough to make the approximation reasonably accurate.* When it is not possible to use this approximation, we will compute the exact confidence intervals based on the binomial distribution. While we will not go into the computational details of this procedure, we will present the necessary results in graphical form because papers often present results based on small numbers of subjects. Examining the confidence intervals as opposed to only the observed proportion of patients with a given attribute is especially useful in thinking about such studies, because a change of *a single patient* from one group to the other often makes a large difference in the observed proportion of patients with the attribute of interest.

*As discussed in Chapter 5, $n\hat{p}$ and $n(1-\hat{p})$ must both exceed about 5, where $\hat{p}$ is the proportion of the observed sample having the attribute of interest.

Just as there was an analogous way to use the t distribution to relate the difference of means and the confidence interval for a single sample mean, it is possible to show that if the sample size is large enough

$$z = \frac{\text{observed proportion} - \text{true proportion}}{\text{standard error of proportion}}$$

In other words

$$z = \frac{\hat{p} - p}{s_{\hat{p}}}$$

approximately follows the normal distribution (in Table 6–4). Hence, we can use this equation to define the $100(1 - \alpha)$ percent confidence interval for the true proportion p with

$$\hat{p} - z_{\alpha}\, s_{\hat{p}} < p < \hat{p} + z_{\alpha}\, s_{\hat{p}}$$

Quality of Evidence Used as a Basis for Interventions to Improve Hospital Antibiotic Prescribing

Despite many efforts to control antibiotic usage and promote optimal prescribing, practitioners continue to prescribe inappropriately, which contributes not only to increased medical costs but also to the development of antibiotic-resistant bacteria. In 1999, the British Society for Antimicrobial Chemotherapy and Hospital Infection Society convened a Working Party to address the problem of antibiotic prescribing in hospitals.* They did an exhaustive literature search and located 306 papers dealing with recommendations for antibiotic use. They then applied the quality criteria of the Cochrane Collaboration, an international effort that promotes high quality systematic reviews of the literature, and found that 91 of the papers met the minimum criteria for inclusion in a Cochrane review. What is the 95 percent confidence interval for the fraction of articles that met this quality criteria?

*C. Ramsay, E. Brown, G. Hartman, and P. Davey, "Room for Improvement: A Systematic Review of the Quality of Evaluations to Improve Hospital Antibiotic Prescribing," *J. Antimicrob. Chemother.* **52:**764–771, 2003.

The proportion of acceptable articles is $\hat{p} = 91/306 = .297$ and the standard error of the proportion is

$$s_{\hat{p}} = \sqrt{\frac{.297(1 - .297)}{306}} = .026$$

Therefore, the 95 confidence interval for the proportion of acceptable articles is

$$.297 - 1.960(.026) < \text{p} < .297 + 1.960(.026)$$
$$.246 < \text{p} < .348$$

In other words, based on this sample, we can be 95 percent confident that the true proportion of papers on antibiotic prescribing guidelines that met the Cochrane criteria was between 26 percent and 35 percent.

Exact Confidence Intervals for Rates and Proportions

When the sample size or observed proportion is too small for the approximate confidence interval based on the normal distribution to be reliable, you have to compute the confidence interval based on the exact theoretical distribution of a proportion, the *binomial distribution.** Since results based on small sample sizes with low observed rates of events turn up frequently in the medical literature, we present the results of computation of confidence intervals using the binomial distribution.

To illustrate how the procedure we followed above can fall apart when $n\hat{p}$ is below about 5, we consider an example. Suppose a surgeon says that he has done 30 operations without a single complication. His observed complication rate $\hat{p}$ is $0/30 = 0$ percent for the 30 specific patients he operated on. Impressive as this is, it is unlikely that the surgeon will continue operating forever without a complication, so the fact that $\hat{p} = 0$ probably reflects good luck in the randomly selected patients who happened to be operated on during the period in question.

*The reason we could use the normal distribution here and in Chapter 5 is that for large enough sample sizes there is little difference between the binomial and normal distributions. This result is a consequence of the central-limit theorem, discussed in Chapter 2.

To obtain a better estimate of p, the surgeon's true complication rate, we will compute the 95 percent confidence interval for p.

Let us try to apply our existing procedure. Since $\hat{p} = 0$,

$$s_{\hat{p}} = \sqrt{\frac{\hat{p}(1 - \hat{p})}{n}} = \sqrt{\frac{0(1 - 0)}{30}} = 0$$

and the 95 percent confidence interval is from zero to zero. This result does not make sense. There is no way that a surgeon can *never* have a complication. Obviously, the approximation breaks down.

Figure 7–5 gives a graphical presentation of the 95 percent confidence intervals for proportions. The upper and lower limits are read off the vertical axis using the pair of curves corresponding to the size of the sample n used to estimate $\hat{p}$ at the point on the horizontal axis corresponding to the observed $\hat{p}$. For our surgeon, $\hat{p} = 0$ and $n = 30$, so the 95 percent confidence interval for his true complication rate is from 0 to .10. In other words, we can be 95 percent confident that his true complication rate, based on the 30 cases we happened to observe, is somewhere between 0 and 10 percent.

Now, suppose the surgeon had a single complication. Then $\hat{p} = 1/30 = 0.033$ and

$$s_{\hat{p}} = \sqrt{.033(1 - .033)/30} = .033$$

so the 95 percent confidence interval for the true complication rate, computed using the approximate method, is

$$.33 - 1.96(.033) < p < .33 + 1.96(.033)$$
$$-.032 < p < .098$$

Think about this result for a moment. There is no way a surgeon can have a *negative* complication rate.

Figure 7–5 gives the exact confidence interval, from 0 to .13, or 0 to 13 percent.* This confidence interval is not too different from that

*When there are no "failures" observed, the approximate upper end of the 95% confidence interval for the true failure rate is approximately $3/n$, where n is the sample size. For a more extensive discussion of interpreting results when there are no "failures," see J. A. Hanley and A. Lippman-Hand, "If Nothing Goes Wrong, Is Everything All Right? Interpreting Zero Numerators," *JAMA* **249:**1743–1745, 1983.

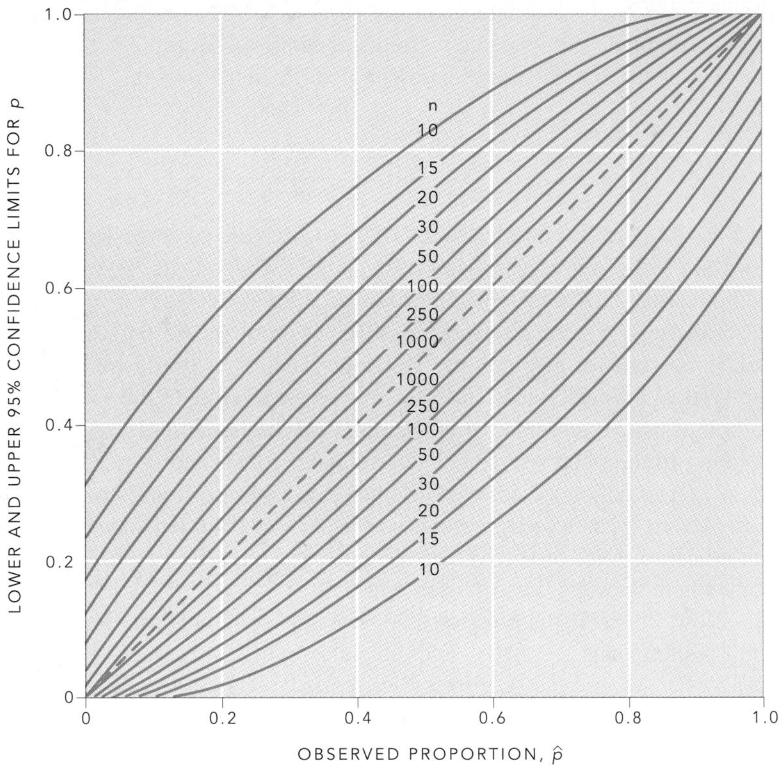

Figure 7–5 Graphical presentation of the exact 95 percent confidence intervals (based on the binomial distribution) for the population proportion. You read this plot by reading the two limits of the lines defined by the sample size at the point on the horizontal axis at the proportion of the sample with the attribute of interest $\hat{p}$. *(Adapted from C. J. Clopper and E. S. Pearson, "The Use of Confidence or Fiducial Limits Illustrated in the Case of the Binomial,"* Biometrika, ***26:****404, 1934.)*

computed when there were no complications, as it should be, since there is little real difference between not having any complications and having only one complication in such a small sample.

Notice how important sample size is, especially for small sample sizes. Had the surgeon been bragging that he had a zero complication rate on the basis of only 10 cases, the 95 percent confidence interval for his true complication rate would have extended from zero all the way to 33 percent!

CONFIDENCE INTERVALS FOR RELATIVE RISK AND ODDS RATIO*

Because the relative risk and odds ratio are ratios, the distributions of the values of these statistics are not normally distributed. It turns out, however, that the logarithm of these ratios is normally distributed. Therefore, we can use approaches similar to those used with proportions to the logarithms of the relative risk and odds ratio, then invert the results to return to the original scale. By convention, statisticians and epidemiologists use the natural logarithm for these calculations.† Using the notation in Table 5–14, the natural logarithm of the relative risk, ln RR, is normally distributed with standard error

$$s_{\ln \mathrm{RR}} = \sqrt{\frac{1 - a/(a+b)}{a} + \frac{1 - c/(c+d)}{c}}$$

Therefore, the $100(1 - \alpha)$ percent confidence interval for the natural logarithm of the true population $\ln \mathrm{RR}_{\text{true}}$ is

$$\ln \mathrm{RR} - z_\alpha\, s_{\ln \mathrm{RR}} < \ln \mathrm{RR}_{\text{true}} < \ln \mathrm{RR} + z_\alpha\, s_{\ln \mathrm{RR}}$$

We convert these estimates back to the original units by applying the exponential function to the terms in this equation to obtain

$$e^{\ln \mathrm{RR} - z_\alpha s_{\ln \mathrm{RR}}} < \mathrm{RR}_{\text{true}} < e^{\ln \mathrm{RR} + z_\alpha s_{\ln \mathrm{RR}}}$$

Thus, you could test the null hypothesis that the true RR = 1, that the treatment (or risk factor) had no effect, by computing this confidence interval and seeing if it included 1.0.

Likewise, the natural logarithm of the odds ratio, OR, is normally distributed. Using the notation in Table 5–15, the standard error is

$$s_{\ln \mathrm{OR}} = \sqrt{\frac{1}{a} + \frac{1}{b} + \frac{1}{c} + \frac{1}{d}}$$

*In an introductory course, this section can be skipped without any loss of continuity.

†The natural logarithm has the base $e = 2.71828\ldots$ rather than 10, which is the base of the common logarithm. Because e is the base, the natural logarithm and exponential functions are *inverses,* i.e., $e^{\ln x} = x$ and $\ln e^x = x$.

and the $100(1 - \alpha)$ percent confidence interval for the true odds ratio is

$$e^{\ln \mathrm{OR} - z_\alpha s_{\ln \mathrm{OR}}} < \mathrm{OR}_{\mathrm{true}} < e^{\ln \mathrm{OR} + z_\alpha s_{\ln \mathrm{OR}}}$$

This confidence interval can also be used to test the null hypothesis that the true OR = 1, that exposure to the risk factor is not associated with an increase in the odds of having the disease.

Difference in Thrombosis with Aspirin in People Receiving Hemodialysis

Earlier in this chapter we saw how to use a confidence interval to test the null hypothesis that there was no difference in the probability of thrombosis in people receiving aspirin or a placebo. We can also test this hypothesis by examining the relative risk of thrombosis in this clinical trial. In Chapter 5, we estimated that the relative risk of a thrombosis was .44 in people receiving aspirin compared to people receiving a placebo. Using the data in Table 5–1, which shows that $a = 6$, $b = 13$, $c = 18$, and $d = 7$, we estimate the standard error of ln RR as

$$s_{\ln \mathrm{RR}} = \sqrt{\frac{1 - 6/(6 + 13)}{6} + \frac{1 - 18/(18 + 7)}{18}} = .360$$

To estimate the 95 percent confidence interval, we note that $z_{.05} = 1.960$ and compute

$$e^{\ln .44 - 1.960 \times .360} < \mathrm{RR}_{\mathrm{true}} < e^{\ln .44 - 1.960 \times .360}$$

$$e^{-1.527} < \mathrm{RR}_{\mathrm{true}} < e^{-.115}$$

$$.22 < \mathrm{RR}_{\mathrm{true}} < .89$$

Hence, we can be 95 percent confident that the true relative risk of thrombosis for people taking aspirin compared with placebo is somewhere between .22 and .89. Because this range does not include 1, we conclude that aspirin significantly changes the risk of thrombosis, and prevents thrombosis.

Passive Smoking and Breast Cancer

We can compute the confidence interval for the odds ratio of a premenopausal woman who is exposed to secondhand smoke developing breast cancer using the data in Table 5–16. To compute the 95 percent confidence interval for this odds ratio, we note that the observed odds ratio is 2.91 and, from Table 5–16, $a = 50$, $b = 14$, $c = 43$, and $d = 35$. Therefore,

$$s_{\ln \mathrm{OR}} = \sqrt{\frac{1}{50} + \frac{1}{14} + \frac{1}{43} + \frac{1}{35}} = .378$$

and, so,

$$e^{\ln 2.91 - 1.960 \times .378} < \mathrm{OR}_{\mathrm{true}} < e^{\ln 2.91 - 1.960 \times .378}$$

$$e^{.327} < \mathrm{OR}_{\mathrm{true}} < e^{1.809}$$

$$1.39 < \mathrm{OR}_{\mathrm{true}} < 6.10$$

Thus, we can be 95 percent confident that the true odds ratio is somewhere between 1.39 and 6.10. Because the 95 percent confidence interval for the true relative risk excludes 1, we conclude that passive smoking significantly increases the odds of breast cancer in premenopausal women.

CONFIDENCE INTERVAL FOR THE ENTIRE POPULATION*

So far computed intervals that we can have a high degree of confidence in will include a *population parameter,* such as μ or p. It is often desirable to determine a confidence interval for the *population itself,* most commonly when defining the normal range of some variable. The most common approach is to take the range defined by 2 standard deviations about the sample mean on the grounds that this interval

*Confidence intervals for the population are also called *tolerance limits*. The procedures derived in this section are appropriate for analyzing data obtained from a population that is normally distributed. If the population follows other distributions, there are alternate procedures for computing confidence intervals for the population.

contains 95 percent of the members of a population that follows the normal distribution (Fig. 2–5). In fact, in carefully worded language Chapter 2 suggested this rule. When the sample used to compute the mean and standard deviation is large (more than 100 to 200 members), this common rule of thumb is reasonably accurate. Unfortunately, most clinical studies are based on much smaller samples (of the order of 5 to 20 individuals). With such small samples, use of this two standard deviations rule of thumb seriously underestimates the range of values likely to be included in the population from which the samples were drawn.

For example, Fig. 2–8 showed the population of the heights of all 200 Martians, together with the results of three random samples of 10 Martians each. Figure 2–8*A* showed that 95 percent of all Martians have heights between 31 and 49 cm. The mean and standard deviation of the heights of population of all 200 Martians are 40 and 5 cm, respectively. The three samples illustrated in Fig. 2–8 yield estimates of the mean of 41.5, 36, and 40 cm, and of the standard deviation of 3.8, 5, and 5 cm, respectively. Suppose we simply compute the range defined by two *sample* standard deviations above and below the *sample* mean with the expectation that this range will include 95 percent of the population. Figure 7–6*A* shows the results of this computation for each of the three samples in Fig. 2–8. The light area defines the range of actual heights that covers 95 percent of the Martians' heights. Two of the three samples yield intervals that do not include 95 percent of the population.

This problem arises because both the sample mean and standard deviation are only *estimates* of the population mean and standard deviation and so cannot be used interchangeably with the population mean and standard deviation when computing the range of population values. To see why, consider the sample in Fig. 2–8*B* that yielded estimates of the mean and standard deviation of 36 and 5 cm, respectively. By good fortune, the estimate of the standard deviation computed from the sample equaled the population standard deviation. The estimate of the population mean, however, was low. As a result, the interval 2 standard deviations above and below the sample mean did not reach high enough to cover 95 percent of the entire population values. Because of the potential errors in the estimates of the population mean and standard deviation, we must be conservative and use a range greater than

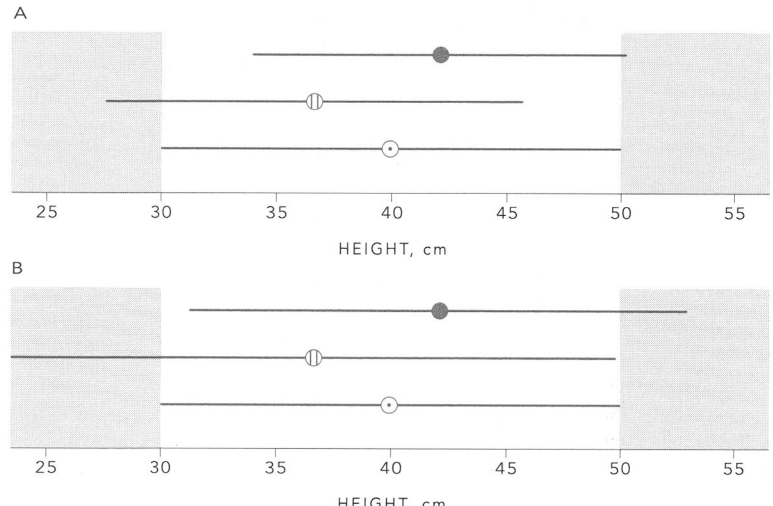

Figure 7-6 ***(A)*** The range defined by the sample mean ±2 standard deviations for the three samples of 10 Martians each shown in Fig. 2-8. Two of the three resulting ranges do *not* cover the entire range that includes 95 percent of the population members (indicated by the white area). ***(B)*** The 95 percent confidence intervals for the population, computed as the sample mean $\pm K_{.05}$ times the sample standard deviation covers the actual range that includes 95 percent of the actual population; 95 percent of all such intervals will cover 95 percent of the actual population range.

2 standard deviations around the sample mean to be sure of including, say, 95 percent of the entire population. However, as the size of the sample used to estimate the mean and standard deviation increases, the certainty with which we can use these estimates to compute the range spanned by the entire population increases, so we do not have to be as conservative (i.e., take fewer multiples of the sample standard deviation) when computing an interval that contains a specified proportion of the population members.

Specifying the confidence interval for the entire population is more involved than specifying the confidence intervals we have discussed so far because you must specify both the *fraction of the population* if you wish the interval to cover and the *confidence you wish to have that any given interval will cover it.* The size of the interval depends on these two things and the size of the sample used to estimate the mean and

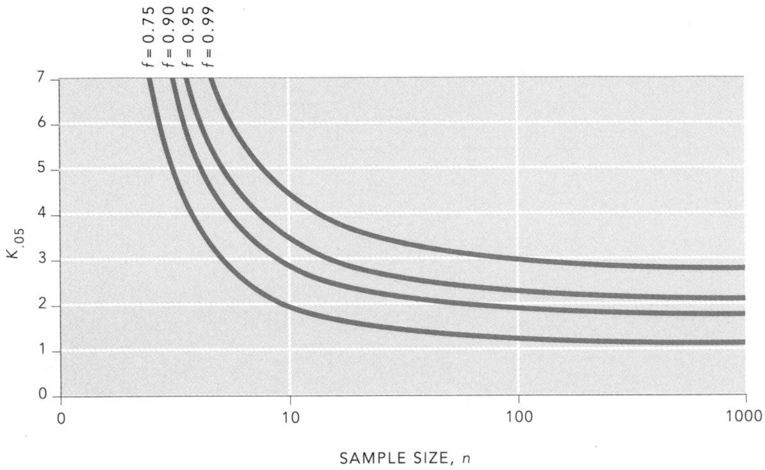

Figure 7–7 $K_{.05}$ depends on the size of the sample n used to estimate the mean and standard deviation and the fraction f of the population you want the interval to include.

standard deviation. The $100(1 - \alpha)$ percent confidence interval for $100f$ percent of the population is

$$\overline{X} - K_\alpha s < X < \overline{X} + K_\alpha s$$

in which $\overline{X}$ and s are the sample mean and standard deviation and K_α is the number of sample standard deviations about the sample mean needed to cover the desired part of the population. Figure 7–7 shows $K_{.05}$ as a function of sample size for various values of f. It plays a role similar to t_α or z_α.

K_α is larger than t_α (which is larger than z_α) because it accounts for uncertainty in the estimates of both the mean *and* standard deviation, rather than the mean alone.*

*For a derivation of K_α that clearly shows how it is related to the confidence limits for the mean and standard deviation, see A. E. Lewis, *Biostatistics*, Reinhold, New York, 1966, chapter 12, "Tolerance Limits and Indices of Discrimination."

Notice that K_α can be much larger than 2 for sample sizes in the range of 5 to 25, which are common in biomedical research. Thus, simply taking 2 standard deviations about the mean may substantially underestimate the range of the population from which the samples were drawn. Figure 7–6*B* shows the 95 percent confidence interval for 95 percent of the population of Martians' heights based on the three samples of 10 Martians each shown in Fig. 2–8. All three of the intervals include 95 percent of the population.

As Chapter 2 discussed, many people confuse the standard error of the mean with the standard deviation and consider the range defined by "sample mean ± 2 standard errors of the mean" to encompass about 95 percent of the population. This error leads them to seriously underestimate the possible range of values in the population from which the sample was drawn. We have seen that, for the relatively small sample sizes common in biomedical research, applying the 2 standard deviations rule may underestimate the range of values in the underlying population as well.

PROBLEMS

7-1 Find the 90 and 95 percent confidence intervals for the mean levels of polychlorinated biphenyl (PCB) levels in Prob. 2-3.

7-2 Find the 95 percent confidence interval for the difference in mean adenosine triphosphate (ATP) production per gram in the two groups of children in Prob. 3-1. Based on this confidence interval is the difference significant with $P < .05$?

7-3 Find the 95 percent confidence intervals for the proportions of adverse outcomes as well as the 95 percent confidence interval for the difference in rates of adverse outcomes in Prob. 5-1. Compare this result with the hypothesis test in Prob. 5-1.

7-4 Find the 95 percent confidence intervals for the mean forced midexpiratory flows for the different test groups in Prob. 3-2. Use this information to identify people with different or similar lung function (as we did with Bonferroni *t* tests in Chapter 4).

7-5 Find the 95 percent confidence intervals for the percentage of articles that reported the results of research based on data collected before deciding on the question to be investigated. Use the data in Prob. 5-6.

7-6 Use the data in Prob. 2-3 to find the 95 percent confidence interval for 90 and 95 percent of the population of PCB concentrations in Japanese adults. Plot these intervals together with the observations.

7-7 Rework Prob. 5-11 using confidence intervals.

7-8 Rework Prob. 5-12 using confidence intervals.

7-9 Rework Prob. 5-13 using confidence intervals.

7-10 Rework Prob. 5-14 using confidence intervals.

Chapter 8

How to Test for Trends

The first statistical problem we posed in this book, in connection with Fig. 1–2*A*, dealt with a drug that was thought to be a diuretic, but that experiment cannot be analyzed using our existing procedures. In it, we selected different people and gave them different doses of the diuretic, then measured their urine output. The people who received larger doses produced more urine. The statistical question is whether the resulting pattern of points relating urine production to drug dose provided sufficient evidence to conclude that the drug increased urine production in proportion to drug dose. This chapter develops the tools for analyzing such experiments. We will estimate how much one variable increases (or decreases) on the average as another variable changes with a *regression line* and quantifies the *strength* of the association with *a correlation coefficient.**

*Simple linear regression is a special case of the more general method of *multiple regression* in which case there are multiple independent variables. For a discussion of multiple regression and related procedures written in the same style as this book, see S. A. Glantz and B. K. Slinker, *Primer of Applied Regression and Analysis of Variance,* (2nd ed). McGraw-Hill, New York, 2001.

MORE ABOUT THE MARTIANS

As in all other statistical procedures, we want to use a sample drawn at random from a population to make statements about the population. Chapters 3 and 4 discussed populations whose members are normally distributed with mean μ and standard deviation σ and used estimates of these parameters to design test statistics (like F and t) that permitted us to examine whether or not some *discrete* treatment was likely to have affected the mean value of a variable of interest. Now, we add another parametric procedure, *linear regression,* to analyze experiments in which the samples were drawn from populations characterized by a mean response varying *continuously* with the size of the treatment. To understand the nature of this population and the associated random samples, we return again to Mars, where we can examine the entire population of 200 Martians.

Figure 2–1 showed that the heights of Martians are normally distributed with a mean of 40 cm and a standard deviation of 5 cm. In addition to measuring the heights of each Martian, let us also weigh each one. Figure 8–1 shows a plot in which each point represents the height x and weight y of one Martian. Since we have observed the *entire population,* there is no question that tall Martians tend to be heavier than short Martians.

There are a number of things we can conclude about the heights and weights of Martians as well as the relationship between these two variables. As noted in Chapter 2, the heights are normally distributed with mean $\mu = 40$ cm and standard deviation $\sigma = 5$ cm. The weights are also normally distributed with mean $\mu = 12$ g and standard deviation $\sigma = 2.5$ g. The most striking feature of Fig. 8–1, however, is that the *mean weight of Martians at each height* increases as height increases.

For example, the Martians who are 32 cm tall weigh 7.1, 7.9, 8.3, and 8.8 g, so the mean weight of Martians who are 32 cm tall is 8 g. The 8 Martians who are 46 cm tall weigh 13.7, 14.5, 14.8, 15.0, 15.1, 15.2, 15.3, and 15.8 g, so the mean weight of Martians who are 46 cm tall is 15 g. Figure 8–2 shows that the mean weight of Martians at each height increases *linearly* as height increases.

This line does not make it possible, however, to predict the weight of *an individual* Martian if you know his or her height. Why not? There is

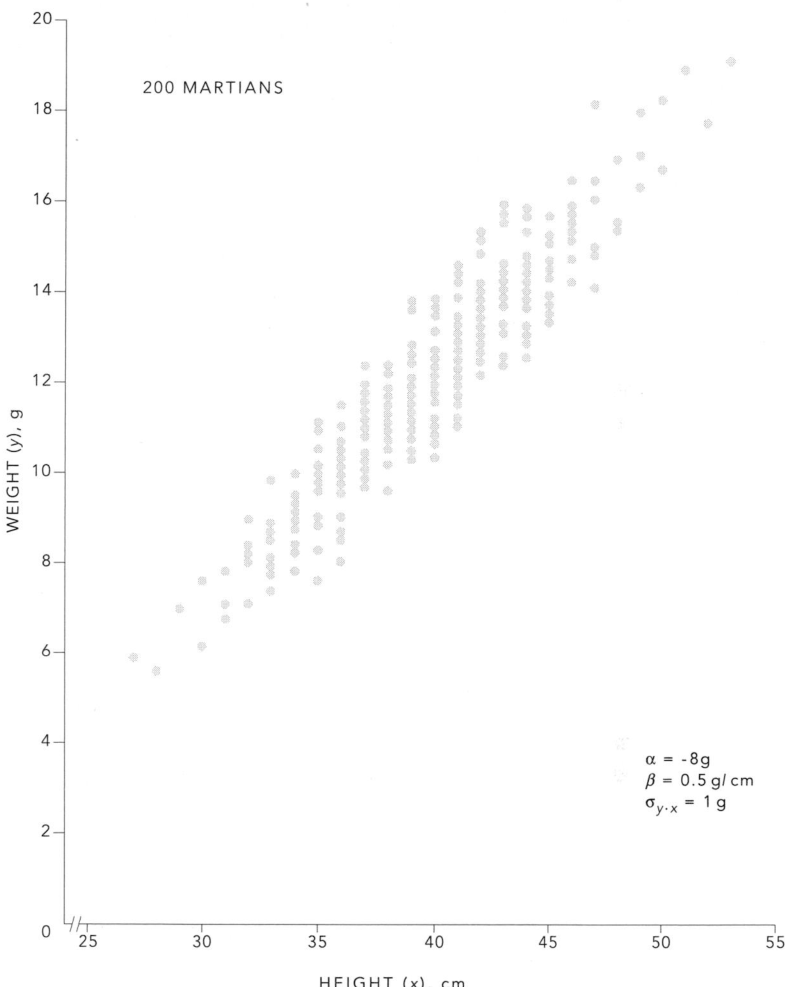

Figure 8–1 The relationship between height and weight in the population of 200 Martians, with each Martian represented by a circle. The weights at any given height follow a normal distribution. In addition, the mean weight of Martians at any given height increases linearly with height, and the variability in weight at any given height is the same regardless of height. A population must have these characteristics to be suitable for linear regression or correlation analysis.

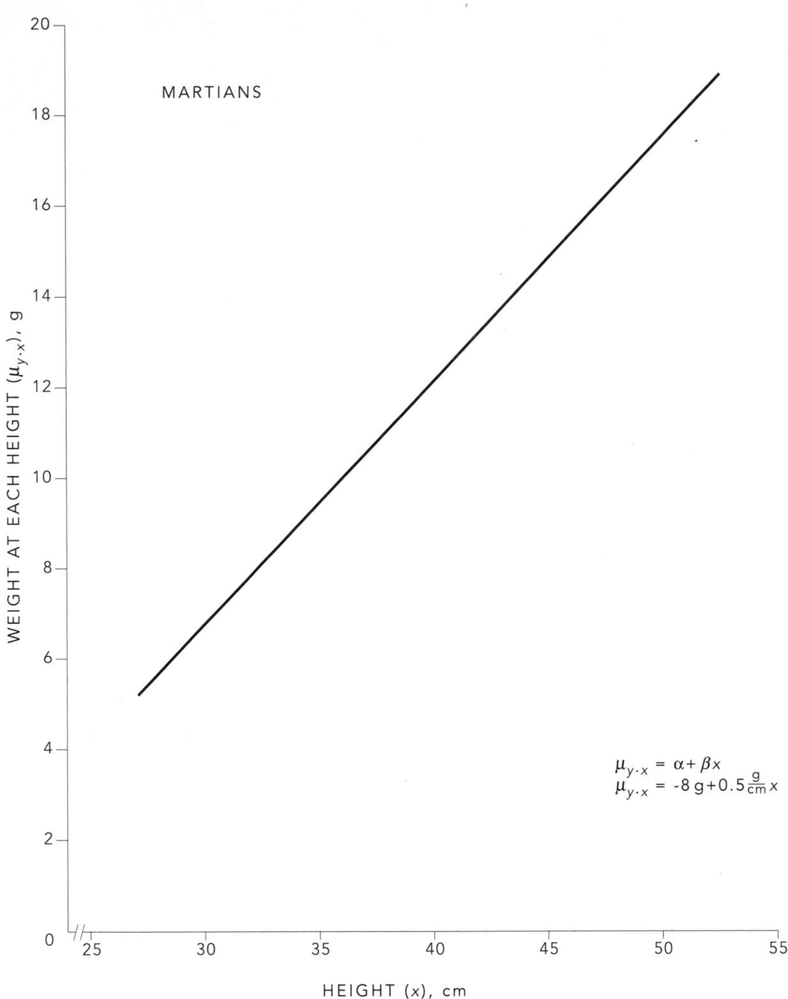

Figure 8–2 The line of means for the population of Martians in Fig. 8–1.

variability in weights among Martians at each height. Figure 8–1 reveals that standard deviation of weights of Martians with *any given height* is about 1 g. We need to distinguish this standard deviation from the standard deviation of weights of *all* Martians computed without regard for the fact that mean weight varies with height.

The Population Parameters

Now, let us define some new terms and symbols so that we can generalize from Martians to other populations with similar characteristics. Since we are considering how weight varies with height, call height the *independent variable* x and weight the *dependent variable* y. In some instances, including the example at hand, we can only *observe* the independent variable and use it to *predict* the expected mean value of the dependent variable. (There is variability in the dependent variable at each value of the independent variable). In other cases, including controlled experiments, it is possible to *manipulate* the independent variable to control, with some uncertainty, the value of the dependent variable. In the first case, it is only possible to identify an *association* between the two variables, whereas in the second case it is possible to conclude that there is a *causal* link.*

For any given value of the independent variable x, it is possible to compute the value of the mean of all values of the dependent variable corresponding to that value of x. We denote this mean $\mu_{y \cdot x}$ to indicate that it is the mean of all the values of y in the population at a given value of x. These means fall along a straight line given by

$$\mu_{y \cdot x} = \alpha + \beta x$$

in which α is the intercept and β is the slope† of the *line of means*. For example, Fig. 8–2 shows that, on the average, the average weight of

*In an observational study, statistical analysis alone only permits identification of an association. In order to identify a causal relationship, one generally requires independent evidence to explain the biological (or other) mechanisms that give rise to the observed association. For example, the fact that several epidemiological studies demonstrated an association between passive smoking and heart disease combined with laboratory studies showing short-term effects of secondhand smoke and secondhand smoke constituents on the heart, led to the conclusion that passive smoking *causes* heart disease. For details on how a variety of such evidence is combined to use observational studies as *part* of the case for a causal relationship, see S. A. Glantz and W. W. Parmley, "Passive Smoking and Heart Disease: Epidemiology, Physiology, and Biochemistry," *Circulation,* **83:**1–12, 1991. Also S. A. Glantz and W. W. Parmley, "Passive Smoking and Heart Disease: Mechanisms and Risk," *JAMA* **273:**1047–1053, 1995.

†It is, unfortunately, statistical convention to use α and β in this way even though the same two Greek letters also denote the size of the Type I and Type II errors in hypothesis testing. The meaning of α should be clear from the context. β always refers to the slope of the line of means in this chapter.

Martians increases by 0.5 g for every 1-cm increase in height, so the slope β of the $\mu_{y \cdot x}$ versus-x line is 0.5 g/cm. The intercept α of this line is -8 g. Hence,

$$\mu_{y \cdot x} = -8 \text{ g} + (0.5 \text{ g/cm})x$$

There is variability about the line of means. For any given value of the independent variable x, the values of y for the population are normally distributed with mean $\mu_{y \cdot x}$ and standard deviation $\sigma_{y \cdot x}$. This notation indicates that $\sigma_{y \cdot x}$ is the standard deviation of weights (y) computed after allowing for the fact that mean weight varies with height (x). As noted above, the residual variation about the line of means for our Martians is 1 g; $\sigma_{y \cdot x} = 1$ g. The amount of this variability is an important factor in determining how useful the line of means is for predicting the value of the dependent variable, for example, weight, when you know the value of the independent variable, for example, height. The methods we develop below require that this standard deviation be *the same* for all values of x. In other words, the variability of the dependent variable about the line of means is the same regardless of the value of the independent variable.

In sum, we will be analyzing the results of experiments in which the observations were drawn from populations with these characteristics:

- *The mean of the population of the dependent variable at a given value of the independent variable increases (or decreases) linearly as the independent variable increases.*
- *For any given value of the independent variable, the possible values of the dependent variable are distributed normally.*
- *The standard deviation of population of the dependent variable about its mean at any given value of the independent variable is the same for all values of the independent variable.*

The parameters of this population are α and β, which define the line of means, the dependent-variable population mean at each value of the independent variable, and $\sigma_{y \cdot x}$, which defines the variability about the line of means. Now let us turn our attention to the problem of estimating these parameters from samples drawn at random from such populations.

HOW TO ESTIMATE THE TREND FROM A SAMPLE

Since we observed the entire population of Mars, there was no uncertainty how weight varied with height. This situation contrasts with real problems, in which we cannot observe all members of a population and must infer things about it from a limited sample which we hope is representative. To understand the information that such samples contain, let us consider a sample of 10 individuals selected at random from the population of 200 Martians. Figure 8–3*A* shows the members of the population that happened to be selected; Fig. 8–3*B* shows what an investigator or reader would see. What do the data in Fig. 8–3*B* allow you to say about the underlying population? How certain can you be about the resulting statements?

Simply looking at Fig. 8–3*B* reveals that weight increases as height increases among the 10 specific individuals in *this* sample. The real question of interest, however, is: Does weight vary with height in the population the sample came from? After all, there is always a chance that we could draw an unrepresentative sample, just as in Fig. 1–2. Before we can test the hypothesis that the apparent trend in the data is due to chance rather than a true trend in the population, we need to estimate the population trend from the sample. This task boils down to estimating the intercept α and slope β of the line of means.

The Best Straight Line through the Data

We will estimate the two population parameters α and β with the intercept and slope, a and b, of a straight line placed through the sample points. Figure 8–4 shows the same sample as Fig. 8–3*B* with four proposed lines, labeled I, II, III, and IV. Line I is obviously not appropriate; it does not even pass through the data. Line II passes through the data but has a much steeper slope than the data suggest is really the case. Lines III and IV seem more reasonable; they both pass along the cloud defined by the data points. Which one is best?

To select the best line and so get our estimates a and b of α and β, we need to define precisely what "best" means. To arrive at such a definition, first think about why line II seems better than line I and line III seems better than line II. The "better" a straight line is, the closer it comes to all the points taken as a group. In other words, we want to select the line that minimizes the total variability between the data and

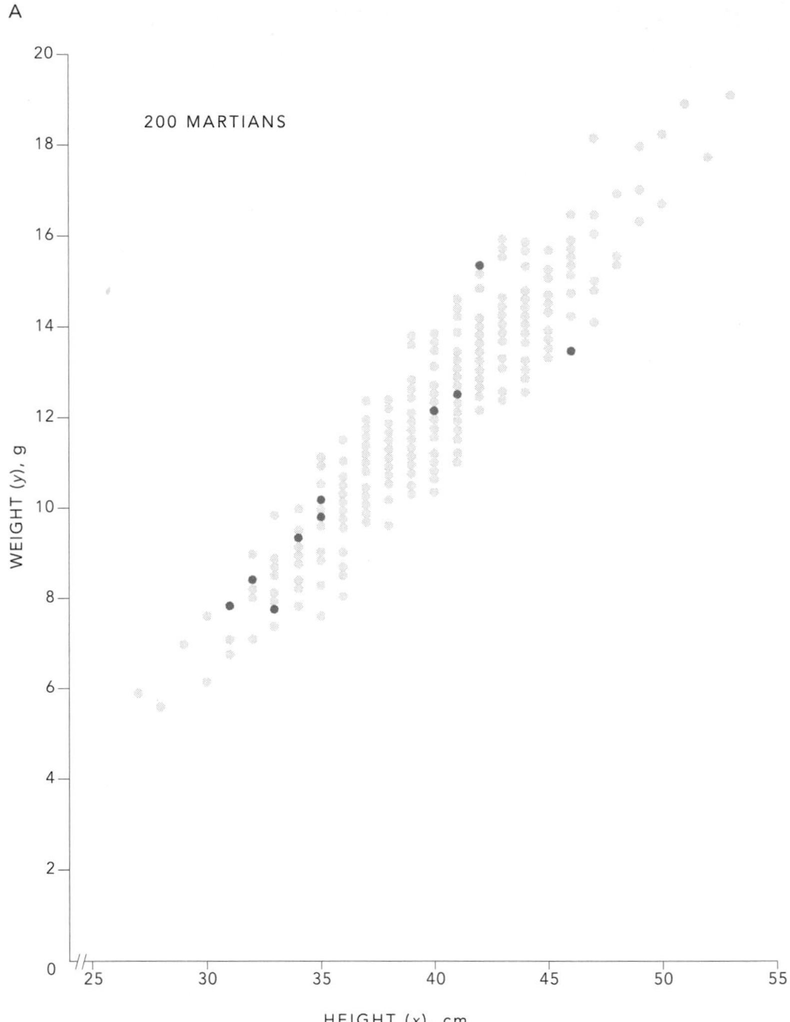

Figure 8–3 A random sample of 10 Martians, showing ***(A)*** the members of the population that were selected together with ***(B)*** the sample as it appears to the investigator.

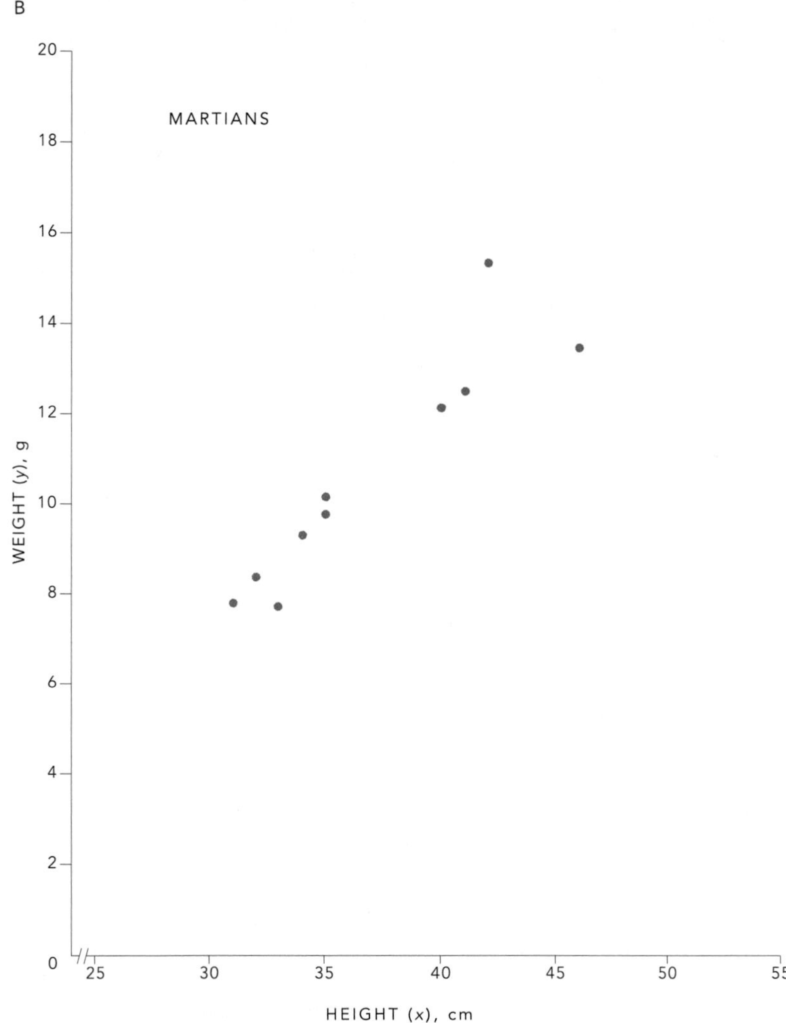

Figure 8–3 *(continued)*

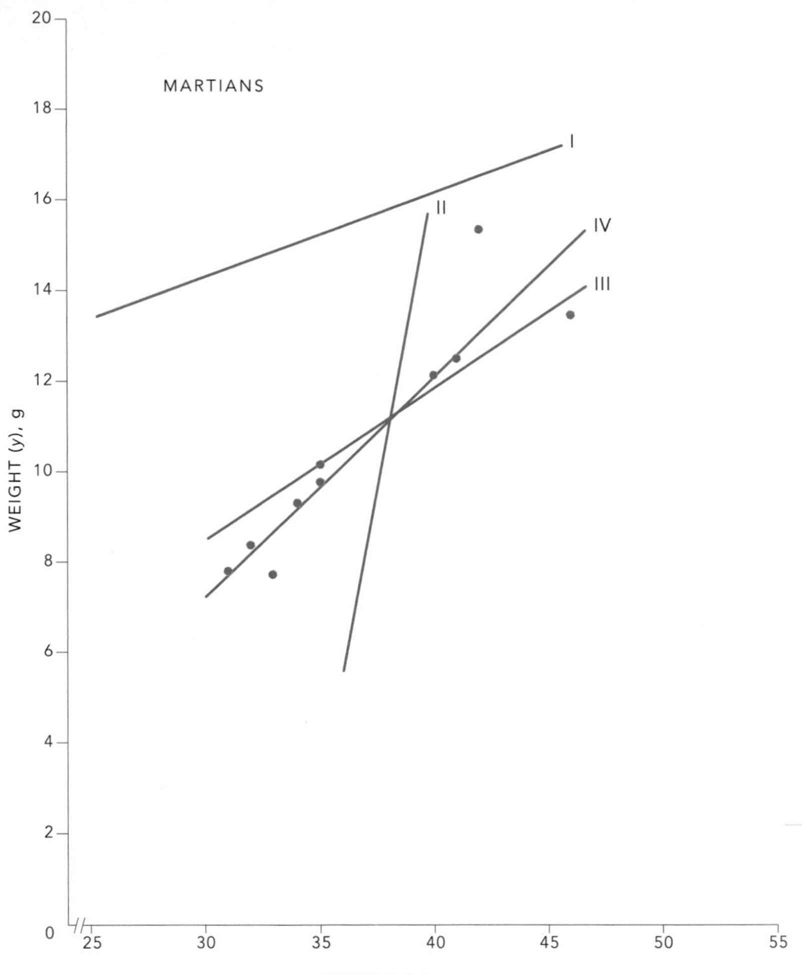

Figure 8–4 Four different possible lines to estimate the line of means from the sample in Fig. 8–3. Lines I and II are unlikely candidates because they fall so far from most of the observations. Lines III and IV are more promising.

the line. The farther any one point is from the line, the more the line varies from the data, so let us select the line that leads to the smallest total variability between the observed values and the values predicted from the straight line.

The problem becomes one of defining a measure of variability, then selecting values of a and b to minimize this quantity. Recall that we quantified variability in a population with the variance (or standard deviation) by computing the sum of the squared deviations from the mean and then divided by the sample size minus 1. Now we will use the same idea and use *sum of the squared differences between the observed values of the dependent variable and the value on the line at the same value of the independent variable* as our measure of how much any given line varies from the data. We square the deviations so that positive and negative deviations contribute equally. Figure 8–5 shows the deviations associated with lines III and IV in Fig. 8–4. The sum of squared deviations is smaller for line IV than line III, so it is the best line. In fact, it is possible to prove mathematically that line IV is the one with the smallest sum of squared deviations between the observations and the line.* For this reason, this procedure is often called the *method of least squares* or *least-squares regression.*

The resulting line is called the *regression line* of y on x (in this case the regression line of weight on height). Its equation is

$$\hat{y} = a + bx$$

$\hat{y}$ denotes the value of y on the regression for a given value of x. This notation distinguishes it from the observed value of the dependent variable Y. The intercept a is given by

$$a = \frac{(\Sigma Y)\,(\Sigma X^2) - (\Sigma X)\,(\Sigma XY)}{n(\Sigma X^2) - (\Sigma X)^2}$$

*For this proof and a derivation of the formulas for the slope and intercept of this line, see S. A. Glantz and B. K. Slinker, *Primer of Applied Regression and Analysis of Variance (2 ed.),* New York: McGraw-Hill, 2001, p. 19.

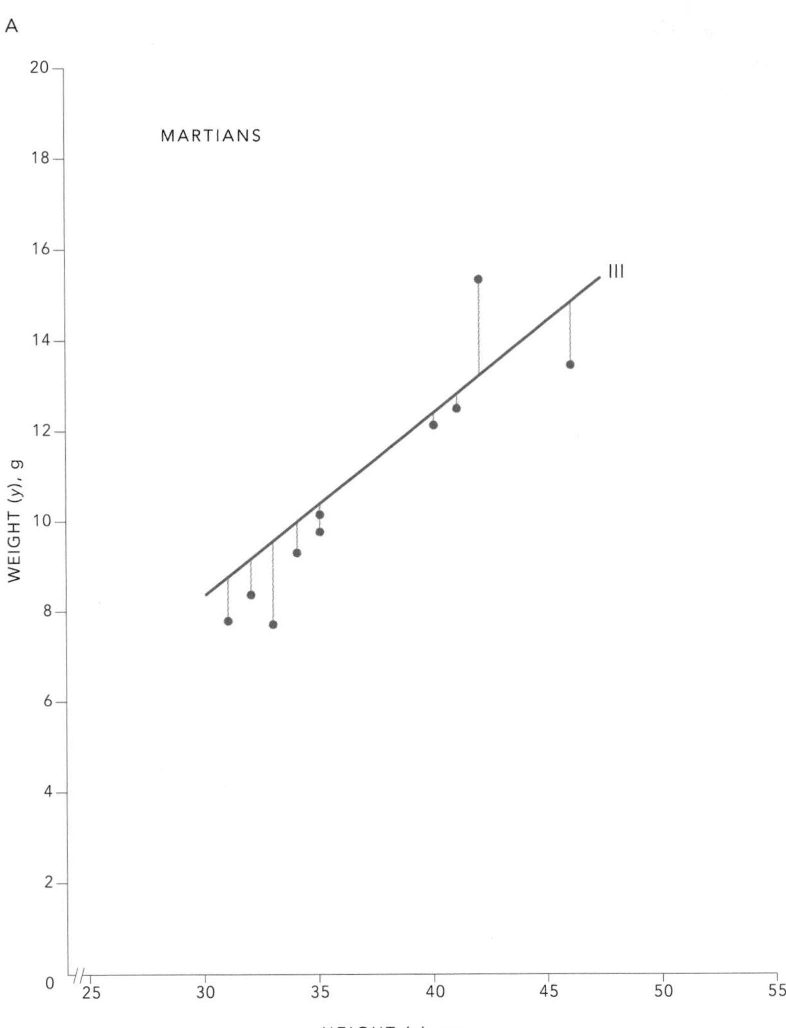

Figure 8–5 Lines III and IV in Fig. 8–4, together with the deviations between the lines and the observations. Line IV is associated with the smallest sum of squared deviations between the regression line and the observed values of the dependent variable. The vertical lines indicate the deviations. The black line is the line of means for the population of Martians in Fig. 8–1. The regression line approximates the line of means but does not precisely coincide with it. Line III in Fig. 8–4 is associated with larger deviations than line IV.

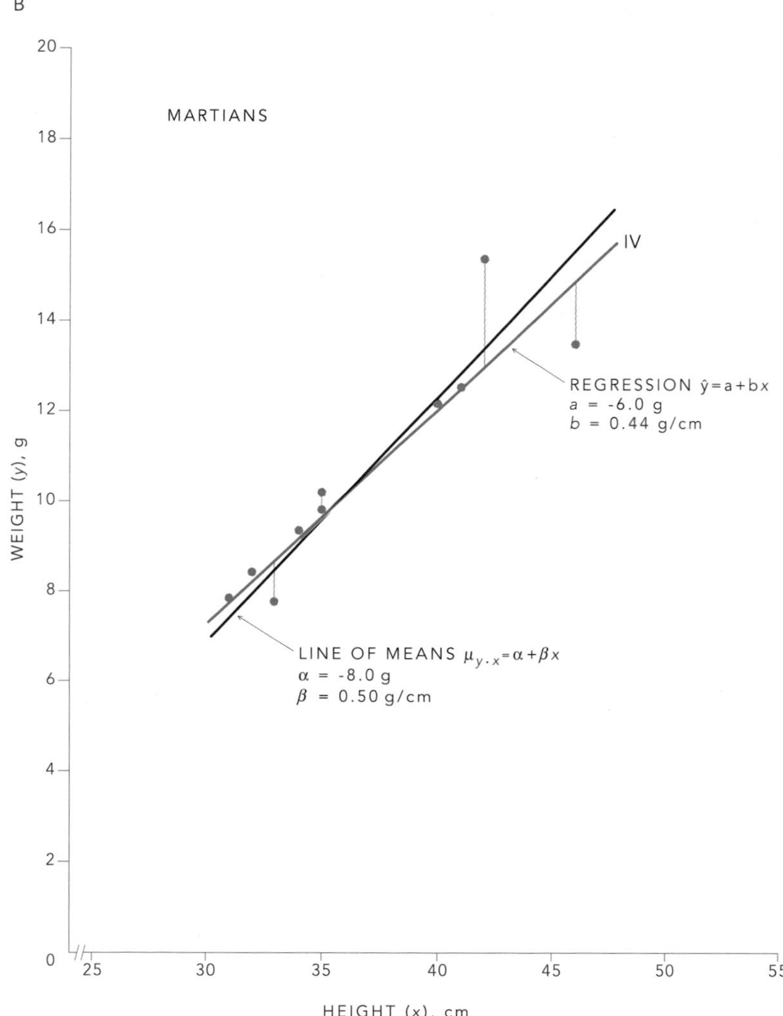

Figure 8–5 *(continued)*

and the slope is given by

$$b = \frac{n(\Sigma XY) - (\Sigma X)(\Sigma Y)}{n(\Sigma X^2) - (\Sigma X)^2}$$

in which X and Y are the coordinates of the n points in the sample.*

Table 8–1 shows these computations for the sample of 10 points in Fig. 8–3*B*. From this table, $n = 10$, $\Sigma X = 369$ cm, $\Sigma Y = 103.8$ g, $\Sigma X^2 =$ 13,841 cm^2, and $\Sigma XY = 3930.1$ g $\times$ cm. Substitute these values into the equations for the intercept and slope of the regression line to find

$$a = \frac{(103.8 \text{ g})(13{,}841 \text{ cm}^2) - (369 \text{ cm})(3930.1 \text{ g}\cdot\text{cm})}{10(13{,}841 \text{ cm}^2) - (369 \text{ cm})^2}$$
$$= -6.0 \text{ g}$$

and

$$b = \frac{10(3930.1 \text{ g}\cdot\text{cm}) - (369 \text{ cm})(103.8 \text{ g})}{10(13{,}841 \text{ cm}^2) - (369 \text{ cm})^2} = 0.44 \text{ g/cm}$$

Table 8–1 Computation of Regression Line in Fig. 8–5*B*

Observed heightX, cm	Observed weight *Y*, g	X^2, cm^2	*XY*, g·cm
31	7.8	961	241.8
32	8.3	1,024	265.6
33	7.6	1,089	250.8
34	9.1	1,156	309.4
35	9.6	1,225	336.0
35	9.8	1,225	343.0
40	11.8	1,600	472.0
41	12.1	1,681	496.1
42	14.7	1,764	617.4
46	13.0	2,116	598.0
369	103.8	13,841	3,930.1

*The calculations can be simplified by computing b first, then finding a from $a = \bar{Y} - b\bar{X}$, in which $\bar{X}$ and $\bar{Y}$ are the means of all observations of the independent and dependent variables, respectively.

Line IV in Figs. 8–4 and 8–5*B* is this regression line.

$$\hat{y} = -6.0 \text{ g} + (0.44 \text{ g/cm})x$$

These two values are estimates of the population parameters, $\alpha = -8$ g and $\beta = 0.5$ g/cm, the intercept and slope of the line of means. The light line in Fig. 8–5*B* shows the line of means.

Variability about the Regression Line

We have the regression line to estimate the line of means, but we still need to estimate the variability of population members about the line of means, $\sigma_{y \cdot x}$. We estimate this parameter by computing the square root of the "average" squared deviation of the data about the regression line

$$s_{y \cdot x} = \sqrt{\frac{\Sigma[Y - (a + bX)]^2}{n - 2}}$$

where $a + bX$ is the value $\hat{y}$ on the regression line corresponding to the observation at X; Y is the actual observed value of y; $Y - (a + bX)$ is the amount that the observation deviates about the regression line; and Σ denotes the sum, over all the data points, of the squares of these deviations $[Y - (a + bX)]^2$. We divide by $n - 2$ rather than n for reasons analogous to dividing by $n - 1$ when computing the sample standard deviation as an estimate of the population standard deviation. Since the sample will not show as much variability as the population, we need to decrease the denominator when computing the "average" squared deviation from the line to compensate for this tendency to underestimate the population variability.

$s_{y \cdot x}$ is called the *standard error of the estimate.* It is related to the standard deviations of the dependent and independent variables and the slope of the regression line according to

$$s_{y \cdot x} = \sqrt{\frac{n - 1}{n - 2}(s_Y^2 - b^2 s_X^2)}$$

where s_Y and s_X are the standard deviations of the dependent and independent variables, respectively.

For the sample shown in Fig. 8–3*B* (and Table 8–1), $s_X - 5.0$ cm and $s_Y = 2.4$ g, so

$$s_{y\cdot x} = \sqrt{\frac{9}{8}[2.4^2 - 0.44^2(5.0^2)]} = 0.96 \text{ g}$$

This number is an estimate of the actual variability about the line of means, $\sigma_{y\cdot x} = 1$ g.

Standard Errors of the Regression Coefficients

Just as the sample mean is only an estimate of the true population mean, the slope and intercept of the regression line are only estimates of the slope and intercept of the line of means in the population. In addition, just as different samples yield different estimates for the population mean, different samples will yield different regression lines. After all, there is nothing special about the sample in Fig. 8–3. Figure 8–6*A* shows another sample of 10 individuals drawn at random from the population of all Martians. Figure 8–6*B* shows what you would see. Like the sample in Fig. 8–3*B*, the results of this sample also suggest that taller Martians tend to be heavier, but the relationship looks a little different from that associated with our first sample. This sample yields estimates of $a = -4.0$ *g* and $b = 0.38$ g/cm as estimates of the intercept and slope of the line of means.

There is a population of possible values of a and b corresponding to all possible samples of a given size drawn from the population in Fig. 8–1. These distributions of all possible values of a and b have means α and β, respectively, and standard deviations σ_a and σ_b called the *standard error of the intercept* and *standard error of the slope,* respectively.

These standard errors can be used just as we used the standard error of the mean and standard error of a proportion. Specifically, we will use them to test hypotheses about, and compute confidence intervals for, the regression coefficients and the regression equation itself.

The standard deviation of the population of all possible values of the regression line intercept, the *standard error of the intercept,* can be estimated from the sample with*

$$s_a = s_{y \cdot x}\sqrt{\frac{1}{n} + \frac{\overline{X}^2}{(n-1)s_X^2}}$$

The *standard error of the slope* of the regression line is the standard deviation of the population of all possible slopes. Its estimate is

$$s_b = \frac{1}{\sqrt{n-1}}\frac{s_{y \cdot x}}{s_X}$$

From the data in Fig. 8–3*B* and Table 8–1 it is possible to compute the standard errors for the slope and intercept as

$$s_a = (0.96\text{ g})\sqrt{\frac{1}{10} + \frac{(36.9\text{ cm})^2}{(10-1)(5.0\text{ cm})^2}} = 2.4\text{ g}$$

and

$$s_b = \frac{1}{\sqrt{10-1}}\frac{0.96\text{ g}}{5.0\text{ cm}} = 0.06\text{ g/cm}$$

Like the sample mean, both *a* and *b* are computed from sums of the observations. Like the distributions of all possible values of the sample mean, the distributions of all possible values of *a* and *b* tend to be normally distributed. (This result is another consequence of the central-limit theorem.) The specific values of *a* and *b* associated with the regression line are then randomly selected from normally distributed populations. Therefore, these standard errors can be used to compute confidence intervals and test hypotheses about the intercept and slope of the line of means using the *t* distribution, just as we did for the sample mean in Chapter 7.

*For a derivation of these formulas, see J. Neter, M. H. Kutner, C. J. Nachtsheim, and W. Wasserman *Applied Linear Statistical Models: Regression, Analysis of Variance, and Experimental Designs,* Boston: WCB McGraw-Hill, 1996, chap. 2, "Inferences in Regression Analysis."

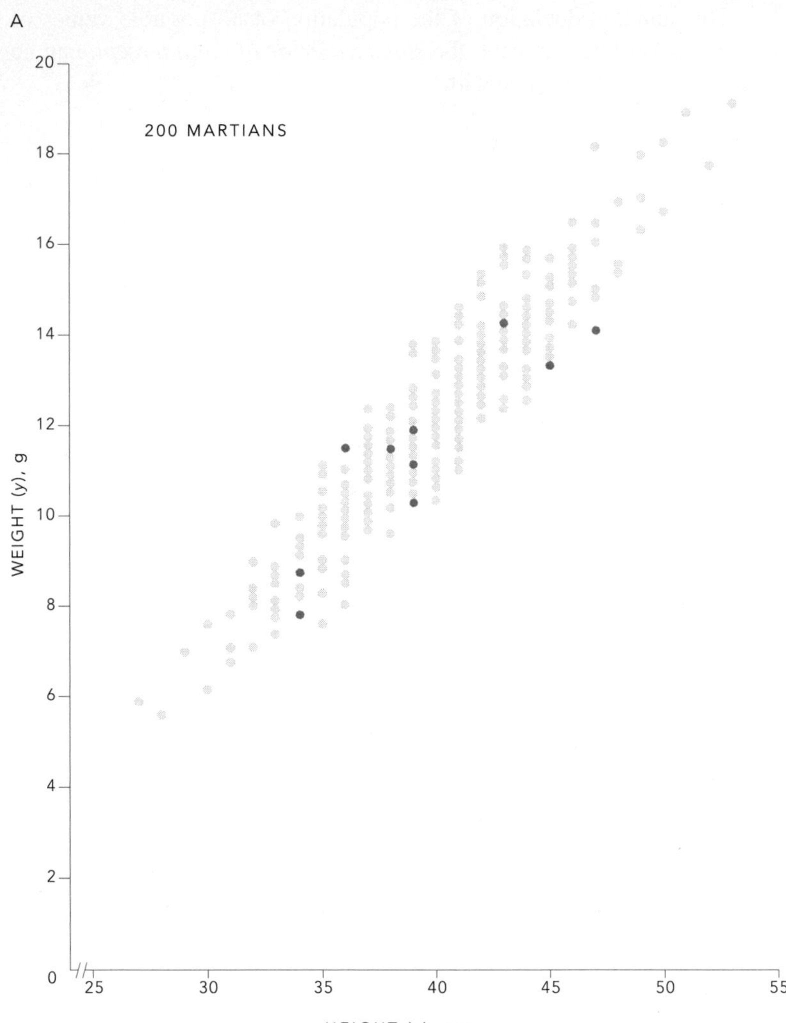

Figure 8–6 This figure illustrates a second random sample of 10 Martians drawn from the population in Fig. 8–1. This sample is associated with a different regression line than that computed from the first sample, shown in Fig. 8–5*A*.

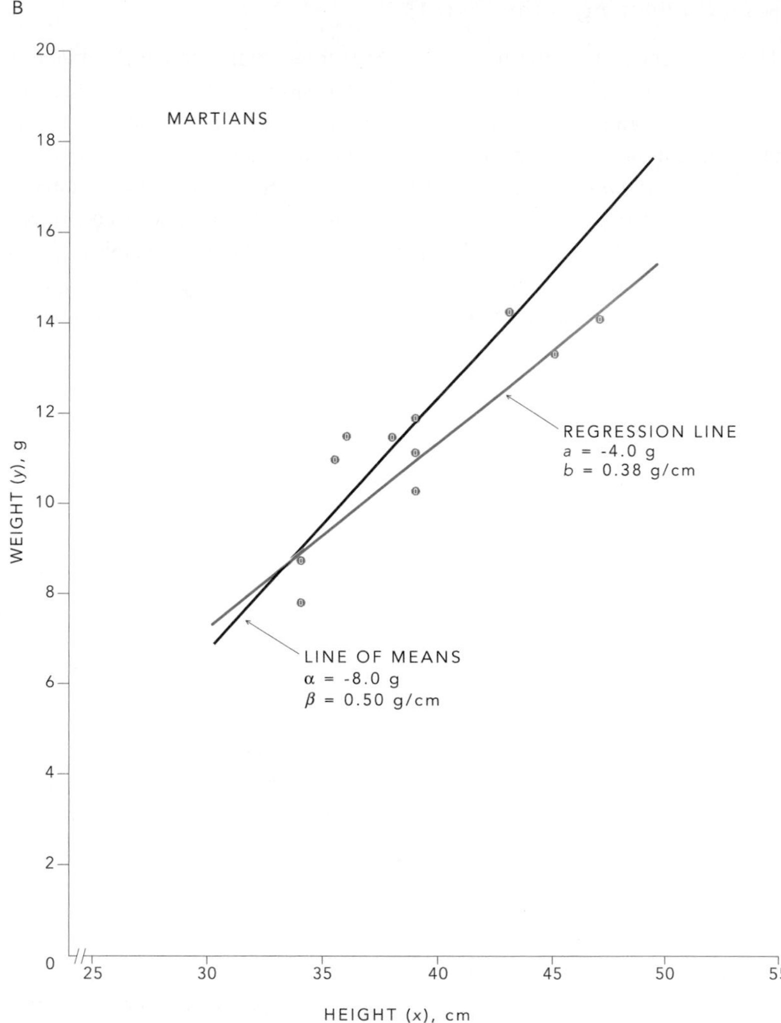

Figure 8–6 *(continued)*

How Convincing Is the Trend?

There are many hypotheses we can test about regression lines, but the most common and important one is that the slope of the line of means is zero. This hypothesis is equivalent to estimating the chance that we would observe a trend as strong or stronger than the data show *when there is actually no relationship* between the dependent and independent variables. The resulting P value quantifies the certainty with which you can reject the hypothesis that there is no *linear* trend relating the two variables.*

Since the population of possible values of the regression slope is approximately normally distributed, we can use the general definition of the t statistic

$$t = \frac{\text{parameter estimate} - \text{true value of population parameter}}{\text{standard error of parameter estimate}}$$

to test this hypothesis. The equivalent mathematical statement is

$$t = \frac{b - \beta}{s_b}$$

This equation permits testing the hypothesis that there is no trend in the population from which the sample was drawn, that is, $\beta = 0$, using either of the approaches to hypothesis testing developed earlier.

To take a classic hypothesis-testing approach (as in Chapter 4), set β to zero in the equation above and compute

$$t = \frac{b}{s_b}$$

then compare the resulting value of t with the critical value t_α defining the 100α percent most extreme values of t that would occur if the hypothesis of no trend in the population was true. (Use the value corresponding to $\nu = n - 2$ degrees of freedom.)

*This restriction is important. As discussed later in this chapter, it is possible for there to be a strong *nonlinear* relationship in the observations and for the procedures we discuss here to miss it.

For example, the data in Fig. 8–3*B* (and Table 8–1) yielded $b = 0.44$ g/cm and $s_b = 0.064$ g/cm from a sample of 10 points. Hence, $t = 0.45/0.057 = 7.894$, which exceeds 5.041, the value of t for $P < .001$ with $\nu = 10 - 2 = 8$ degrees of freedom (from Table 4–1). Hence, it is unlikely that this sample was drawn from a population in which there was no relationship between the independent and dependent variables, that is, height and weight. We can use these data to assert that as height increases, weight increases ($P < .001$).

Of course, like all statistical tests of hypotheses, this small P value does not guarantee that there is really a trend in the population. For example, the sample in Fig. 1–2*A* is associated with $P < .001$. Nevertheless, as Fig. 1–2*B* shows, there is no trend in the underlying population.

If we wish to test the hypothesis that there is no trend in the population using confidence intervals, we use the definition of t above to find the $100(1 - \alpha)$ percent confidence interval for the slope of the line of means,

$$b - t_\alpha s_b < \beta < b + t_\alpha s_b$$

We can compute the 95 percent confidence interval for β by substituting the value of $t_{.05}$ with $\nu = n - 2 = 10 - 2 = 8$ degrees of freedom, 2.306, into this equation together with the observed values of b and s_b

$$.44 - 2.306(.06) < \beta < .44 + 2.306(.06)$$
$$0.30 \text{ g/cm} < \beta < 0.58 \text{ g/cm}$$

Since this interval does not contain zero, we can conclude that there is a trend in the population ($P < .05$).* Note that the interval contains the true value of the slope of the line of means, $\beta = 0.5$ g/cm.

It is likewise possible to test hypotheses about, or compute confidence intervals for, the intercept using the fact that

$$t = \frac{a - \alpha}{s_a}$$

*The 99.9 percent confidence interval does not contain zero either, so we could obtain the same P value (.001) as with the first method using confidence intervals.

is distributed according to the t distribution with $\vartheta = n - 2$ degrees of freedom. For example, the 95 percent confidence interval for the intercept based on the observations in Fig. 8–3B is

$$a - t_{.05}\, s_a < \alpha < a + t_{.05}\, s_a$$
$$-6.2 - 2.306(2.4) < \alpha < -6.2 + 2.306(2.4)$$
$$-11.3 \text{ g} < \alpha < -1.1 \text{ g}$$

which includes the true intercept of the line of means, $\alpha = -8$ g.

A number of other useful confidence intervals associated with regression analysis, such as the confidence interval for the line of means, will be discussed next.

Confidence Interval for the Line of Means

There is uncertainty in the estimates of the slope and intercept of the regression line. The standard errors of the slope and the intercept, s_a and s_b, quantify this uncertainty. These standard errors are $s_a = 2.4$ g and $s_b = 0.06$ g/cm for the regression of height or weight for the Martians in the sample in Fig. 8–3. Thus, the line of means could lie slightly above or below the observed regression line or have a slightly different slope. It nevertheless is likely that the line of means lies within a band surrounding the observed regression line. Figure 8–7A shows this region. It is wider at the ends than in the middle because the regression line must be straight and must go through the point defined by the means of the independent and dependent variables.

There is a distribution of possible values for the regression line at each value of the independent variable x. Since these possible values are normally distributed about the line of means, it makes sense to talk about the standard error of the regression line. (This is another consequence of the central-limit theorem.) Unlike the other standard errors we have discussed so far, this standard error is not constant but depends on the value of the independent variable x:

$$s_{\hat{y}} = s_{y \cdot x}\sqrt{\frac{1}{n} + \frac{(x - \overline{X})^2}{(n - 1)s_X^2}}$$

Since the distribution of possible values of the regression line is normally distributed, we can compute the $100(1 - \alpha)$ percent confidence interval for the regression line with

$$\hat{y} - t_\alpha s_{\hat{y}} < y < \hat{y} + t_\alpha s_{\hat{y}}$$

in which t_α has $\nu = n - 2$ degrees of freedom and $\hat{y}$ is the point on the regression line for each value of x,

$$\hat{y} = a + bx$$

Figure 8–7*A* shows the *95 percent confidence interval for the line of means.* It is wider at the ends than the middle, as it should be. Note also that it is much narrower than the range of the data because it is the confidence interval for the line of means, not the population as a whole.

It is not uncommon for investigators to present the confidence interval for the regression line and discuss it as though it were the confidence interval for the population. This practice is analogous to reporting the standard error of the mean instead of the standard deviation to describe population variability. For example, Fig. 8–7*A* shows that we can be 95 percent confident that the *mean* weight of all 40-cm tall Martians is between 11.0 and 12.5 g. We cannot be 95 percent confident that the weight of any one Martian that is 40 cm tall falls in this narrow range.

Confidence Interval for an Observation

To compute a confidence interval for an individual observation, we must combine the total variability that arises from the variation in the underlying population about the line of means, estimated with $s_{y \cdot x}$, *and* the variability due to uncertainty in the location of the line of means $s_{\hat{y}}$. Since the variance of a sum is the sum of the variances, the standard deviation of the predicted value of the observation will be

$$s_{Y\text{new}} = \sqrt{s_{y \cdot x}^2 + s_{\hat{y}}^2}$$

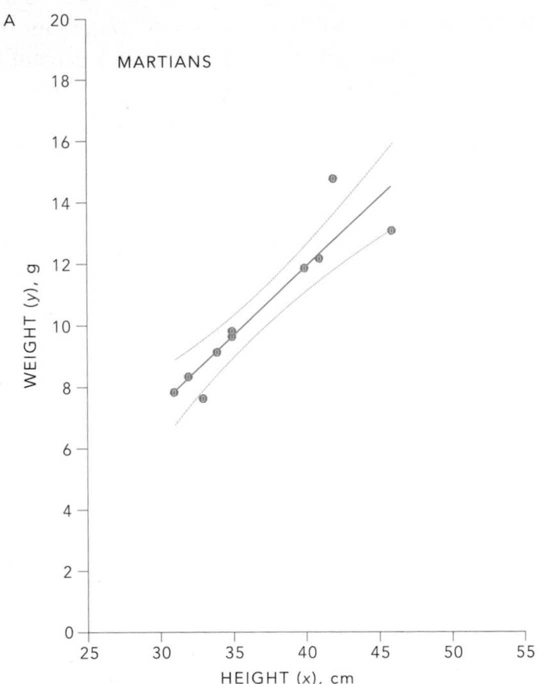

Figure 8–7 ***(A)*** The 95 percent confidence interval for the regression line relating Martian weight or height using the data in Fig. 8–3. ***(B)*** The 95 percent confidence interval for an additional observation of Martian weight at a given height. This is the confidence interval that should be used to estimate true weight from height to be 95 percent confident that the range includes the true weight.

We can eliminate $s_{\hat{y}}$ from this equation by replacing it with the equation for $s_{\hat{y}}$ in the last section

$$s_{Y\text{new}} = s_{y \cdot x}\sqrt{1 + \frac{1}{n} + \frac{(x - \overline{X})^2}{(n - 1)s_X^2}}$$

This standard error can be used to define the $100(1 - \alpha)$ percent confidence interval for an observation according to

$$\hat{y} - t_\alpha\, s_{Y\text{new}} < y < \hat{y} + t_\alpha\, s_{Y\text{new}}$$

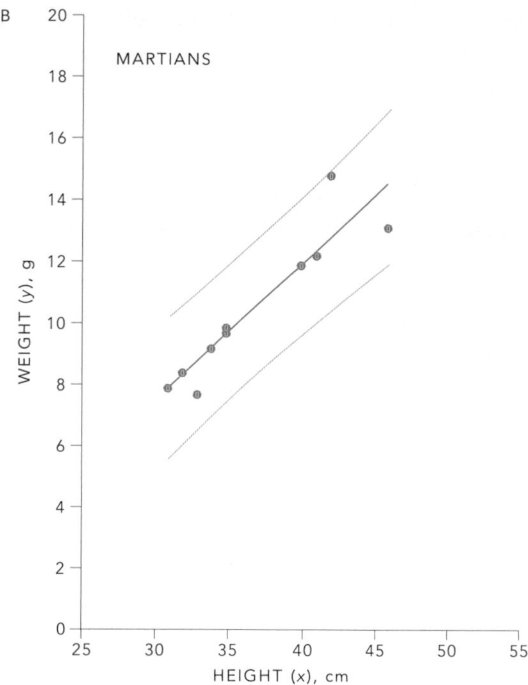

Figure 8–7 *(continued)*

(Remember that both $\hat{y}$ and $s_{Y_{\text{new}}}$ depend on the value of the independent variable x.)

The two lines around the regression line in Fig. 8–7*B* show the 95 percent confidence interval for an additional observation. This band includes both the uncertainty due to random variation in the population and variation due to uncertainty in the estimate of the true line of means. Notice that most members of the sample fall in this band. It quantifies the uncertainty in using Martian height to estimate weight, and hence, the uncertainty in the true weight of a Martian of a given height. For example, it shows that we can be 95 percent confident that the true weight of a 40-cm tall Martian is between 9.5 and 14.0 g. This confidence interval describes the precision with which it is possible to estimate the true weight. This information is much more useful than the fact that there is a statistically significant* relationship between the Martian weight and height ($P < .001$).

HOW TO COMPARE TWO REGRESSION LINES†

The situation often arises in which one wants to compare two regression lines. There are actually three possible comparisons one might want to make:

- *Test for a difference in slope (without regard for the intercepts).*
- *Test for a difference in intercept (without regard for the slopes).*
- *Make an overall test of coincidence, in which we ask if the lines are different.*

The procedures for comparing two slopes or intercepts is a direct extension of the fact that the observed slopes and intercepts follow the t distribution. For example, to test the hypothesis that two samples were drawn from populations with the same slope of the line of means, we compute

$$t = \frac{\text{difference of regression slopes}}{\text{standard error of difference of regression slopes}}$$

or, in mathematical terms,

$$t = \frac{b_1 - b_2}{s_{b_1 - b_2}}$$

*$t = b/s_b = .44/.060 = 7.333$ for the data in Fig. 8–3. $t_{.001}$ for $\nu = 10 - 2 = 8$ degrees of freedom is 5.041.

†This section deals with more advanced material and can be skipped without loss of continuity. It is also possible to test for differences between more than three regression lines using techniques which are generalizations of regression and analysis of variance; See J. H. Zar, *Biostatistical Analysis* (4th ed.) Prentice-Hall, Upper Saddle River, NJ, 1999, chapter 18, "Comparing Simple Linear Regression Equations." For a discussion of how to use multiple regression models to compare several regression lines, including how to test for parallel shifts between regression lines, see S. Glantz and B. Slinker, *Primer of Applied Regression and Analysis of Variance* (2nd ed.), McGraw-Hill, New York, 2001, chapter 3, "Regression with Two or More Independent Variables."

where the subscripts 1 and 2 refer to data from the first and second regression data samples. This value of t is compared to the critical value of the t distribution with $\nu = n_1 + n_2 - 4$ degrees of freedom. This test is exactly analogous to the definition of the t test to compare two sample means.

If the two regressions are based on the same number of data points, the standard error of the difference of two regression slopes is

$$s_{b_1 - b_2} = \sqrt{s_{b_1}^2 + s_{b_2}^2}$$

If there are a different number of points, use the pooled estimate of the difference of the slopes. Analogous to the pooled estimate of the variance in the t test in Chapter 4, compute a pooled estimate of the variation about the regression lines as

$$s_{y \cdot x_p}^2 = \frac{(n_1 - 2)s_{y \cdot x_1}^2 + (n_2 - 2)s_{y \cdot x_2}^2}{n_1 + n_2 - 4}$$

and use this value to compute

$$s_{b_1 - b_2} = \sqrt{\frac{s_{y \cdot x_p}^2}{(n_1 - 1)s_{x_1}^2} + \frac{s_{y \cdot x_p}^2}{(n_2 - 1)s_{x_2}^2}}$$

Likewise, to compare the intercepts of two regression lines, we compute

$$t = \frac{a_1 - a_2}{s_{a_1 - a_2}}$$

where

$$s_{a_1 - a_2} = \sqrt{s_{a_1}^2 + s_{a_2}^2}$$

if there are the same number of points for each regression equation, and we use a formula based on the pooled variance estimate if there are unequal number of points in the two regressions.

Overall Test for Coincidence of Two Regression Lines

It is also possible to test the null hypothesis that two regressions are *coincident,* that is, have the same slope and intercept. Recall that we computed the slope and intercept of the regression line by selecting the values that minimized the total sum of squared differences between the observed values of the dependent variable and the value on the line at the same value of the independent variable (residuals). The square of the standard error of the estimate, $s_{y \cdot x}$, is the estimate of this residual variance around the regression line and it is a measure of how closely the regression line fits the data. We will use this fact to construct our test, by examining whether fitting the two sets of data with separate regression lines (in which the slopes and intercepts can be different) produces smaller residuals than fitting all the data with a single regression line (with a single slope and intercept).

The specific procedure for testing for coincidence of two regression lines is:

- *Fit each set of data with a separate regression line.*
- *Compute the pooled estimate of the variance around the two regression lines,* $s^2_{y \cdot x_p}$, *using the previous equations. This statistic is a measure of the overall variability about the two regression lines, allowing the slopes and intercepts of the two lines to be different.*
- *Fit all the data with one regression line, and compute the variance around this one "single" regression line,* $s^2_{y \cdot x_s}$. *This statistic is a measure of the overall variability observed when the data are fit by assuming that they all fall along one line of means.*
- *Compute the "improvement" in the fit obtained by fitting the two data sets with separate regression lines compared to fitting them with a single regression line using*

$$s^2_{y \cdot x_{\text{imp}}} = \frac{(n_1 + n_2 - 2)s^2_{y \cdot x_s} - (n_1 + n_2 - 4)s^2_{y \cdot x_p}}{2}$$

- *The numerator in this expression is the reduction in the total sum of squared differences between the observations and regression line that occurs when the two lines are allowed to have different slopes and intercepts. It can also be computed as*

$$s^2_{y \cdot x_{\text{imp}}} = \frac{SS_{\text{res}_s} - SS_{\text{res}_p}}{2}$$

where SS_{res} are the sum of squared residuals about the regressions.

- *Quantify the relative improvement in the fit obtained by fitting the two sets of data separately with the residual variation about the regression line obtained by fitting the two lines separately, using the* F *test statistic,*

$$F = \frac{s^2_{y \cdot x_{\text{imp}}}}{s^2_{y \cdot x_p}}$$

- *Compare the observed value of the F test statistic with the critical values of* F *for $\nu_n = 2$ numerator degrees of freedom and $\nu_d = n_1 + n_2 - 4$ denominator degrees of freedom.*

If the observed value of F exceeds the critical value of F, it means that we obtain a significantly better fit to the data (measured by the residual variation about the regression line) by fitting the two sets of data with separate regression lines than we do by fitting all the data with a single line. We reject the null hypothesis of a single line of means and conclude that the two sets of data were drawn from populations with different lines of means.

Relationship between Weakness and Muscle Wasting in Rheumatoid Arthritis

Rheumatoid arthritis is a disease in which a person's joints become inflamed so that movement becomes painful, and people find it harder to complete mechanical tasks, such as holding things. At the same time, as people age, they often lose muscle mass. As a result, P. S. Helliwell

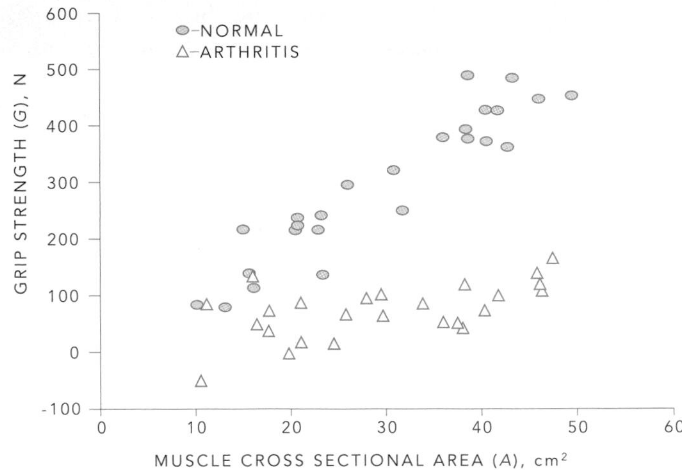

Figure 8–8 This plot shows the grip strength as a function of muscle cross-sectional area in 25 normal people and 25 people with arthritis. The question is: Are the relationships between these two variables the same in both groups of people?

and S. Jackson* wondered whether the reduction in grip strength noted in people who had arthritis was due to the arthritic joints or simply a reflection of a reduction in mass of muscle.

To investigate this question, they measured the cross sectional area (in cm^2) of the forearms of a group of normal people and a group of similar people with arthritis as well as the force (in newtons) with which they could grip a test device. Figure 8–8 shows the data from such an experiment, using different symbols with the two groups of people indicated. The question is: Is the relationship between muscle cross sectional area and grip strength different for the normal people (circles) and the people with arthritis (triangles)?

We will answer this question by first doing a test for overall coincidence of the two regressions. Figure 8–9*A* shows the same data as in Fig. 8–8, with separate regression equations fit to the two sets of data and Table 8–2 presents the results of fitting these two regression equations. Using the formula presented earlier,

*P. S. Helliwell and S. Jackson, Relationship between weakness and muscle wasting in rheumatoid arthritis, *Ann. Rheum. Dis.* **53:**726–728, 1994.

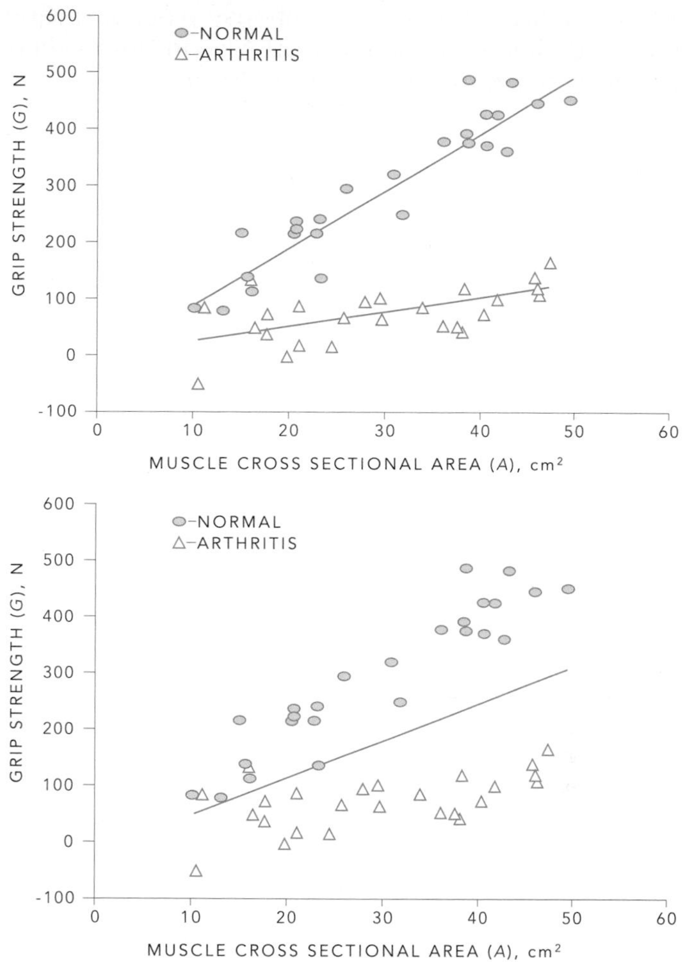

Figure 8–9 In order to test whether the two groups of people (normal subjects and people with arthritis) have a similar relationship between muscle cross-sectional area and grip strength, we first fit the data for the two groups separately **(*A*)**, then together **(*B*)**. If the null hypothesis that there is no difference between the two groups is true, then the variation about the regression lines fit separately will be approximately the same as the variation when the two sets of data are fit separately.

Table 8–2 Comparison of the Relationship between Grip Strength and Muscle Cross-Sectional Area in Normal People and People with Arthritis (See Figs. 8–8 and 8–9)

	Normal	Arthritis	All People
Sample size n	25	25	50
Intercept a (s_a), N	−7.3 (25.3)	3.3 (22.4)	−23.1 (50.5)
Slope b (s_b), N/cm^2	10.19 (.789)	2.41 (.702)	6.39 (1.579)
Standard error of the estimate $s_{y \cdot x}$, N	45.7	40.5	129.1

the pooled estimate of the variance about the two regression lines fit separately is

$$s^2_{\text{grip}\cdot\text{area}_p} = \frac{(n_{\text{normal}} - 2)s^2_{\text{grip}\cdot\text{area}_{\text{normal}}} + (n_{\text{arthritis}} - 2)s^2_{\text{grip}\cdot\text{area}_{\text{arthritis}}}}{n_{\text{normal}} + n_{\text{arthritis}} - 4}$$

$$= \frac{(25 - 2)45.7^2 + (25 - 2)40.5^2}{25 + 25 - 4} = 1864N^2$$

Next, fit all the data to a single regression equation, without regard for the group to which each person belongs; Figure 8–9*B* shows this result, with the results of fitting the single regression equation as the last column in Table 8–2. The total variance of the observations about the single regression line is $s^2_{\text{grip}\cdot\text{area}_s} = (129.1)^2 = 16{,}667N^2$. This value is larger than that observed when the two curves were fit separately. To estimate the improvement (reduction) in variance associated with fitting the two curves separately, we compute

$$s^2_{\text{grip}\cdot\text{area}_{\text{imp}}}$$

$$= \frac{(n_{\text{normal}} + n_{\text{arthritis}} - 2)s^2_{\text{grip}\cdot\text{area}_s} - (n_{\text{normal}} + n_{\text{arthritis}} - 4)s^2_{\text{grip}\cdot\text{area}_p}}{2}$$

$$= \frac{(25 + 25 - 2)16{,}667 - (25 + 25 - 4)1864}{2} = 714{,}263N^2$$

Finally, we compare the improvement in the variance about the regression line obtained by fitting the two groups separately with that obtained by fitting them separately (which yields the smallest residual variance) with the F test

$$F = \frac{s^2_{\text{grip}\cdot\text{area}_{\text{imp}}}}{s^2_{\text{grip}\cdot\text{area}_p}} = \frac{714{,}263}{1864} = 383.188$$

This value exceeds 5.10, the critical value of F for $P < .01$ with $\nu_d = 2$ and $\nu_d = n_{\text{normal}} + n_{\text{arthritis}} - 4 = 25 + 25 - 4 = 46$ degrees of freedom, so we conclude that the relationship between grip force and cross sectional area is different for normal people and people with arthritis.

The next question that arises is where the difference comes from. Are the intercepts or slopes different? To answer this question, we compare the intercepts and slopes of the two regression equations. We begin with the intercepts. Substituting the results from Table 8–2 into the equations above for the case of equal sample sizes,

$$s_{a_{\text{normal}} - a_{\text{arthritis}}} = \sqrt{s^2_{a_{\text{normal}}} + s^2_{a_{\text{arthritis}}}} = \sqrt{(25.3)^2 + (22.4)^2} = 33.8N$$

and

$$t = \frac{a_{\text{normal}} - a_{\text{arthritis}}}{s_{a_{\text{normal}} - a_{\text{arthritis}}}} = \frac{(-7.3) - (3.3)}{33.8} = -.314$$

which does not come near exceeding 2.013 in magnitude, the critical value of t for $P < .05$ for $\nu = n_{\text{normal}} + n_{\text{arthritis}} - 4 = 46$ degrees of freedom. Therefore, we do not conclude that the intercepts of the two lines are significantly different.

A similar analysis comparing the slopes yields $t = 7.367$, so we do conclude that the slopes are different ($P < .001$). Hence the increase in grip force per unit increase in cross sectional muscle area is smaller for people with arthritis than normal people.

CORRELATION AND CORRELATION COEFFICIENTS

Linear regression analysis of a sample provides an estimate of how, on the average, a dependent variable changes when an independent variable changes and an estimate of the variability in the dependent variable about the line of means. These estimates, together with their standard errors, permit computing confidence intervals to show the certainty with which you can predict the value of the dependent variable for a given value of the independent variable. In some experiments, however, two variables are measured that change together, but neither can be considered to be the dependent variable. In such experiments, we abandon all premise of making a statement about causality and simply seek to describe the strength of the relationship between the two variables. The *correlation coefficient*, a number between -1 and $+1$, is often used to quantify the strength of this association. Figure 8–10 shows that the tighter the relationship

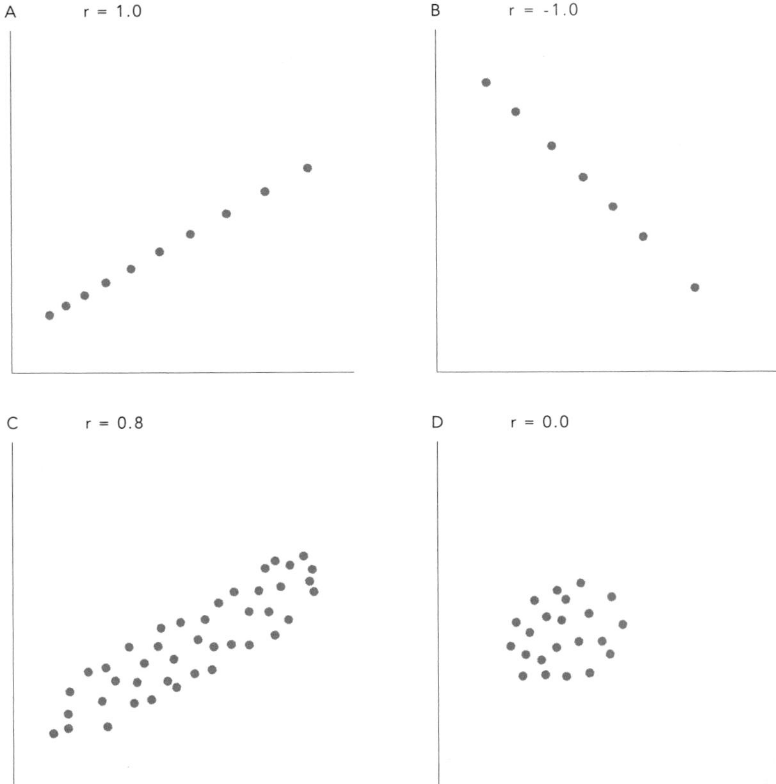

Figure 8–10 The closer the magnitude of the correlation coefficient is to 1, the less scatter there is in the relationship between the two variables. The closer the correlation coefficient is to 0, the weaker the relationship between the two variables.

between the two variables, the closer the magnitude of r to 1; the weaker the relationship between the two variables, the closer r is to 0. We will examine two different correlation coefficients.

The first, called the *Pearson product-moment correlation coefficient,* quantifies the strength of association between two variables that are normally distributed like those in Fig. 8–1. It, therefore, provides an alternative perspective on the same data we analyzed using linear regression. When people refer to *the* correlation coefficient, they almost always mean the Pearson product-moment correlation coefficient.

The second, called the *Spearman rank correlation coefficient,* is used to quantify the strength of a trend between two variables that are measured on an *ordinal scale.* In an ordinal scale responses can be graded, but there is no arithmetic relationship between the different possible responses. For example, Pap smears, the common test for cervical cancer, are graded according to this scale: (1) normal, (2) cervicitis (inflammation, usually due to infection), (3) mild to moderate dysplasia (abnormal but noncancerous cells), (4) moderate to severe dysplasia, and (5) cancerous cells present. In this case, a rating of 4 denotes a more serious condition than a rating of 2, but it *is not* necessarily *twice* as serious. This situation contrasts with observations quantified on an *interval scale* where there are arithmetic relationships between the responses. For example, a Martian who weighs 16 g *is* twice as heavy as one who weighs 8 g. Ordinal scales often appear in clinical practice when conditions are ranked according to seriousness.

The Pearson Product-Moment Correlation Coefficient

The problem of describing the strength of association between two variables is closely related to the linear-regression problem, so why not simply arbitrarily make one variable dependent on the other? Figure 8–11 shows that reversing the roles of the two variables when computing the regression line results in *different* regression lines. This situation arises because in the process of computing the slope and intercept of the regression line we minimize the sum of squared deviations between the regression line and the observed values of the *dependent* variable. If we reverse the roles of the two variables, there is a different dependent variable, so different values of the regression line intercept and slope minimize the sum of squared deviations. We need

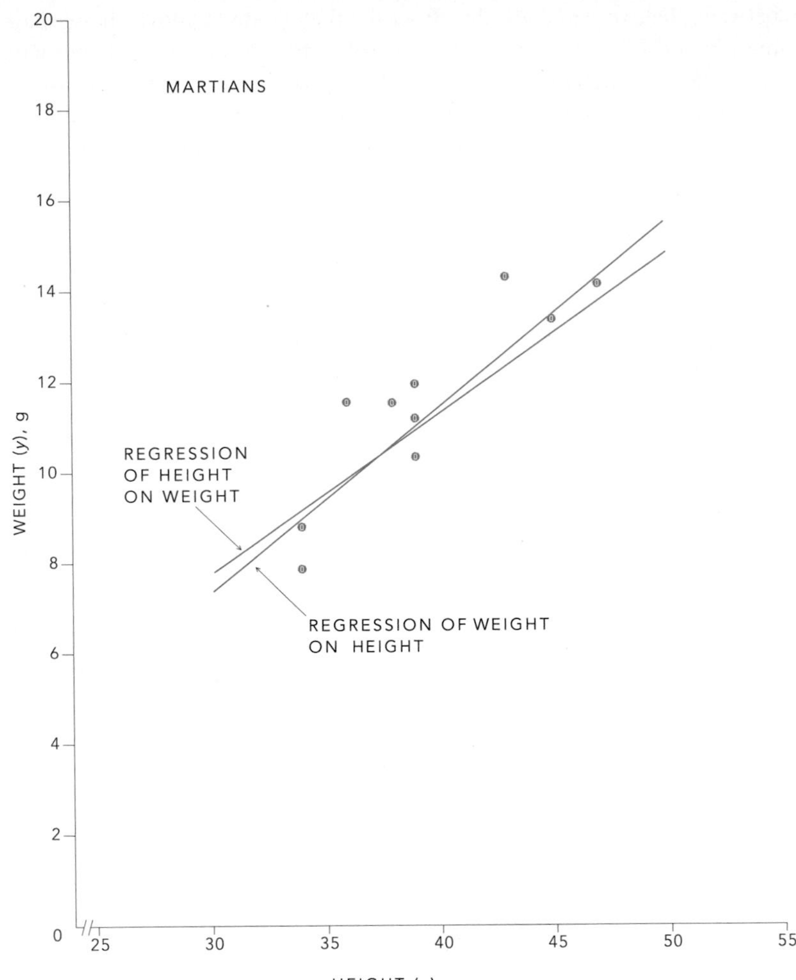

Figure 8–11 The regression of y on x yields a different regression line than the regression of x on y for the same data. The correlation coefficient is the same in either case.

a measure of association that does not require arbitrarily deciding that one of the variables is the independent variable.

The Pearson product-moment correlation coefficient r, defined by

$$r = \frac{\Sigma(X - \overline{X})(Y - \overline{Y})}{\sqrt{\Sigma X - \overline{X})^2 \Sigma(Y - \overline{Y})^2}}$$

in which the sums are over all the observed (X, Y) points, has this property. Its value does not depend on which variable we call x and y. The magnitude of r describes the *strength of the association* between the two variables, and sign of r tells the direction of this association: $r = +1$ when the two variables increase together (Fig. 8–10*A*), and $r = -1$ when one decreases as the other increases (Fig. 8–10*B*). Figure 8–10*C* also shows the more common case of two variables that are correlated, though not perfectly. Figure 8–10*D* shows two variables that do not appear to relate to each other at all; $r = 0$.

Table 8–3 illustrates how to compute the correlation coefficient using the sample of 10 points in Fig 8–3*B*. (These are the same data used to illustrate the computation of the regression line in Table 8–1 and Fig. 8–5*B*.) From Table 8–3, $n = 10$, $\overline{X} = \Sigma X/n = 369/10$ cm $=$ 36.9 cm, and $\overline{Y} = \Sigma Y/n = 103.8/10$ g $= 10.38$ g, so $\Sigma(X - \overline{X})(Y - \overline{Y}) =$

Table 8–3 Computation of Correlation Coefficient for Sample in Fig. 8–3*B*

Observed height X, cm	Observed weight Y, g	$(X - \overline{X})$, cm	$(Y - \overline{Y})$, g	$(X - \overline{X})(Y - \overline{Y})$, cm · g	$(X - \overline{X})^2$, cm^2	$(Y - \overline{Y})^2$, g^2
31	7.8	−5.9	−2.6	15.2	34.8	6.7
32	8.3	−4.9	−2.1	10.2	24.0	4.3
33	7.6	−3.9	−2.8	10.8	15.2	7.7
34	9.1	−2.9	−1.3	3.7	8.4	1.6
35	9.6	−1.9	−0.8	1.5	3.6	0.3
35	9.8	−1.9	−0.6	1.1	3.6	2.0
40	11.8	3.1	1.4	4.4	9.6	2.0
41	12.1	4.1	1.7	7.1	16.8	3.0
42	14.7	5.1	4.3	22.0	26.0	18.7
46	13.0	9.1	2.6	23.8	82.8	6.9
369	103.8	0.0	0.0	99.9	224.9	51.8

99.9 g × cm, $\Sigma(X - \bar{X})^2 = 224.9\ \text{cm}^2$, and $\Sigma(Y - \bar{Y})^2 = 51.8\ \text{g}^2$. Substitute these numbers into the definition of the correlation coefficient to obtain

$$r = \frac{99.9\ \text{g}\cdot\text{cm}}{\sqrt{224.9\ \text{cm}^2 \cdot 51.8\ \text{g}^2}} = 0.925$$

To gain more feeling for the meaning to the magnitude of a correlation coefficient, Table 8–4 lists the values of the correlation coefficients for the observations in Figs. 8–2 and 8–8.

The Relationship between Regression and Correlation

Obviously, it is possible to compute a correlation coefficient for any data suitable for linear regression analysis. Indeed, the correlation coefficients in Table 8–3 all were computed from the same examples we used to illustrate regression analysis. In the context of regression analysis it is possible to add to the meaning of the correlation coefficient. Recall that we selected the regression equation that minimized the sum of squared deviations between the points on the regression line and the value of the dependent variable at each observed value of the independent variable. It can be shown that the correlation coefficient also equals

$$r = \sqrt{1 - \frac{\text{sum of squared deviations from regression line}}{\text{sum of squared deviations from mean}}}$$

where the deviations are all measured for the dependent variable.

Table 8–4 Correlations between Variables in Examples

Figure	Variables	Correlation coefficient, r	Sample size, n
8–7	Height and weight of Martians	.925	10
8–9*A*	Grip force and muscle cross-sectional area in normal people	.938	25
8–9*B*	Grip force and muscle cross-sectional area in normal people	.581	25

Let SS_{res} equal the sum of squared deviations (residuals) from the regression line and SS_{tot} equal the total sum of squared deviations from the mean of the dependent variable. Then

$$r = \sqrt{1 - \frac{SS_{res}}{SS_{tot}}}$$

When there is no variation in the observations about the regression line $SS_{res} = 0$, the correlation coefficient equals 1 (or -1), indicating the dependent variable can be predicted with no uncertainty from the independent variable. On the other hand, when the residual variation about the regression line is the same as the variation about the mean value of the dependent variable, $SS_{res} = SS_{tot}$, there is no trend in the data and $r = 0$. The dependent variable cannot be predicted at all from the independent variable.

The square of the correlation coefficient, r^2, is known as the *coefficient of determination.* Since, from the preceding equation,

$$r^2 = 1 - \frac{SS_{res}}{SS_{tot}}$$

and SS_{tot} is a measure of the total variation in the dependent variable, people say that the coefficient of determination is the fraction of the total variance in the dependent variable "explained" by the regression equation. This is rather unfortunate terminology, because the regression line does not "explain" anything in the sense of providing a mechanistic understanding of the relationship between the dependent and independent variables. Nevertheless, the coefficient of determination is a good description of how clearly a straight line describes the relationship between the two variables.

Likewise, the sum of squared deviations from the regression line, SS_{res}, is just $(n - 2)s_{y \cdot x}^2$ and the sum of squared deviations about the mean, SS_{tot}, is just $(n - 1)s_Y^2$. (Recall the definition of sample variance or standard deviation.) Hence the correlation coefficient is related to the results of regression analysis according to

$$r = \sqrt{1 - \frac{n-2}{n-1} \frac{s_{y \cdot x}^2}{s_Y^2}}$$

Thus, as the standard deviation of the residuals about the regression line $s_{y\cdot x}$ decreases with respect to the total variation in the dependent variable, quantified with s_Y, the ratio $s_{y\cdot x}/s_Y$ decreases and the correlation coefficient increases. Thus, the greater the value of the correlation coefficient, the more precisely the dependent variable can be predicted from the independent variable.

This approach must be used with caution, however, because the absolute uncertainty as described with the confidence interval is usually more informative in that it allows you to gauge the size of the uncertainty in the prediction relative to the size of effect that is of clinical or scientific importance. As Fig. 8–7 showed, it is possible to have correlations well above 0.9 (generally considered quite respectable in biomedical research) and still have substantial uncertainty in the value of an additional observation for a given value of the independent value.

The correlation coefficient is also related to the slope of the regression equation according to

$$r = b\frac{s_X}{s_Y}$$

We can use the following intuitive argument to justify this relationship: When there is no relationship between the two variables under study, both the slope of the regression line and the correlation coefficient are zero.

How to Test Hypotheses about Correlation Coefficients

Earlier in this chapter we tested for a trend by testing the hypothesis that the slope of the line of means was zero using the t test

$$t = \frac{b}{s_b}$$

with $\nu = n - 2$ degrees of freedom. Since we have just noted that the correlation coefficient is zero when the slope of the regression line is zero, we will test the hypothesis that there is no trend relating two variables by testing the hypothesis that the correlation coefficient is zero with the t test

$$t = \frac{r}{\sqrt{(1 - r^2)/(n - 2)}}$$

with $\nu = n - 2$ degrees of freedom. While this statistic looks quite foreign, it is just another way of writing the t statistic used to test the hypothesis that $\beta = 0$.*

Journal Size and Selectivity

As part of an assessment of medical journals' policies regarding how the editors handle the peer review of statistical aspects of manuscripts submitted to their journals, Steven Goodman and his colleagues† surveyed a sample of medical journals. In addition to asking the editors

*To see this, recall that

$$r = \sqrt{1 - \frac{n - 2}{n - 1} \frac{s_{y \cdot x}^2}{s_Y^2}}$$

so

$$s_{y \cdot x}^2 = \frac{n - 1}{n - 2}(1 - r^2)s_Y^2$$

Use this result to eliminate $s_{y \cdot x}$ from

$$s_b = \frac{1}{\sqrt{n - 1}} \frac{s_{y \cdot x}}{s_x}$$

to obtain

$$s_b = \frac{s_Y}{s_X} \sqrt{\frac{1 - r^2}{n - 2}}$$

Substitute this result together with $b = r(s_y/s_x)$ into $t = b/s_b$ to obtain the t test for the correlation coefficient

$$t = \frac{r(s_Y/s_X)}{(s_Y/s_X)\sqrt{(1 - r^2)/(n - 2)}} = \frac{r}{\sqrt{(1 - r^2)/(n - 2)}}$$

†S. N. Goodman, D. G. Altman, S. L. George, "Statistical Reviewing Policies of Medical Journals," *J. Gen. Intern. Med.* **13:**753–756, 1998.

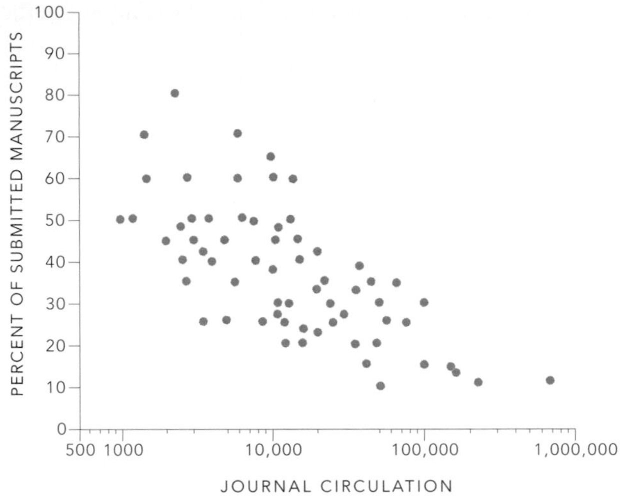

Figure 8–12 There appears to be a relationship between the fraction of submitted papers journals select for publication and the (logarithm of) journal circulation, with larger journals being more selective. *(Based on Fig. 1 of S. N. Goodman, D. G. Altman, S. L. George, "Statistical Reviewing Policies of Medical Journals,"* J. Gen. Intern. Med. ***13:****753–756, 1998.)*

about their policies on statistical review, Goodman and his colleagues also collected data on the percentage of submitted manuscripts that were ultimately accepted for publication and the size of the journals' circulation. Figure 8–12 shows data relating these two variables, which makes it possible to test whether the larger journals are more selective.

Note that rather than plotting the publication rate against the circulation, Fig. 8–12 plots it against the logarithm of the circulation. The reason for this *variable transformation* is to adjust the scale so that the line more closely met the assumptions of correlation, which require that the data be scattered around a straight line. (The Spearman rank correlation coefficient, discussed in the following section, does not require making this assumption.) Variable transformations are a common tool in more advanced statistical methods to account for failures of normality or linearity.*

*For a more detailed discussion of variable transformations, see S. A. Glantz and B. K. Slinker, *Primer of Applied Regression and Analysis of Variance (2nd ed),* New York: McGraw-Hill, 2001, pp 150–153, 163–166.

Logarithmic transformations are particularly useful when the observations span several orders of magnitude, as is the case here. This situation often arises in dose-ranging studies of drugs.

The correlation between acceptance rate and (logarithm of) journal circulation, based on the 113 journals in the sample in Figure 8–12, is 0.64. To test the null hypothesis that there is no linear relationship between acceptance rate and logarithm of journal circulation, compute

$$t = \frac{0.64}{\sqrt{(1 - 0.64^2) / (113 - 2)}} = 8.78$$

The computed value of t exceeds $t_{.001} = 3.38$ for $\nu = 113 - 2 = 111$ degrees of freedom, so we conclude that there is a correlation between journal size and selectivity ($P < .001$).

Does this result *prove* that increasing circulation makes journals more selective? No. An investigator could not manipulate the size of the circulation of the sample of 113 different journals in Figure 8.12, so these data are the results of an observational rather than an experimental study. These two variables could be related to some third underlying *confounding variable* that makes both the observed variables change simultaneously. Indeed, in this case, the underlying confounding variable is probably perceived quality of the journal, with authors willing to submit their manuscripts to more competitive journals because they are more prestigious, and because of the higher quality, more people are willing to subscribe to the journal.

When interpreting the results of regression analysis, it is important to keep the distinction between observational and experimental studies in mind. When investigators can actively manipulate the independent variable and observe changes in the dependent variable, they can draw strong conclusions about how changes in the independent variable *cause* changes in the dependent variable. On the other hand, when investigators only observe the two variables changing together, they can only observe an *association* between them in which one changes as the other changes. It is impossible to rule out the possibility that both variables are independently responding to some third factor and that the independent variable does not causally affect the dependent variable.

THE SPEARMAN RANK CORRELATION COEFFICIENT

It is often desirable to test the hypothesis that there is a trend in a clinical state, measured on an ordinal scale, as another variable changes. The Pearson product-moment correlation coefficient is a parametric statistic designed to be used on data distributed normally along interval scales, so it cannot be used. It also requires that the trend relating the two variables be linear. When the sample suggests that the population from which both variables were drawn from does not meet these criteria, it is possible to compute a measure of association based on the *ranks* rather than the values of the observations. This new correlation coefficient, called the *Spearman rank correlation coefficient* r_s, is based on ranks and can be used for data quantified with an ordinal scale.* The Spearman rank correlation coefficient is a *nonparametric* statistic because it does not require that the observations be drawn from a normally distributed population.†

The idea behind the Spearman rank correlation coefficient is simple. The values of the two variables are ranked in ascending (or descending) order, taking into account the signs of the values. For example, ranking 1,

*Another rank correlation coefficient, known as the *Kendall rank correlation coefficient* τ, can be generalized to the case in which there are multiple independent variables. For problems involving only two variables it yields conclusions identical to the Spearman rank correlation coefficient, although the value of τ associated with a given set of observations differs from the value of r_s associated with the same observations. For a discussion of both procedures, see S. Siegel and N. J. Castellar, Jr., *Nonparametric Statistics for the Behavioral Sciences* (2d ed.), McGraw-Hill, New York, 1988, chap. 9, "Measures of Association and Their Tests of Significance."

†In addition to being explicitly designed to analyze data measured on a rank scale, nonparametric methods can be used in cases where the normality assumptions that underlie the parametric methods are not met or you do not want to assume that they are met. When the assumptions of parametric methods are not met, the nonparametric methods are appropriate. When either nonparametric or parametric methods are appropriate, the nonparametric methods generally have lower power than the parametric methods. In the case of Pearson (parametric) and Spearman (nonparametric) correlations, this difference is very small. For example, sizes above 10, the power of the Spearman rank order correlation coefficient is computed exactly the same as for the Pearson product-correlation, except that σ_Z is computed as

$$\sigma_Z = \sqrt{\frac{1.060}{n - 3}}$$

i.e., with 1.060 in the numerator instead of 1.000.

-1, and 2 (from the smallest value -1 to the largest value, 2) yields the ranks 2, 1, and 3, respectively. Next, the Pearson product-moment correlation between the *ranks* (as opposed to the observations) is computed using the same formula as before. A mathematically equivalent formula for the Spearman rank correlation coefficient that is easier to compute is

$$r_s = 1 - \frac{6\Sigma d^2}{n^3 - n}$$

in which d is the difference of the two ranks associated with each point. The resulting correlation coefficient can then be compared with the population of all possible values it would take on if there were in fact no association between the two variables. If the value of r_s associated with the data is larger than this critical value, we conclude that the observations are not compatible with the hypothesis of no association between the two variables.

Table 8–5 illustrates how to compute r_s for the observations in Fig. 8–3. Both the variables (height and weight) are ranked from 1 to 10 (since there are 10 data points), 1 being assigned to the smallest value and 10 to the largest value. When there is a tie, as there is when

Table 8–5 Computation of Spearman Rank Correlation Coefficient for Observations in Fig. 8–3

Height		Weight		
Value, cm	Rank*	Value, g	Rank*	Difference of ranks d
31	1	7.7	2	−1
32	2	8.3	3	−1
33	3	7.6	1	2
34	4	9.1	4	0
35	5.5	9.6	5	0.5
35	5.5	9.9	6	−0.5
40	7	11.8	7	0
41	8	12.2	8	0
42	9	14.8	9	0
46	10	15.0	10	0

*1 = smallest value; 10 = largest value.

the height equals 35 cm, both values are assigned the mean of the ranks that would be used if there were no tie. Since the weight tends to increase as height increases, the ranks of both variables increase together. The Pearson correlation of these two lists of ranks is the Spearman rank correlation coefficient.

The Spearman rank correlation coefficient for the data in Table 8–5 is

$$r_s = 1 - \frac{6[(-1)^2 + (-1)^2 + 2^2 + 0^2 + 0.5^2 + (-0.5)^2 + 0^2 + 0^2 + 0^2 + 0^2]}{10^3 - 10}$$

$$= 0.96$$

Table 8–6 gives various risks of making a Type I error. The observed value of r_s exceeds .903, the critical value for the most extreme .1 percent of values when there are $n = 10$ data points, so we can report that there is an association between weight and height ($P < .001$).

Table 8–6 Critical Values for Spearman Rank Correlation Coefficient*

	Probability of greater value *P*								
n	.50	.20	.10	.05	.02	.01	.005	.002	.001
4	.600	1.000	1.000						
5	.500	.800	.900	1.000	1.000				
6	.371	.657	.829	.886	.943	1.000	1.000		
7	.321	.571	.714	.786	.893	.929	.964	1.000	1.000
8	.310	.524	.643	.738	.833	.881	.905	.952	.976
9	.267	.483	.600	.700	.783	.833	.867	.917	.933
10	.248	.455	.564	.648	.745	.794	.830	.879	.903
11	.236	.427	.536	.618	.709	.755	.800	.845	.873
12	.217	.406	.503	.587	.678	.727	.769	.818	.846
13	.209	.385	.484	.560	.648	.703	.747	.791	.824
14	.200	.367	.464	.538	.626	.679	.723	.771	.802
15	.189	.354	.446	.521	.604	.654	.700	.750	.779
16	.182	.341	.429	.503	.582	.635	.679	.729	.762
17	.176	.328	.414	.485	.566	.615	.662	.713	.748
18	.170	.317	.401	.472	.550	.600	.643	.695	.728
19	.165	.309	.391	.460	.535	.584	.628	.677	.712
20	.161	.299	.380	.447	.520	.570	.612	.662	.696

(continued)

Table 8–6 Critical Values for Spearman Rank Correlation Coefficient* (*Continued*)

	Probability of greater value *P*								
n	.50	.20	.10	.05	.02	.01	.005	.002	.001
21	.156	.292	.370	.435	.508	.556	.599	.648	.681
22	.152	.284	.361	.425	.496	.544	.586	.634	.667
23	.148	.278	.353	.415	.486	.532	.573	.622	.654
24	.144	.271	.344	.406	.476	.521	.562	.610	.642
25	.142	.265	.337	.398	.466	.511	.551	.598	.630
26	.138	.259	.331	.390	.457	.501	.541	.587	.619
27	.136	.255	.324	.382	.448	.491	.531	.577	.608
28	.133	.250	.317	.375	.440	.483	.522	.567	.598
29	.130	.245	.312	.368	.433	.475	.513	.558	.589
30	.128	.240	.306	.362	.425	.467	.504	.549	.580
31	.126	.236	.301	.356	.418	.459	.496	.541	.571
32	.124	.232	.296	.350	.412	.452	.489	.533	.563
33	.121	.229	.291	.345	.405	.446	.482	.525	.554
34	.120	.225	.287	.340	.399	.439	.475	.517	.547
35	.118	.222	.283	.335	.394	.433	.468	.510	.539
36	.116	.219	.279	.330	.388	.427	.462	.504	.533
37	.114	.216	.275	.325	.383	.421	.456	.497	.526
38	.113	.212	.271	.321	.378	.415	.450	.491	.519
39	.111	.210	.267	.317	.373	.410	.444	.485	.513
40	.110	.207	.264	.313	.368	.405	.439	.479	.507
41	.108	.204	.261	.309	.364	.400	.433	.473	.501
42	.107	.202	.257	.305	.359	.395	.428	.468	.495
43	.105	.199	.254	.301	.355	.391	.423	.463	.490
44	.104	.197	.251	.298	.351	.386	.419	.458	.484
45	.103	.194	.248	.294	.347	.382	.414	.453	.479
46	.102	.192	.246	.291	.343	.378	.410	.448	.474
47	.101	.190	.243	.288	.340	.374	.405	.443	.469
48	.100	.188	.240	.285	.336	.370	.401	.439	.465
49	.098	.186	.238	.282	.333	.366	.397	.434	.460
50	.097	.184	.235	.279	.329	.363	.393	.430	.456

*For sample sizes greater than 50, use

$$t = \frac{r_s}{\sqrt{(1 - r_s^2)/(n - 2)}}$$

with $\nu = n - 2$ degrees of freedom to obtain the approximate *P* value.

Source: Adapted from J. H. Zar, *Biostatistical Analysis*. Prentice-Hall, Englewood Cliffs, N.J., 1974, p. 498. Used by permission.

In this example, of course, we could just as well have used the Pearson product-moment correlation. Had we been dealing with data measured on an ordinal scale, we would have had to use the Spearman rank correlation coefficient.

Variation among Interns in Use of Laboratory Tests: Relation to Quality of Care

Is extensive use of laboratory tests a mark of a careful and thorough physician or one who carelessly wastes the patients' money? To study this question, Steven Schroeder and colleagues* studied the use of laboratory tests among 21 medical interns. Each intern's clinical ability was ranked with respect to the rest of the interns by a panel of faculty members. These ranks form an ordinal scale. The intern who was judged to have the most clinical ability was ranked 1, and the one judged to have the least clinical ability was ranked 21. The investigators measured intensity of laboratory use by computing the total cost of laboratory services ordered by each intern during the patients' first 3 days of hospitalization, when the intern would be most actively formulating a diagnosis. Mean costs of laboratory use were computed for each intern's group of patients and ranked in order of increasing cost. Figure 8–13 shows the results of this procedure. Schroeder and his colleagues report that the Spearman rank order correlation for these two sets of ranks was −.13. This value does not exceed .435, the critical value for r_s to be considered "big" with $P < .05$.

Does this mean that there is no apparent relationship between the quality of an intern and the amount of money spent on laboratory tests? No. Figure 8–13*B* shows that there is probably a relationship between quality of care and amount of money spent on laboratory tests. The less skilled interns tend to fall at the ends of the cost spectrum; they order many fewer or many more tests than the better interns.

What caused this apparent error? Correlation analysis, whether based on the Pearson or Spearman correlation coefficient, is based on the assumption that if the two variables are related to each other, the relationship takes the form of a consistently upward or downward trend. When

*S. A. Schroeder, A. Schliftman, and T. E. Piemine, "Variation among Physicians in Use of Laboratory Tests: Relation to Quality of Care." *Med. Care,* **12:**709–713, 1974.

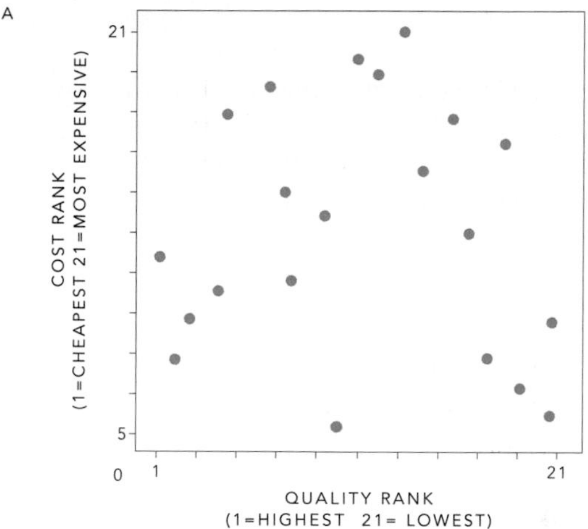

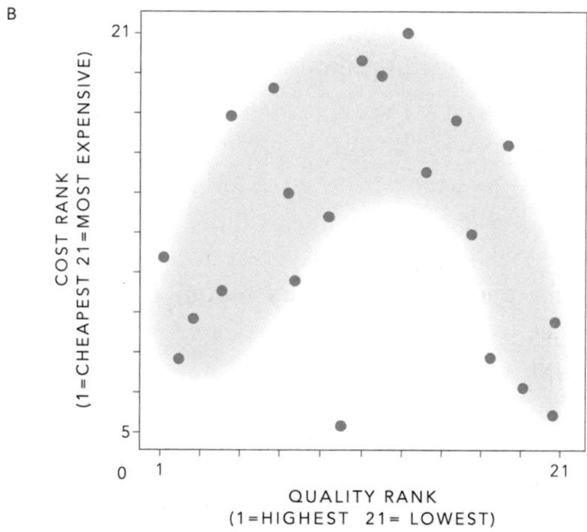

Figure 8–13 ***(A)*** Relationship between the relative clinical skill of 21 interns and the relative amount of money each spent on laboratory tests during the first 3 days of a patient's hospitalization. The Spearman rank correlation coefficient for these data is only −.13, which could be interpreted as showing that there is no relationship between clinical skill and expenditures for laboratory tests. ***(B)*** Closer examination of the data, however, suggests that the best and the worst interns spend less money than those closer to the midrange of skill. Since correlation techniques generally fail to detect such U-shaped relationships, it is important always to examine the raw data as well as the numerical results of a regression or correlation analysis. (*Adapted from fig. 1 of S. A. Schroeder, A. Schliftman, and T. E. Piemine, "Variation Among Physicians in Use of Laboratory Tests: Relation to Quality of Care,"* Med. Care, ***12:****709–713, 1974.*)

the relationship is U-shaped (as in Fig. 8–13) correlation procedures will fail to detect the relationship.

This example illustrates an important rule that should be scrupulously observed when using any form of regression or correlation analysis: Do not just look at the numbers. *Always look at a plot of the raw data* to make sure the data are consistent with the assumptions behind the method of analysis.

POWER AND SAMPLE SIZE IN REGRESSION AND CORRELATION

Power and sample-size computations for regression and correlation are straightforward, based on the fact that testing for a slope significantly different from zero is equivalent to testing for a correlation coefficient significantly different from zero.

The key to these computations is transforming the correlation coefficient according to

$$Z = \frac{1}{2} \ln \left(\frac{1 + r}{1 - r} \right)$$

Z is normally distributed with standard deviation

$$\sigma_Z = \sqrt{\frac{1}{n - 3}}$$

Thus,

$$z = \frac{Z}{\sigma_Z}$$

follows the standard normal distribution if there is no correlation between the dependent and independent variables in the underlying population. If there is a correlation in the underlying population of ρ, then

$$z = \frac{Z - Z_\rho}{\sigma_Z}$$

will be normally distributed, where

$$Z_\rho = \frac{1}{2} \ln \left(\frac{1 + \rho}{1 - \rho} \right)$$

We will use this fact to compute power analogously to the way we did it for the t test.*

For example, let us compute the power of a regression analysis to detect a correlation of $\rho = .9$ in the underlying population with 95 percent confidence based on a sample size of 10 observations. We first compute

$$Z_\rho = \frac{1}{2} \ln \left(\frac{1 + \rho}{1 - \rho} \right) = \frac{1}{2} \ln \left(\frac{1 + .9}{1 - .9} \right) = 1.472$$

and

$$\sigma_Z = \sqrt{\frac{1}{n - 3}} = .378$$

Therefore, if the actual correlation in the underlying population is .9, the distribution of z is centered on $Z_\rho / \sigma_Z = 1.472/.378 = 3.894$ (Figure 8–14; compare with Fig. 6–6).

If we use $\alpha = 0.05$ to require 95 percent confidence in asserting that the correlation is different from zero, then we will reject the null hypothesis when the value of z associated with the data exceeds $z_{\alpha(2)} = 1.960$, the (two-tail) value that defines the most extreme values of the normal distribution (from Table 4–1). This value is

*This fact can also be used as an alternative technique to test the hypothesis that the correlation coefficient is zero by computing the confidence interval for the observed correlation coefficient as

$$Z - z_\alpha \sigma_Z < Z_\rho < Z + z_\alpha \sigma_Z$$

then converting the upper and lower limits of Z back to correlations by inverting the transformation of r to Z.

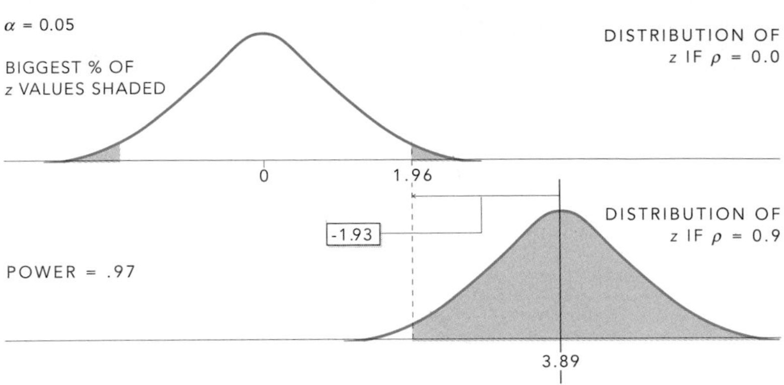

Figure 8–14 The power of a correlation to detect a correlation in the population of $\rho = .9$ with a sample size of 10 and 95 percent confidence is the area under the actual distribution of the z test statistic above $z_\alpha = 1.960$. If $\rho = 0.9$ the actual distribution of z will be centered on 3.894.

$1.960 - 3.894 = -1.934$ below the center of the actual distribution of z. From Table 6–2, .97 of the possible z values is to the right of -1.934. Thus, the power of a linear regression or correlation of .9 with 95 percent confidence and a sample size of 10 is 97 percent.

This process can be reduced to a simple equation. The power of linear regression or correlation to detect a correlation of ρ is the area of the standard normal distribution to the right of

$$z_{1-\beta(\text{upper})} = z_{\alpha(2)} - \frac{Z_\rho}{\sqrt{\dfrac{1}{n-3}}}$$

To obtain the sample size necessary to detect a specified correlation with a specified power to a specified level of confidence comes from solving this equation for n

$$n = \left(\frac{z_{\alpha(2)} - z_{1-\beta(\text{upper})}}{Z_\rho}\right)^2 + 3$$

COMPARING TWO DIFFERENT MEASUREMENTS OF THE SAME THING: THE BLAND-ALTMAN METHOD*

The need often arises, particularly in clinical studies, to compare two different ways of measuring the same thing, when neither method is perfect. For example, as medical technology progresses, less invasive procedures for measuring physiological parameters are developed. The question that arises in the process of developing these new techniques is: How well do they agree with older, more invasive, techniques? Similar questions arise when assessing the repeatability of a measurement: If I measure the same thing twice, how much do the measurements vary? Why not simply compute a regression equation or correlation coefficient for the two sets of observations?

First, neither variable is a natural independent variable, and the choice of independent variable affects the results in a regression equation. The situation in comparing two imperfect clinical measurements of the same thing differs from the *calibration* problem that is common in laboratory science, in which one compares measured values with a known standard. For example, one could mix a known amount of salt with a known amount of distilled water to obtain a given saline concentration, then measure the salt concentrations with some device. It would then be possible to plot the measured salt concentration against the actual salt concentration to obtain a calibration curve. The standard error of the estimate would represent a good measure of uncertainty in the measurement. When comparing two imperfect clinical measurements, there is no such standard.

Second, the correlation coefficient measures the strength of agreement against the null hypothesis of no relationship. When comparing two measurements of the same thing, there will almost always be a relationship between these two measures, so the null hypothesis of no relationship that is implicit in correlation analysis makes no sense.

Third, correlation depends on the range of data in the sample. All else being equal, the wider the range of the observations, the higher the correlation. The presence of an outlier can lead to a high correlation even if there is a good deal of scatter among the rest of the observations.

*This section deals with more advanced material and can be skipped with no loss of continuity.

J. Martin Bland and Douglas Altman* developed a simple descriptive technique to assess the agreement between two imperfect clinical measurements or repeatability of duplicate observations. The idea is quite simple: The most straightforward measure of disagreement between the two observations is the difference, so simply compute the differences between all the pairs of observations. Next, compute the mean and standard deviation of the differences. The mean difference is a measure of the *bias* between the two observations and the standard deviation is a measure of the variation between the two observations. Finally, because both observations are equally good (or bad), our best estimate of the true value of the variable being measured is the mean of the two different observations. Plotting the difference against the mean gives an indication of whether there are any systematic differences between the two measurement techniques as a function of the magnitude of the thing being measured.

We will now illustrate the Bland-Altman method with an example.

Assessing Mitral Regurgitation with Echocardiography

The heart pumps blood around the body. The blood goes from the right heart to the lungs, where it takes up oxygen and releases waste gases, to the left heart, where it is pumped to the body, then back to the right heart. This pumping requires that there be valves inside the heart to keep the blood going in the correct direction when the heart contracts. The valve between the lungs and the left heart, known as the mitral valve, prevents blood from being pushed back into the lungs when the left heart is contracting to push the blood to the body. When this valve becomes diseased, it allows blood to be pushed back toward the lungs when the left heart contracts, a situation called *mitral regurgitation*. Mitral regurgitation is bad because it reduces the forward flow of blood

*For a more detailed discussion of the Bland-Altman method, see D. G. Altman and J. M. Bland, "Measurement in Medicine: The Analysis of Method Comparison Studies," *Statistician* **32:**307–317, 1983, or J. M. Bland and D. G. Altman, "Statistical Methods for Assessing Agreement Between Two Measures of Clinical Measurement," *Lancet* **1**(8476):307–310, 1986.

from the heart to the body and also has adverse effects on the lungs. If it gets bad enough, it becomes necessary to do open heart surgery to replace the valve. Hence, measuring the amount of mitral regurgitation is an important clinical problem.

The amount of regurgitation is quantified with the *regurgitant fraction,*

$$\text{Regurgitant fraction} = \frac{\text{mitral flow (into the left heart)} - \text{aortic flow (out to the body)}}{\text{mitral flow}}$$

If the mitral valve is working properly, all the mitral flow into the left heart will appear as flow out into the aorta, and the regurgitant fraction will be 0. As the valve becomes more and more incompetent, the regurgitant fraction will increase towards 1.

The traditional way to measure regurgitant fraction has been to do a cardiac catheterization, in which a small tube (called a catheter) is threaded from an artery in the person's arm or leg into the heart; then, a chemical known as a contrast agent that appears opaque on an x-ray is injected into the heart so that the regurgitant flow can be seen in an x-ray motion picture taken while the contrast agent is being injected. This is an unpleasant, expensive, and potentially dangerous procedure.

Andrew MacIsaac and colleagues* proposed using a noninvasive procedure known as Doppler echocardiography to replace cardiac catheterization as a way to measure regurgitant fraction. Doppler echocardiography involves placing a device that sends high frequency sound waves into the heart and records the reflections on the chest of a person. This information can be used to measure flows into and out of the heart, much as weather radar measures flows of air to track storms and other weather patterns. They compared their method with traditional cardiac catheterization to assess the level of agreement between the two methods.

Table 8–7 shows the results of their study and Figure 8–15*A*

*A. I. MacIsaac, I. G. McDonald, R. L. G. Kirsner, S. A. Graham, R. W. Gill, "Quantification of Mitral Regurgitation by Integrated Doppler Backscatter Power," *J. Am. Coll. Cardiol.* **24:**690–695, 1994. Data used with permission.

Table 8–7 Mitral Value Regurgitant Fraction Measured with Doppler Echocardiography and Cardiac Catheterization in 20 People

Observations			
Doppler	Catheterization	Difference	Mean
.49	.62	−.13	.56
.83	.72	.11	.78
.71	.63	.08	.67
.38	.61	−.23	.50
.57	.49	.08	.53
.68	.79	−.11	.74
.69	.72	−.03	.71
.07	.11	−.04	.09
.75	.66	.09	.71
.52	.74	−.22	.63
.78	.83	−.05	.81
.71	.66	.05	.69
.16	.34	.18	.25
.33	.50	−.17	.42
.57	.62	−.05	.60
.11	.00	.11	.06
.43	.45	−.02	.44
.11	.06	.05	.85
.31	.46	−.15	.39
.20	.03	.17	.12
.47	.50	−.03	.49
		Mean = −.03	
		SD = .12	

shows a plot of the two measurements against each other, with each person in the study contributing one point. The correlation between the two methods is .89. This fact indicates reasonable agreement, but does not tell us anything about the quantitative nature of the agreement in terms of how well the two methods quantify mitral regurgitant fraction.

Table 8–7 also shows the computations necessary to construct a Bland-Altman description of how well the two methods agree. The third column in the table represents the differences between the two determinations of regurgitant fraction, and the last column is the mean

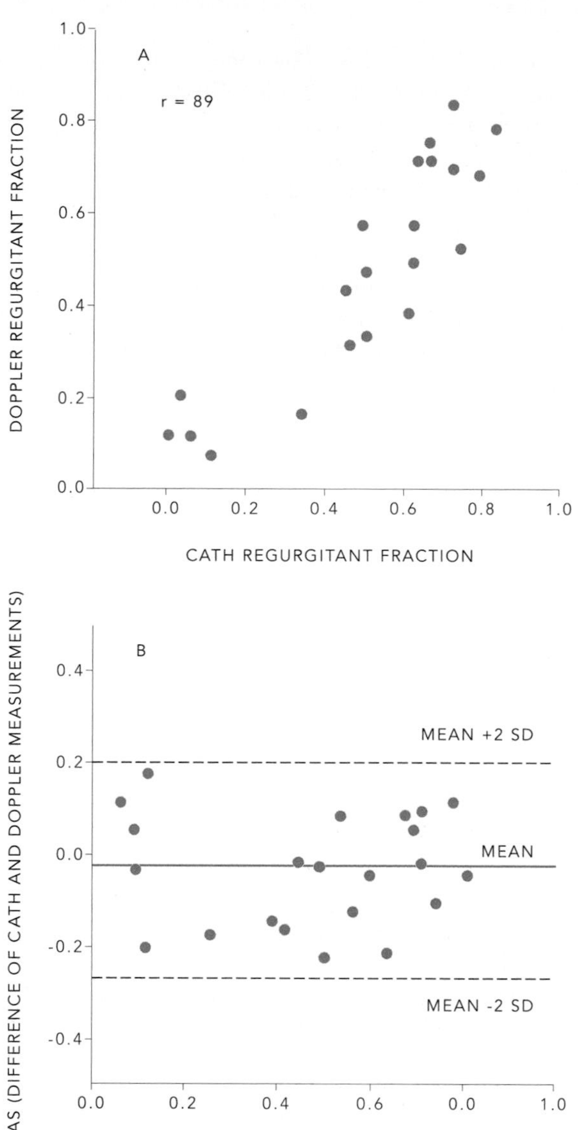

Figure 8–15 ***(A)*** Relationship between mitral regurgitant fraction measured with cardiac catheterization and Doppler echocardiography in 20 people. ***(B)*** Bland-Altman curve for the data in panel ***A.*** Note that there is little systematic difference between the two measurements.

of the two methods. Figure 8–15*B* shows a plot of the differences against the mean responses. There are several points to be made from this information. First, the mean difference in regurgitant fraction between the two methods is only −.03, which indicates that there is no systemic bias between the two different methods. Next, the standard deviation of the differences is .12, which is small compared to the levels of regurgitation observed (which range up to .83). There also does not appear to be a relationship between the difference between the two observations and the mean mitral regurgitation. Taking the range two standard deviations above and below the mean difference gives a measure of the extent of disagreement between the two methods. These results lead to the conclusion that Doppler echocardiography appears to yield a measure of mitral regurgitation that is as good as the more invasive cardiac catheterization procedure.

Similar procedures could be used to quantify repeatability of two observations of the same thing by different observers or even repeat observations by the same observer.

SUMMARY

The methods described in this chapter allow us to quantify the relationship between two variables. The basic approach is the same as in earlier statistical methods: we described the nature of the underlying population, summarized this information with appropriate statistical parameters, then developed procedures for estimating these parameters and their standard errors from one or more samples. When relating two variables with regression or correlation, it is particularly important to examine a graph of the data to see that the assumptions underlying the statistical method you are using is reasonably satisfied by the data you have collected.

PROBLEMS

8-1 Plot the data and compute the linear regression of Y on X and correlation coefficient for each of the following sets of observations.

a

X	Y
30	40
37	50
30	40
47	60

b

X	Y
30	20
37	25
30	20
47	35
40	50

c

X	Y
30	50
37	62
30	50
47	72
40	10

b

X	Y
50	62
40	50
60	72

c

X	Y
50	13
40	10
60	23
20	60
25	74
20	60
35	84

In each case, draw the regression line on the same plot as the data. What stays the same and what changes? Why?

8-2 Plot the data and compute the linear regression of Y on X and correlation coefficient for each of the following sets of observations.

a

X	Y
15	31
19	25
15	41
29	30
20	37
25	30
20	47
35	60
25	40

b

X	Y
20	40
21	75
20	40
31	85
30	50
18	65
30	50
28	75
40	60
15	55
40	60
25	65

In each case, draw the regression line on the same plot as the data. Discuss the results.

8-3 The plots below show data from four different experiments. Compute the regression and correlation coefficients for each of these four sets of data. Discuss the similarities and differences among these sets of data. Include an examination of the assumptions made in linear regression and correlation analyses. (This example is from F. J. Anscombe, "Graphs in Statistical Analysis," *Am. Stat.*, **27**:17–21, 1973.) The data are listed on the top of the next page.

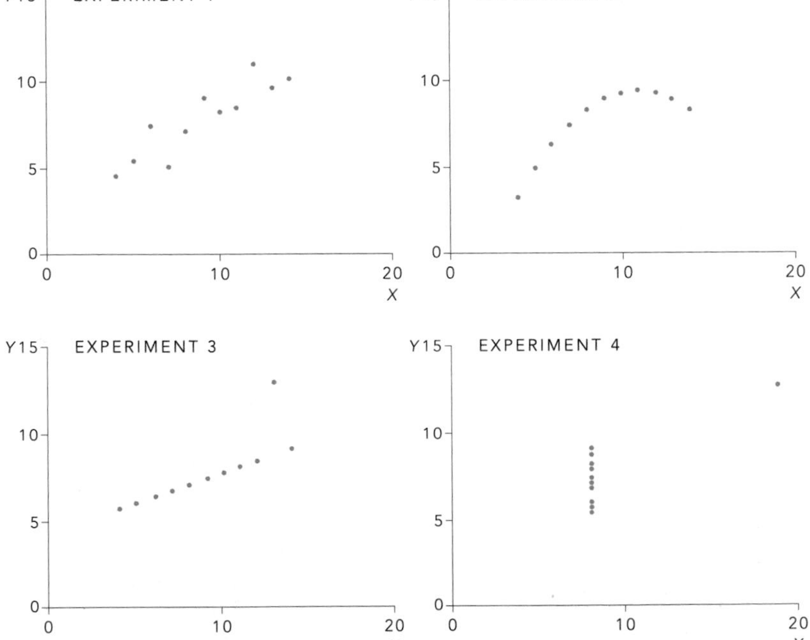

Experiment 1		Experiment 2		Experiment 3		Experiment 4	
X	Y	X	Y	X	Y	X	Y
10	8.04	10	9.14	10	7.46	8	6.58
8	6.95	8	8.14	8	6.77	8	5.76
13	7.58	13	8.74	13	12.74	8	7.71
9	8.81	9	8.77	9	7.11	8	8.84
11	8.33	11	9.26	11	7.81	8	8.47
14	9.96	14	8.10	14	8.84	8	7.04
6	7.24	6	6.13	6	6.08	8	5.25
4	4.26	4	3.10	4	5.39	19	12.50
12	10.84	12	9.13	12	8.15	8	5.56
7	4.82	7	7.26	7	6.42	8	7.91
5	5.68	5	4.74	5	5.73	8	6.89
ΣX	99		99		99		99
ΣY	82.5		82.5		82.5		82.5
ΣX^2	1001		1001		1001		1001
ΣY^2	660		660		660		660
ΣXY	797.5		797.5		797.5		797.5

8-4 Polychlorinated biphenyls (PCBs) are compounds that were once used as an insulating material in electrical transformers before being banned in the United States during the 1970s because of concerns about their toxicity. Despite the ban, PCBs can still be detected in most people because they are persistent in the environment and tend to accumulate in fat tissue as animals that absorb PCBs eat other animals that have absorbed PCBs. One of the major current sources of human PCB exposure is eating fatty fish caught from contaminated waters. In the early 1980s, the husband and wife team of Joseph Jacobsen and Sandra Jacobsen ("Intellectual Impairment in Children Exposed to Polychlorinated Biphenyls In Utero," *N. Engl. J. Med.*, **335:**783–789, 1996) began a prospective study to examine the relationship between PCB levels in a group of women who ate Lake Michigan fish and the intellectual development of their children. The amount of PCBs (ng/g of fat) detected in maternal milk was used as an indicator of prenatal exposure to PCBs. The Jacobsens then administered the Wechsler Intelligence Scale for Children IQ test to the children when they were 11 years old. Is there any association between maternal PCB level and the childrens' IQ score?

Maternal milk PCB level (ng/g of fat)	Full Scale IQ
539	116
1093	108
1665	94
476	127
550	122
999	97
974	85
1205	115
604	112
850	108
596	112
547	105
1164	95
905	108

8-5 The ability to measure hormone levels based on a blood spot (like that used by diabetics for glucose monitoring) has several advantages over measurements based on a blood draw. First, blood spots allow for repeated measurements over the time course of minutes and hours. Second, they can be collected with minimal training by a research assistant or the subject. Finally, they are easy to store in a variety of experimental conditions. The low levels of hormone in both blood spots and blood draws are currently measured by a technique called the radioimmunoassay (RIA), an assay based on binding of a radioactively labeled hormone to a specific antibody. Elizabeth Shirtcliff and colleagues ("Assaying Estradiol in Biobehavioral Studies Using Saliva and Blood Spots: Simple Radioimmunoassay Protocols, Reliability and Comparative Validity," *Horm. Behav.* **38:**137–147, 2000) used a modification of a commercially available RIA to detect estradiol (the primary estrogen found in humans) in blood spots and compared the results to those obtained by blood draw. How good is the agreement between the volumes measured using these two techniques? Here are her results:

Estradiol measurements	
Blood spot estradiol (pg/mL)	Blood draw estradiol (pg/mL)
17	25
18	29
21	24
22	33
27	35
30	40
34	40
35	45
36	58
40	63
44	70
45	60
49	70
50	95
52	105
53	108
57	95
58	90
72	130
138	200

8-6 Arteries adjust their size on a minute-to-minute basis to meet the needs of the body for blood to carry oxygen to the tissues and to remove waste products. A substantial part of this response is mediated by the one cell thick lining of the arteries known as the vascular endothelium responding to nitric oxide that the endothelium produces from the amino acid L-arginine. As part of an investigation of the effect of secondhand smoke on the ability of the endothelium to dilate arteries, Stuart Hutchison and his colleagues ("Secondhand Tobacco Smoke Impairs Rabbit Pulmonary Artery Endothelium-Dependent Relaxation," *Chest* **120:**2004–2012, 2001) examined the relationship between how much segments of arteries relaxed after being exposed to different levels of L-arginine and subjected to two different stimuli, acetylcholine and a drug, A23187. Is there a relationship between relaxation and L-arginine level in the presence of these two different relaxing agents? (Note: To "linearize" the data, take logarithms of the arginine levels before doing the analysis.) Here are the data:

Acetylcholine		A23187	
Arginine level	Relaxation Force (%)	Arginine level	Relaxation Force (%)
.02	−10	.03	−2
.03	−21	.04	−47
.1	−48	.10	−36
.5	−52	.13	−27
.6	−41	.5	−43
.7	−52	.6	−56
.9	−67	.6	−50
.9	−58	.7	−77
.9	−32	.8	−67
1.2	−58	.8	−42
1.3	−29	1.2	−60
		1.2	−36
		1.6	−68

8-7 Erectile dysfunction is widely recognized to be associated with diabetes and cardiovascular disease. To investigate whether erectile dysfunction was associated with lower urinary tract infections, Wo-Sik Chung and colleagues ("Lower Urinary Tract Symptoms and Sexual Dysfunction in Community-Dwelling Men," *Mayo Clin. Proc.* **79:**745–749, 2004) administered standard questionnaires to men between ages 40 and 70 years to assess the presence of lower urinary tract infections as well as questions regarding erectile function, with higher scores on the questionnaires indicating more serious problems with urinary tract infections and better erectile function, respectively. Is there evidence for a relationship between urinary tract infections and erectile dysfunction? Here are the data:

Urinary Tract Infection Score	Erectile Function Score
1	14
0	15
9	6
6	11
5	12
5	10
0	11

(continued)

Urinary Tract Infection Score	Erectile Function Score
4	12
8	10
7	8
0	14
10	3
8	9
4	12
16	3
8	9
2	13
13	2
10	4
18	4

8-8 Mouthwashes that contain chlorhexidine have been shown to be effective in preventing formation of dental plaque, but they taste terrible and may stain the teeth. Ammonium chloride mouth rinses taste better and do not generally stain the teeth, so they are used in several commercially available mouthwashes even though they are not thought to effectively inhibit plaque formation. In light of the continuing use of ammonium chloride-based mouthwashes, F. P. Ashley and colleagues ("Effect of a 0.1% Cetylpyridinium Chloride Mouthrinse on the Accumulation and Biochemical Composition of Dental Plaque in Young Adults," *Caries Res.*, **18**:465–471, 1984) studied the use of such a rinse. Two treatments were studied: a control inactive rinse over a 48-hour period and an active rinse over a 48-hour period. Each subject received both treatments in random order. The amount of plaque was assessed by a clinical score after 24 and 48 hours and by measuring the weight of the plaque accumulation after 48 hours. To see if the clinical scores could be effectively used to assess plaque buildup at 24 hours (when the actual weight of plaque was not measured), these workers correlated the clinical scores and amount of plaque obtained at 48 hours. Do these data suggest that there is a strong association between the clinical score and the amount of plaque?

Clinical score	Dry weight of plaque (mg)
25	2.7
32	1.2
45	2.7
60	2.1
60	3.5
65	2.8
68	3.7
78	8.9
80	5.8
83	4.0
83	4.0
100	5.1
110	5.1
120	4.8
125	5.8
140	11.7
143	8.5
143	11.1
145	7.1
148	14.2
153	12.2

8-9 As part of a study of the nature of cancers of the gum and lower jaw, Eiji Nakayama and his colleagues ("The Correlation of Histological Features with a Panoramic Radiography Pattern and a Computed Tomography Pattern of Bone Destruction in Carcinoma of the Mandibular Gingiva," *Oral Surg., Oral Med., Oral Path., Oral Radiol, and Endodontics* **96:**774–782, 2003) were interested in relating the extent of cancer invasion, determined by direct histological investigation with the levels of invasion measured on a computed tomographic scan of people with cancer. They measured both variables on an ordinal scale as follows:

1. Erosive
2. Erosive and Partially Mixed
3. Mixed
4. Mixed and Partially Invasive
5. Invasive

Is there a relationship between these two ways of quantifying the extent of cancer between these two ways of assessing the disease severity? Is the relationship strong enough to use these two methods interchangeably? Here are the data:

Histology	Computed Tomography
3	5
3	2
1	1
4	5
3	3
3	3
5	4
4	3
4	3
3	3
5	5
4	3
4	4
2	2
3	5
1	3
3	2
2	3
4	3
2	3
3	2
2	3
3	3
3	3
2	5

8-10 What is the power of the study of journal circulation and selectivity described in Fig. 8–12 to detect a correlation of .6 with 95 percent confidence? (There are 113 journals in the sample.)

8-11 What sample size is necessary to have an 80 percent power for detecting a correlation between journal circulation and selectivity with 95 percent confidence if the actual correlation in the population is .6?

8-12 Clinical and epidemiologic studies have demonstrated an association between high blood pressure, diabetes, and high levels of lipids measured in blood. In addition, several studies demonstrated that people with high blood pressure have lower insulin sensitivity than people with normal blood pressure, and that physical fitness affects insulin sensitivity. To investigate whether there is a genetic component of the relationship between high blood pressure and insulin sensitivity, Tomas Endre and colleagues ("Insulin Resistance Is Coupled to Low Physical Fitness in Normotensive Men with a Family History of Hypertension," *J. Hypertens.* **12:**81–88, 1994) investigated the relationship between insulin sensitivity and a measure of physical fitness in two groups of men with normal blood pressure, one with immediate relatives who have high blood pressure and a similar group of men from families with normal blood pressure. They used the waist-to-hip ratio of the men as a measure of physical fitness and examined the relationship between it and insulin sensitivity index in these two groups of men. Is the relationship the same in these two groups of men? (Use the logarithm of the insulin sensitivity index as the dependent variable in order to linearize the relationship between the two variables.)

Controls (no immediate family member with high blood pressure)			Relatives (immediate family member with high blood pressure)		
Waist/hip ratio, R	Insulin sensitivity	Log (insulin sensitivity), I	Waist/hip ratio, R	Insulin sensitivity	Log (insulin sensitivity) I
0.775	21.0	1.322	0.800	10.0	1.000
0.800	20.0	1.301	0.810	5.0	0.699
0.810	13.5	1.130	0.850	9.5	0.978
0.800	8.5	0.929	0.875	2.5	0.398
0.850	10.5	1.021	0.850	4.0	0.602
0.860	10.0	1.000	0.870	5.8	0.760
0.925	12.8	1.106	0.910	9.8	0.989
0.900	9.0	0.954	0.925	8.0	0.903
0.925	6.5	0.813	0.925	6.0	0.778
0.945	11.0	1.041	0.940	4.3	0.628
0.945	10.5	1.021	0.945	8.5	0.929
0.950	9.5	0.978	0.960	9.0	0.954
0.975	5.5	0.740	1.100	8.5	0.929
1.050	6.0	0.778	1.100	4.5	0.653
1.075	3.8	0.574	0.990	2.3	0.352

Chapter 9

Experiments When Each Subject Receives More Than One Treatment

The procedures for testing hypotheses discussed in Chapters 3 to 5 apply to experiments in which the control and treatment groups contain *different* subjects (individuals). It is often possible to design experiments in which *each* experimental subject can be observed *before* and *after* one or more treatments. Such experiments are generally more sensitive because they make it possible to measure how the treatment *affects each individual.* When the control and treatment groups consist of different individuals, the changes due to the treatment may be masked by variability between experimental subjects. This chapter shows how to analyze experiments in which each subject is repeatedly observed under different experimental conditions.

We will begin with the *paired t test* for experiments in which the subjects are observed before and after receiving a single treatment. Then, we will generalize this test to obtain *repeated-measures analysis of variance,* which permits testing hypotheses about any number of treatments whose effects are measured repeatedly in the same subjects.

We will explicitly separate the total variability in the observations into three components: variability between the experimental subjects, variability in each individual subject's response, and variability due to the treatments. Like all analyses of variance (including *t* tests), these procedures require that the observations come from normally distributed populations. (Chapter 10 presents methods based on ranks that do not require this assumption.) Finally, we will develop *McNemar's test* to analyze data measured on a nominal scale and presented in contingency tables.

EXPERIMENTS WHEN SUBJECTS ARE OBSERVED BEFORE AND AFTER A SINGLE TREATMENT: THE PAIRED *t* TEST

In experiments in which it is possible to observe each experimental subject *before* and *after* administering a single treatment, we will test a hypothesis about the average *change* the treatment produces instead of the difference in average responses with and without the treatment. This approach reduces the variability in the observations due to differences between individuals and yields a more sensitive test.

Figure 9–1 illustrates this point. Panel *A* shows daily urine production in *two* samples of 10 different people each; one sample group took a placebo and the other took a drug. Since there is little difference in the mean response relative to the standard deviations, it would be hard to assert that the treatment produced an effect on the basis of these observations. In fact, *t* computed using the methods of Chapter 4 is only 1.33, which comes nowhere near $t_{.05} = 2.101$, the critical value for $\nu = n_{\text{pla}} + n_{\text{drug}} - 2 = 10 + 10 - 2 = 18$ degrees of freedom.

Now consider Fig. 9–1*B*. It shows urine productions identical to those in Fig. 9–1*A* but for an experiment in which urine production was measured in *one* sample of 10 individuals *before* and *after* administering the drug. A straight line connects the observations for each individual. Figure 9–1*B* shows that the drug increased urine production in 8 of the 10 people in the sample. This result suggests that the drug *is* an effective diuretic.

By concentrating on the *change* in each individual that accompanied taking the drug (in Fig. 9–1*B*), we could detect an effect that was

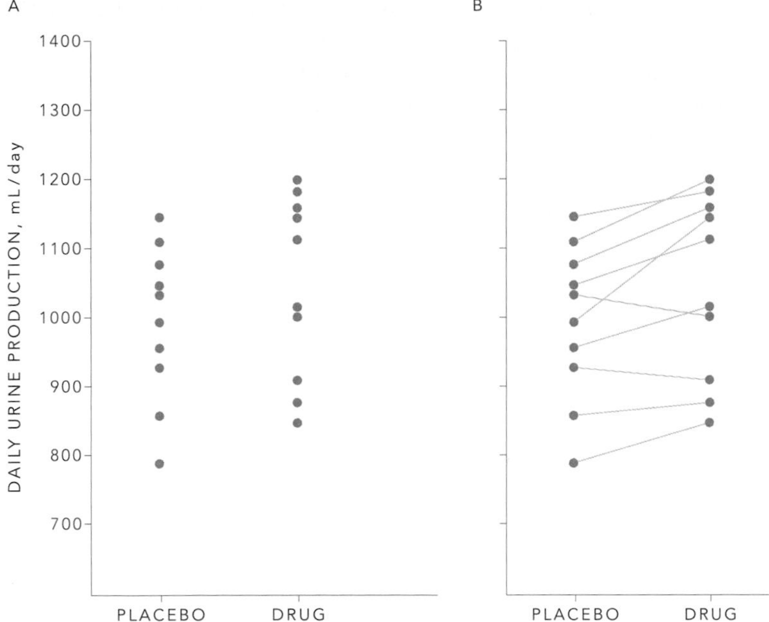

Figure 9–1 ***(A)*** Daily urine production in two groups of 10 different people. One group of 10 people received the placebo and the other group of 10 people received the drug. The diuretic does not appear to be effective. ***(B)*** Daily urine production in a single group of 10 people before and after taking a drug. The drug appears to be an effective diuretic. The observations are identical to those in panel ***A***; by focusing on changes in each individual's response rather than the response of all the people taken together, it is possible to detect a difference that was masked by the between-subjects variability in panel ***A***.

masked by the variability between individuals when different people received the placebo and the drug (in Fig. 9–1*A*).

Now, let us develop a statistical procedure to quantify our subjective impression in such experiments. The *paired t test* can be used to test the hypothesis that there is, on the average, no change in each individual after receiving the treatment under study. Recall that the general definition of the t statistic is

$$t = \frac{\text{parameter estimate} - \text{true value of population parameter}}{\text{standard error of parameter estimate}}$$

The parameter we wish to estimate is the average difference in response δ *in each individual* due to the treatment. If we let d equal the observed change in each individual that accompanies the treatment, we can use $\bar{d}$, the mean change, to estimate δ. The standard deviation of the observed differences is

$$s_d = \sqrt{\frac{\Sigma(d - \bar{d})^2}{n - 1}}$$

So the standard error of the difference is

$$s_{\bar{d}} = \frac{s_d}{\sqrt{n}}$$

Therefore,

$$t = \frac{\bar{d} - \delta}{s_{\bar{d}}}$$

To test the hypothesis that there is, on the average, no response to the treatment, set $\delta = 0$ in this equation to obtain

$$t = \frac{\bar{d}}{s_{\bar{d}}}$$

The resulting value of t is compared with the critical value of $\nu = n - 1$ degrees of freedom.

To recapitulate, when analyzing data from an experiment in which it is possible to observe each individual before and after applying a single treatment:

- *Compute the change in response that accompanies the treatment in each individual d.*
- *Compute the mean change $\bar{d}$ and the standard error of the mean changes $s_{\bar{d}}$.*
- *Use these numbers to compute* $t = \frac{\bar{d}}{s_{\bar{d}}}$.
- *Compare this* t *with the critical value for $\nu = n - 1$ degrees of freedom, where* n *is the number of experimental subjects.*

Note that the number of degrees of freedom, ν, associated with the paired-t test is $n - 1$, less than the $2(n - 1)$ degrees of freedom associated with analyzing these data using an unpaired t test. This loss of degrees of freedom increases the critical value of t that must be exceeded to reject the null hypothesis of no difference. While this situation would seem undesirable, because of the typical biological variability that occurs between individuals, this loss of degrees of freedom is virtually always more than compensated for by focusing on *differences within subjects,* which reduces the variability in the results used to compute t. All other things being equal, paired designs are almost always more powerful for detecting effects in biological data than unpaired designs.

Finally, the paired-t test, like all t tests, is predicated on a normally distributed population. In the t test for unpaired observations developed in Chapter 4, responses needed to be normally distributed. In the paired t test the changes associated with the treatment need to be normally distributed.

Cigarette Smoking and Platelet Function

Smokers are more likely to develop diseases caused by abnormal blood clots (thromboses), including heart attacks and occlusion of peripheral arteries, than nonsmokers. Platelets are small bodies that circulate in the blood and stick together to form blood clots. Since smokers experience more disorders related to undesirable blood clots than nonsmokers, Peter Levine* drew blood samples in 11 people before and after they smoked a single cigarette and measured the extent to which platelets aggregated when exposed to a standard stimulus. This stimulus, adenosine diphosphate, makes platelets release their granular contents, which, in turn, makes them stick together and form a blood clot.

Figure 9–2 shows the results of this experiment, with platelet stickiness quantified as the maximum percentage of all the platelets that aggregated after being exposed to adenosine diphosphate. The *pair* of observations made in each individual before and after smoking the cigarette is connected by straight lines. The mean percentage aggregations were 43.1 before smoking and 53.5 after smoking, with

*P. H. Levine, "An Acute Effect of Cigarette Smoking on Platelet Function: A Possible Link between Smoking and Arterial Thrombosis," *Circulation*, **48:**619–623, 1973.

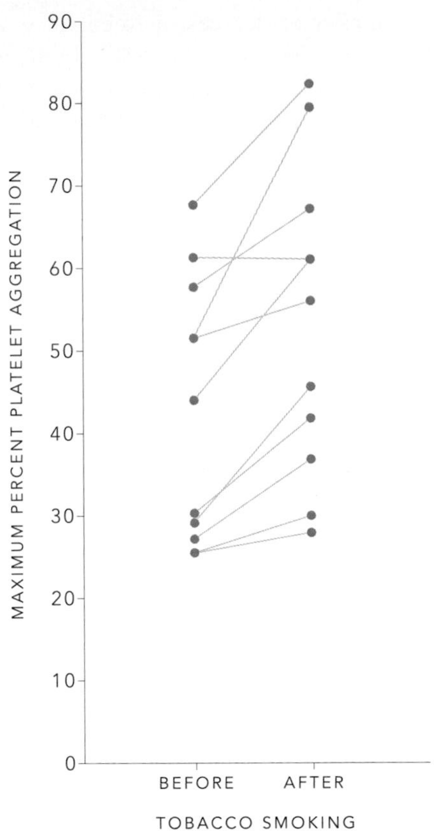

Figure 9–2 Maximum percentage platelet aggregation before and after smoking a tobacco cigarette in 11 people. (*Adapted from fig. 1 of P. H. Levine, "An Acute Effect of Cigarette Smoking on Platelet Function: A Possible Link between Smoking and Arterial Thrombosis,"* Circulation, ***48:****619–623, 1973. By permission of the American Heart Association, Inc.*)

standard deviations of 15.9 and 18.7 percent, respectively. Simply looking at these numbers does not suggest that smoking had an effect on platelet aggregation. This approach, however, omits an important fact about the experiment: the platelet aggregations were not measured in two different groups of people, smokers and nonsmokers, but in a single group of people who were observed both before and after smoking the cigarette.

In all but one individual, the maximum pattern aggregation increased after smoking the cigarette, suggesting that smoking facilitates thrombus formation. The means and standard deviations of platelet aggregation before and after smoking for all people taken together did not suggest this pattern because the variability between individuals masked the variability in platelet aggregation that was due to smoking the cigarette. When we took into account the fact that the observations actually consisted of pairs of observations done before and after smoking in each individual, we could focus on the *change* in response and so remove the variability that was due to the fact that different people have different platelet-aggregation tendencies regardless of whether they smoked a cigarette or not.

The changes in maximum percent platelet aggregation that accompany smoking are (from Fig. 9–2) 2, 4, 10, 12, 16, 15, 4, 27, 9, −1, and 15 percent. Therefore, the mean change in percent platelet aggregation with smoking in these 11 people is $\bar{d} = 10.3$ percent. The standard deviation of the change is 8.0 percent, so the standard error of the change is $S_{\bar{d}} = 8.0/\sqrt{11} = 2.41$ percent. Finally, our test statistic is

$$t = \frac{\bar{d}}{s_{\bar{d}}} = \frac{10.3}{2.41} = 4.27$$

This value exceeds 3.169, the value that defines the most extreme 1 percent of the t distribution with $\nu = n - 1 = 11 - 1 = 10$ degrees of freedom (from Table 4–1). Therefore, we report that smoking increases platelet aggregation ($P < .01$).

How convincing is this experiment that a constituent specific to *tobacco* smoke, as opposed to other chemicals common to smoke in general (e.g., carbon monoxide), or even the stress of the experiment produced the observed change? To investigate this question, Levine also had his subjects "smoke" an unlit cigarette and a lettuce leaf cigarette that contained no nicotine. Figure 9–3 shows the results of these experiments, together with the results of smoking a standard cigarette (from Fig. 9–2).

When the experimental subjects merely pretended to smoke or smoked a non-nicotine cigarette made of dried lettuce, there was no

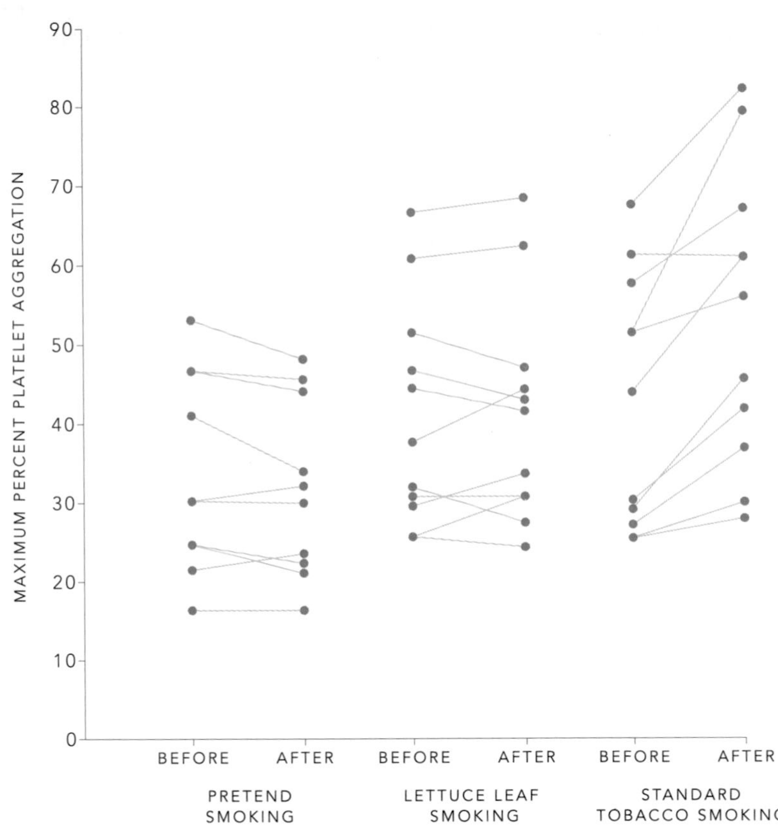

Figure 9–3 Maximum percentage platelet aggregation in 11 people before and after pretending to smoke ("sham smoking"), before and after smoking a lettuce-leaf cigarette that contained no nicotine, and before and after smoking a tobacco cigarette. These observations, taken together, suggest that it was something in the tobacco smoke, rather than the act of smoking or other general constituents of smoke, that produced the change in platelet aggregation. (*Redrawn from fig. 1 of P. H. Levine, "An Acute Effect of Cigarette Smoking on Platelet Function: A Possible Link between Smoking and Arterial Thrombosis,"* Circulation, ***48:****619–623, 1973. By permission of the American Heart Association, Inc.)*

discernible change in platelet aggregation. This situation contrasts with the increase in platelet aggregation that followed smoking a single tobacco cigarette. This experimental design illustrates an important point:

> *In a well-designed experiment, the only difference between the treatment group and the control group, both chosen at random from a population of interest, is the treatment.*

In this experiment the treatment of interest was tobacco constituents in the smoke, so it was important to compare the results with observations obtained after exposing the subjects to non-tobacco smoke. This step helped ensure that the observed changes were due to the tobacco rather than smoking in general. The more carefully the investigator can isolate the treatment effect, the more convincing the conclusions will be.

There are also subtle biases that can cloud the conclusions from an experiment. Most investigators, and their colleagues and technicians, want the experiments to support their hypothesis. In addition, the experimental subjects, when they are people, generally want to be helpful and wish the investigator to be correct, especially if the study is evaluating a new treatment that the experimental subject hopes will provide a cure. These factors can lead the people doing the study to tend to slant judgment calls (often required when collecting the data) toward making the study come out the way everyone wants. For example, the laboratory technicians who measure platelet aggregation might read the control samples on the low side and the smoking samples on the high side without even realizing it. Perhaps some psychological factor among the experimental subjects (analogous to a placebo effect) led their platelet aggregation to increase when they smoked the tobacco cigarette. Levine avoided these difficulties by doing the experiments in a *double-blind* manner in which the investigator, the experimental subject, and the laboratory technicians who analyzed the blood samples did not know the content of the cigarettes being smoked until after all experiments were complete and specimens analyzed. As discussed in Chapter 2, double-blind studies are the most effective way to eliminate bias due to both the observer and experimental subject.

In *single-blind* studies one party, usually the investigator, knows which treatment is being administered. This approach controls biases due to the placebo effect but not observer biases. Some studies are also partially blind, in which the participants know something about the treatment but do not have full information. For example, the blood platelet study might be considered partially blind because both the subject and the investigator obviously knew when the subject was only pretending to smoke. It was possible, however, to withhold this information from the laboratory technicians who actually analyzed the blood samples to avoid biases in their measurements of percent platelet aggregation.

The paired t test can be used to test hypotheses when observations are taken before and after administering a single treatment to a group of individuals. To generalize this procedure to experiments in which the same individuals are subjected to a number of treatments, we now develop *repeated-measures analysis of variance.*

To do so, we must first introduce some new nomenclature for analysis of variance. To ease the transition, we begin with the analysis of variance presented in Chapter 3, in which each treatment was applied to *different* individuals. After reformulating this type of analysis of variance, we will go on to the case of repeated measurements on the same individual.

ANOTHER APPROACH TO ANALYSIS OF VARIANCE*

When we developed analysis of variance in Chapter 3, we assumed that all the samples were drawn from a single population (i.e., that the treatments had no effect), estimated the variability in that population from the variability within the sample groups and between the sample groups, then compared these two estimates to see how compatible they were with the original assumption that all the samples were drawn from a single population. When the two estimates of variability were unlikely to arise if the samples had been drawn from a single population, we rejected the null hypothesis of no effect and concluded that at least one of the samples represented a different population

*This and the following section, which develops repeated-measures analysis of variance (the multitreatment generalization of the paired t test), are more mathematical than the rest of the text. Some readers may wish to skip this section until they encounter an experiment that should be analyzed with repeated-measures analysis of variance. Despite the fact that such experiments are common in the biomedical literature, this test is rarely used. This decision leads to the same kinds of multiple-t-test errors discussed in Chapters 3 and 4 for the unpaired t test.

(i.e., that at least one treatment had an effect). We used estimates of the population *variance* to quantify variability.

In Chapter 8, we used a slightly different method to quantify the variability of observed data points about a regression line. We used the *sum of squared deviations* about the regression line to quantify variability. The variance and sum of squared deviations, of course, are intimately related. One obtains the variance by dividing the sum of squared deviations by the appropriate number of degrees of freedom. We now will recast analysis of variance using sums of squared deviations to quantify variability. This new nomenclature forms the basis of all forms of analysis of variance, including repeated-measures analysis of variance.

In Chapter 3, we considered the following experiment. To determine whether diet affected cardiac output in people living in a small town, we randomly selected four groups of seven people each. People in the control group continued eating normally; people in the second group ate only spaghetti; people in the third group ate only steak; and people in the fourth group ate only fruit and nuts. After 1 month, each person was catheterized and his cardiac output measured. Figure 3–1 showed that diet did not, in fact, affect cardiac output. Figure 3–2 showed the results of the experiment as they would appear to you as an investigator or reader. Table 9–1 presents the same data in tabular form. The four different groups did show some variability in cardiac output. The question is: How consistent is this observed variability with the hypothesis that diet did not have any effect on cardiac output?

Some New Notation

Tables 9–1 and 9–2 illustrate the notation we will now use to answer this question; it is required for more general forms of analysis of variance. The four different diets are called the *treatments* and are represented by the columns in the table. We denote the four different treatments with the numbers 1 to 4 (1 = control, 2 = spaghetti, 3 = steak, 4 = fruit and nuts). Seven *different* people receive each treatment. Each particular experimental subject (or, more precisely, the observation or data point associated with each subject) is represented by X_{ts}, where t represents the treatment and s represents a specific

Table 9–1 Cardiac Output (L/min) in Different Groups of Seven People Fed Different Diets

	Treatment			
	Control	Spaghetti	Steak	Fruit and nuts
	4.6	4.6	4.3	4.3
	4.7	5.0	4.4	4.4
	4.7	5.2	4.9	4.5
	4.9	5.2	4.9	4.9
	5.1	5.5	5.1	4.9
	5.3	5.5	5.3	5.0
	5.4	5.6	5.6	5.6
Treatment (column) means	4.96	5.23	4.93	4.80
Treatment (column) sums of squares	0.597	0.734	1.294	1.200
Grand mean = 4.98		Total sum of squares = 4.501		

Table 9–2 Notation for One-Way Analysis of Variance in Table 9–1

	Treatment			
	1	2	3	4
	X_{11}	X_{21}	X_{31}	X_{41}
	X_{12}	X_{22}	X_{32}	X_{42}
	X_{13}	X_{23}	X_{33}	X_{43}
	X_{14}	X_{24}	X_{34}	X_{44}
	X_{15}	X_{25}	X_{35}	X_{45}
	X_{16}	X_{26}	X_{36}	X_{46}
	X_{17}	X_{27}	X_{37}	X_{47}
Treatment (column) means	$\bar{X}_1$	$\bar{X}_2$	$\bar{X}_3$	$\bar{X}_4$
Treatment (column) sums of squares	$\sum_s (X_{1s} - \bar{X}_1)^2$	$\sum_s (X_{2s} - \bar{X}_2)^2$	$\sum_s (X_{3s} - \bar{X}_3)^2$	$\sum_s (X_{4s} - \bar{X}_4)^2$
Grand mean = $\bar{X}$		Total sum of squares = $\sum_t \sum_s (X_{ts} - \bar{X})^2$		

subject in that treatment group. For example, $X_{11} = 4.6$ L/min represents the observed cardiac output for the first subject ($s = 1$) who received the control diet ($t = 1$). $X_{35} = 5.1$ L/min represents the fifth subject ($s = 5$) who had the steak diet ($t = 3$).

Tables 9–1 and 9–2 also show the mean cardiac outputs for all subjects (in this case, people) receiving each of the four treatments, labeled $\overline{X}_1$, $\overline{X}_2$, $\overline{X}_3$, and $\overline{X}_4$. For example, $\overline{X}_2 = 5.23$ L/min is the mean cardiac output observed among people who were treated with spaghetti. The tables also show the variability within each of the treatment groups, quantified by the *sum of squared deviations about the treatment mean,*

> Sum of squares for treatment t = sum, over all subjects who received treatment t, of (value of observation for subject−mean response of all individuals who received treatment t)^2

The equivalent mathematical statement is

$$SS_t = \sum_s (X_{ts} - \overline{X}_t)^2$$

The summation symbol, Σ, has been modified to indicate that we sum over all s subjects who received treatment t. We need this more explicit notation because we will be summing up the observations in different ways. For example, the sum of squared deviations from the mean cardiac output for the seven people who ate the control diet ($t = 1$) is

$$\begin{aligned} SS_1 &= \sum_s (X_{1s} - \overline{X}_1)^2 \\ &= (4.6 - 4.96)^2 + (4.7 - 4.96)^2 + (4.7 - 4.96)^2 \\ &\quad + (4.9 - 4.96)^2 + (5.1 - 4.96)^2 + (5.3 - 4.96)^2 \\ &\quad + (5.4 - 4.96)^2 = 0.597\ (\text{L/min})^2 \end{aligned}$$

Recall that the definition of sample variance is

$$s^2 = \frac{\Sigma(X - \overline{X})^2}{n - 1}$$

where n is the size of the sample. The expression in the numerator is just the sum of squared deviations from the sample mean, so we can write

$$s^2 = \frac{\text{SS}}{n - 1}$$

Hence, the variance in treatment group t equals the sum of squares for that treatment divided by the number of individuals who received the treatment (i.e., the sample size) minus 1.

$$s_t^2 = \frac{\text{SS}_t}{n - 1}$$

In Chapter 3, we estimated the population variance from within the groups for our diet experiment with the average of the variances computed from within each of the four treatment groups

$$s_{\text{wit}}^2 = \tfrac{1}{4}(s_{\text{con}}^2 + s_{\text{spa}}^2 + s_{\text{st}}^2 + s_{\text{fn}}^2)$$

In the notation of Table 9–1, we can rewrite this equation as

$$s_{\text{wit}}^2 = \tfrac{1}{4}(s_1^2 + s_2^2 + s_3^2 + s_4^2)$$

Now, replace each of the variances in terms of sums of squares.

$$s_{\text{wit}}^2 = \frac{1}{4}\left[\frac{\sum_s (X_{1s} - \overline{X}_1)^2}{n - 1} + \frac{\sum_s (X_{2s} - \overline{X}_2)^2}{n - 1} + \frac{\sum_s (X_{3s} - \overline{X}_3)^2}{n - 1} + \frac{\sum_s (X_{4s} - \overline{X}_4)^2}{n - 1}\right]$$

or

$$s_{\text{wit}}^2 = \frac{1}{4}\left(\frac{\text{SS}_1}{n-1} + \frac{\text{SS}_2}{n-1} + \frac{\text{SS}_3}{n-1} + \frac{\text{SS}_4}{n-1}\right)$$

in which $n = 7$ represents the size of each sample group. Factor $n - 1$ out of the four expressions for variance computed from within each of the four separate treatment groups, and let $m = 4$ represent the number of treatments (diets), to obtain

$$s_{\text{wit}}^2 = \frac{1}{m}\,\frac{\text{SS}_1 + \text{SS}_2 + \text{SS}_3 + \text{SS}_4}{n-1}$$

The numerator of this fraction is just the total of the sums of squared deviations of the observations about the means of their respective treatment groups. Call it the *within-treatments (or within-groups) sum of squares* SS_{wit}. Note that the within-treatments sum of squares is a measure of variability in the observations that is independent of whether or not the mean responses to the different treatments are the same.

For the data from our diet experiment in Table 9–1

$$\text{SS}_{\text{wit}} = .597 + .734 + 1.294 + 1.200 = 3.825\ (\text{L/min})^2$$

Given our definition of SS_{wit} and the equation s_{wit}^2 above, we can write

$$s_{\text{wit}}^2 = \frac{\text{SS}_{\text{wit}}}{m(n-1)}$$

s_{wit}^2 appears in the denominator of the F ratio associated with $\nu_d = m(n-1)$ degrees of freedom. Using this notation for analysis-of-variance, degrees of freedom are often denoted by DF rather than ν, so let us replace $m(n-1)$ with DF_{wit} in the equation for s_{wit}^2 to obtain

$$s_{\text{wit}}^2 = \frac{\text{SS}_{\text{wit}}}{\text{DF}_{\text{wit}}}$$

For the diet experiment, $DF_{wit} = m(n - 1) = 4(7 - 1) = 24$ degrees of freedom.

Finally, recall that in Chapter 2 we defined the variance as the "average" squared deviation from the mean. In this spirit, statisticians call the ratio SS_{wit}/DF_{wit} the within-groups *mean square* and denote it MS_{wit}. This notation is clumsy, since SS_{wit}/DF_{wit} is not really a mean in the standard statistical meaning of the word, and it obscures the fact that MS_{wit} is the estimate of the variance computed from within the groups (that we have been denoting s^2_{wit}). Nevertheless, it is so ubiquitous that we will adopt it. Therefore, we will estimate the variance from within the sample groups with

$$MS_{wit} = \frac{SS_{wit}}{DF_{wit}}$$

We will replace s^2_{wit} in the definition of F with this expression.

For the data in Table 9–1,

$$MS_{wit} = \frac{3.825}{24} = 0.159 \text{ (L/min)}^2$$

Next, we need to do the same thing for the variance estimated from between the treatment groups. Recall that we estimated this variance by computing the standard deviation of the sample means as an estimate of the standard error of the mean, then estimated the population variance with

$$s^2_{bet} = ns^2_{\overline{X}}$$

The square of the standard deviation of treatment means is

$$s^2_{\overline{X}} = \frac{(\overline{X}_1 - \overline{X})^2 + (\overline{X}_2 - \overline{X})^2 + (\overline{X}_3 - \overline{X})^2 + (\overline{X}_4 - \overline{X})^2}{m - 1}$$

in which m again denotes the number of treatment groups (4) and $\overline{X}$ denotes the means of *all* the observations (which also equals the mean of the sample means when the samples are all the same size). We can write this equation more compactly as

$$s_{\overline{X}}^2 = \frac{\sum_t (\overline{X}_t - \overline{X})^2}{m - 1}$$

so that

$$s_{\text{bet}}^2 = \frac{n \sum_t (\overline{X}_t - \overline{X})^2}{m - 1}$$

(Notice that we are now summing over treatments rather than experimental subjects.) The between-groups variance can be written as the sum of squared deviations of the treatment means about the mean of all observations times the sample size divided by $m - 1$. Denote this sum of squares the *between-groups* or *treatment* sum of squares

$$SS_{\text{bet}} = SS_{\text{treat}} = n \sum_t (\overline{X}_t - \overline{X})^2$$

The treatment sum of squares is a measure of the variability between the groups, just as the within-groups sum of squares is a measure of the variability within the groups.

For the data for the diet experiment in Table 9–1

$$\begin{aligned} SS_{\text{treat}} &= n \sum_t (\overline{X}_t - \overline{X})^2 \\ &= 7[(4.96 - 4.98)^2 + (5.23 - 4.98)^2 + (4.93 - 4.98)^2 \\ &\quad + (4.80 - 4.98)^2] = 0.685 \text{ (L/min)}^2 \end{aligned}$$

The treatment (between-groups) variance appears in the numerator of the F ratio and is associated with $\nu = m - 1$ degrees of freedom; we therefore denote $m - 1$ with

$$DF_{\text{bet}} = DF_{\text{treat}} = m - 1$$

in which case

$$s^2_{\text{bet}} = \frac{\text{SS}_{\text{bet}}}{\text{DF}_{\text{bet}}} = \frac{\text{SS}_{\text{treat}}}{\text{DF}_{\text{treat}}}$$

Just as statisticians call the ratio SS_{wit} the within-groups mean square, they call the estimate of the variance from between the groups (or treatments) the *treatment (or between-groups) mean square* MS_{treat} (or MS_{bet}). Therefore,

$$\text{MS}_{\text{bet}} = \frac{\text{SS}_{\text{bet}}}{\text{DF}_{\text{bet}}} = \frac{\text{SS}_{\text{treat}}}{\text{DF}_{\text{treat}}} = \text{MS}_{\text{treat}}$$

For the data in Table 9–1, $\text{DF}_{\text{treat}} = m - 1 = 4 - 1 = 3$, so

$$\text{MS}_{\text{treat}} = \frac{0.685}{3} = 0.228\ (\text{L/min})^2$$

We can write the F-test statistic as

$$F = \frac{\text{MS}_{\text{bet}}}{\text{MS}_{\text{wit}}} = \frac{\text{MS}_{\text{treat}}}{\text{MS}_{\text{wit}}}$$

and compare it with the critical value of F for numerator degrees of freedom, DF_{treat} (or DF_{bet}), and denominator degrees of freedom, DF_{wit}.

Finally, for the data in Table 9–1

$$F = \frac{\text{MS}_{\text{treat}}}{\text{MS}_{\text{wit}}} = \frac{.228}{.159} = 1.4$$

the same value of F we obtained from these data in Chapter 3.

We have gone far afield into a computational procedure that is more complex and, on the surface, less intuitive than the one developed in Chapter 3. This approach is necessary, however, to analyze the results obtained in more complex experimental designs. Surprisingly, there are intuitive meanings which can be attached to these sums of squares and which are very important.

Accounting for All the Variability in the Observations

The sums of squares within and between the treatment groups, SS_{wit} and SS_{treat}, quantify the variability observed within and between the treatment groups. In addition, it is possible to describe the total variability observed in the data by computing the *sum of squared deviations of all observations about the grand mean* $\overline{X}$ *of all the observations,* called *the total sum of squares*

$$SS_{tot} = \sum_t \sum_s (X_{ts} - \overline{X})^2$$

The two summation symbols indicate the sums over all subjects in all treatment groups.

The total number of degrees of freedom associated with this sum of squares is $DF_{tot} = mn - 1$, or 1 less than the total sample size (m treatment groups times n subjects in each treatment group). For the observations in Table 9–1,

$$SS_{tot} = 4.501\ (\text{L/min})^2 \quad \text{and} \quad DF_{tot} = 4(7) - 1 = 27$$

Notice that the variance estimated from all the observations, without regard for the fact that there are different experimental groups, is just

$$\frac{\sum_t \sum_s (X_{ts} - \overline{X})^2}{mn - 1} = \frac{SS_{tot}}{mn - 1}$$

The three sums of squares discussed so far are related in a very simple way.

> *The total sum of squares is the sum of the between-groups (treatment) sum of squares and the within-groups sum of squares*

$$SS_{tot} = SS_{bet} + SS_{wit}$$

In other words, the total variability, quantified with appropriate sums of squared deviations, can be *partitioned* into two components, one due to variability between the experimental groups and another component due to variability within the groups.* It is common to summarize all these computations in an *analysis-of-variance table* such as Table 9–3. Notice that the between-groups and within-groups sums of squares do indeed add up to the total sum of squares.

F is the ratio of MS_{bet} over MS_{wit} and should be compared with the critical value of F with DF_{bet} and DF_{wit} degrees of freedom for the numerator and denominator, respectively, to test the hypothesis that all the samples were drawn from a single population.

Note also that the treatment and within-groups degrees of freedom also add up to the total number of degrees of freedom. This is not

*To see why this is true, first decompose the amount that any given observation deviates from the grand mean, $X_{ts} - \overline{X}$, into two components, the deviation of the treatment group mean from the grand mean and the deviation of the observation from the mean of its treatment group.

$$(X_{ts} - \overline{X}) = (\overline{X}_t - \overline{X}) + (X_{ts} - \overline{X}_t)$$

Square both sides

$$(X_{ts} - \overline{X})^2 = (\overline{X}_t - \overline{X})^2 + (X_{ts} - \overline{X}_t)^2 + 2(\overline{X}_t - \overline{X})(X_{ts} - \overline{X}_t)$$

and sum over all observations to obtain the total sum of squares

$$SS_{tot} = \sum_t \sum_s (X_{ts} - \overline{X})^2$$

$$= \sum_t \sum_s (\overline{X}_t - \overline{X})^2 + \sum_t \sum_s (X_{ts} - \overline{X}_t)^2 + \sum_t \sum_s 2(\overline{X}_t - \overline{X})(X_{ts} - \overline{X}_t)$$

Since $(\overline{X}_t - \overline{X})$ does not depend on which of the n individuals in each sample are being summed over,

$$\sum_s (\overline{X}_t - \overline{X})^2 = n(\overline{X}_t - \overline{X})^2$$

The first term on the right of the equals sign can be written

$$\sum_t \sum_s (\overline{X}_1 - \overline{X})^2 = n \sum_t (\overline{X}_t - \overline{X})^2$$

which is just SS_{bet}. Furthermore, the second term on the right of the equals sign is just SS_{wit}.

It only remains to show that the third term on the right of the equals sign equals zero. To do this, note again that $\overline{X}_t - \overline{X}$ does not depend on which member of each sample is being summed, so we can factor it out of the sum over the member of each sample, in which case

$$\sum_t \sum_s 2(\overline{X}_t - \overline{X})(X_{ts} - \overline{X}_t) = 2 \sum_t (\overline{X}_t - \overline{X}) \sum_s (X_{ts} = \overline{X}_t)$$

Table 9–3 Analysis-of-Variance Table for Diet Experiment

Source of variation	SS	DF	MS
Between groups	0.685	3	0.228
Within groups	3.816	24	0.159
Total	4.501	27	

$$F = \frac{MS_{bet}}{MS_{wit}} = \frac{0.228}{0.159} = 1.4$$

a chance occurrence; it will always be the case. Specifically, if there are m experimental groups with n members each,

$$DF_{bet} = m - 1; \qquad DF_{wit} = m(n - 1); \qquad DF_{tot} = mn - 1$$

so that

$$\begin{aligned} DF_{bet} + DF_{wit} &= (m - 1) + m(n - 1) \\ &= m - 1 + mn - m = mn - 1 = DF_{tot} \end{aligned}$$

In other words, just as it was possible to partition the total sum of squares into components due to between-group (treatment) and within-group variability, it is possible to partition the degrees of freedom. Figure 9–4 illustrates how the sums of squares and degrees of freedom are partitioned in this analysis of variance.

Now we are ready to attack the original problem, that of developing an analysis of variance suitable for experiments in which each experimental subject receives more than one treatment.

But $\bar{X}_t$ is the mean of the n members of treatment group t, so

$$\begin{aligned} \sum_s (X_{ts} - \bar{X}_t) &= \sum_s X_{ts} - \sum_s \bar{X}_t = \sum_s X_{ts} - n\bar{X}_t \\ &= n\left(\sum_s X_{ts}/n - \bar{X}_t\right) = n(\bar{X}_t - \bar{X}_t) = 0 \end{aligned}$$

Therefore,

$$SS_{tot} = SS_{bet} + SS_{wit} + 0 = SS_{bet} + SS_{wit}$$

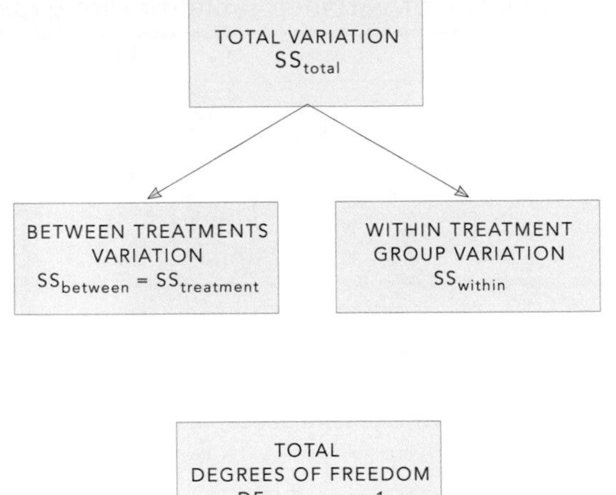

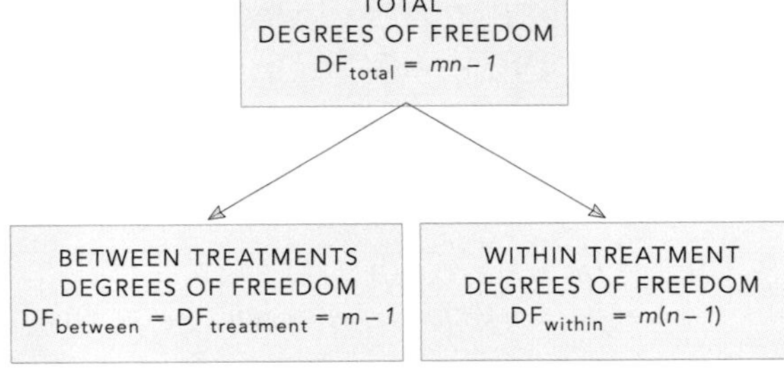

Figure 9–4 Partitioning of the sums of squares and degrees of freedom for a one-way analysis of variance.

EXPERIMENTS WHEN SUBJECTS ARE OBSERVED AFTER MANY TREATMENTS: REPEATED-MEASURES ANALYSIS OF VARIANCE

When each experimental subject receives more than one treatment, it is possible to partition the total variability in the observations into three mutually exclusive components: variability between all the experimental subjects, variability due to the treatments, and variability within the subjects' response to the treatments. The last component of variability represents the fact that there is some random variation in how a given individual responds to a given treatment, together with measurement errors. Figure 9–5 shows this breakdown. The resulting procedure is called a *repeated-measures* analysis of variance because

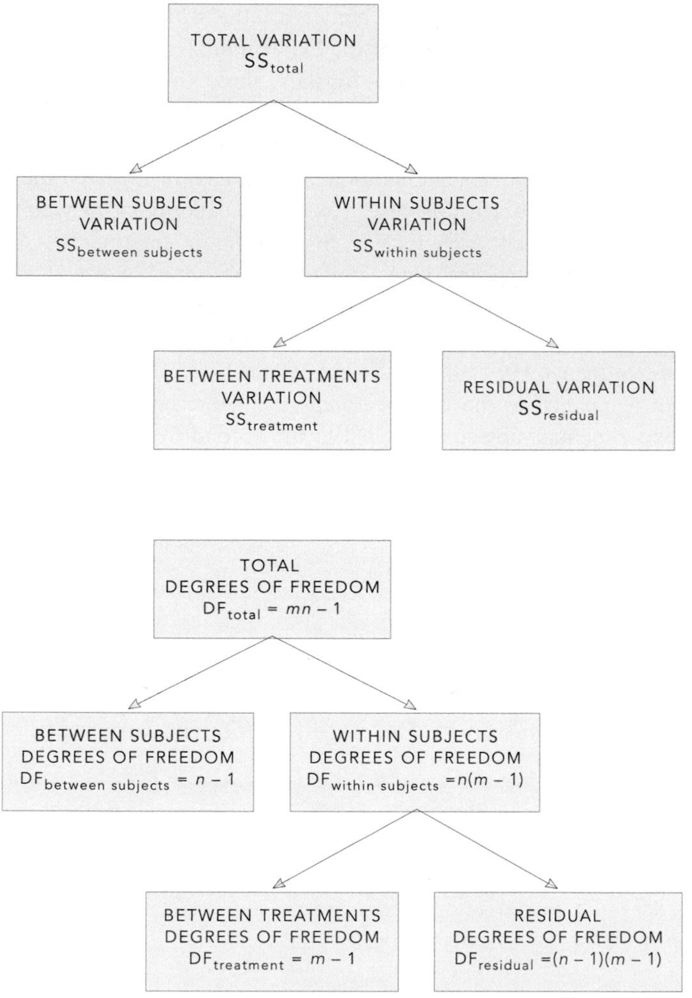

Figure 9–5 Partitioning of the sums of squares and degrees of freedom for a repeated-measures analysis of variance. Notice that this procedure allows us to concentrate on the variation within experimental subjects.

the measurements are repeated under all the different experimental conditions (treatment) in each of the experimental subjects.

Now, let us write expressions for these three kinds of variability. As Fig. 9–5 suggests, the first step is to divide the total variability into variability within subjects and between subjects.

Table 9–4 illustrates the notation we will use for repeated-measures analysis of variance. (In this case it is for an experiment in which four experimental subjects each receive three different treatments). At first glance, this table appears quite similar to Table 9–2, used to analyze experiments in which *different* subjects received each of the treatments. There is one important difference: in Table 9–4 the *same* subjects receive all the treatments. For example, X_{11} represents how the first experimental subject responded to the first treatment; X_{21} represents how the (same) first experimental subject responded to the second treatment. In general, X_{ts} is the response of the sth experimental subject to the t th treatment.

$\bar{S}_1$, $\bar{S}_2$, $\bar{S}_3$, and $\bar{S}_4$ are the mean responses of each of the four subjects to all (three) treatments

$$\bar{S}_s = \frac{\sum_t X_{ts}}{m}$$

Table 9–4 Notation for Repeated-Measures Analysis of Variance

Experimental subject, $n = 4$	Treatment, $m = 3$: 1	2	3	Subject: Mean	SS
1	X_{11}	X_{21}	X_{31}	$\bar{S}_1$	$\sum_t (X_{t1} - \bar{S}_1)^2$
2	X_{12}	X_{22}	X_{32}	$\bar{S}_2$	$\sum_t (X_{t2} - \bar{S}_2)^2$
3	X_{13}	X_{23}	X_{33}	$\bar{S}_3$	$\sum_t (X_{t3} - \bar{S}_3)^2$
4	X_{14}	X_{24}	X_{34}	$\bar{S}_4$	$\sum_t (X_{t4} - \bar{S}_4)^2$
Treatment mean	$\bar{T}_1$	$\bar{T}_2$	$\bar{T}_3$		

Grand mean $\bar{X} = \dfrac{\sum_t \sum_s X_{ts}}{mn}$ $\quad SS_{tot} = \sum_t \sum_s (X_{ts} - \bar{X})^2$

in which there are $m = 3$ treatments. Likewise, $\overline{T}_1$, $\overline{T}_2$, and $\overline{T}_3$ are the mean responses to each of the three treatments of all (four) experimental subjects.

$$\overline{T}_t = \frac{\sum_s X_{ts}}{n}$$

in which there are $n = 4$ experimental subjects.

As in all analyses of variance, we quantify the total variation with the total sum of squared deviations of all observations about the grand mean. The grand mean of all the observations is

$$\overline{X} = \frac{\sum_t \sum_s X_{ts}}{mn}$$

and the total sum of squared deviations from the grand mean is

$$SS_{tot} = \sum_t \sum_s (X_{ts} - \overline{X})^2$$

This sum of squares is associated with $DF_{tot} = mn - 1$ degrees of freedom.

Next, we partition this total sum of squares into variation within subjects and variation between subjects. The variation of observations within subject 1 about the mean observed for subject 1, $\overline{S}_1$, is

$$SS_{\text{wit subj 1}} = \sum_t (X_{t1} - \overline{S}_1)^2$$

Likewise, the variation in observations within subject 2 about the mean observed in subject 2 is

$$SS_{\text{wit subj 2}} = \sum_t (X_{t2} - \overline{S}_2)^2$$

We can write similar sums for the other two experimental subjects. The total variability observed within all subjects is just the sum of the variability observed within each subject

$$\text{SS}_{\text{wit subjs}} = \text{SS}_{\text{wit subj 1}} + \text{SS}_{\text{wit subj 2}} + \text{SS}_{\text{wit subj 3}} + \text{SS}_{\text{wit subj 4}}$$
$$= \sum_s \sum_t (X_{ts} - \bar{S}_s)^2$$

Since the sum of squares within each subject is associated with $m - 1$ degrees of freedom (where m is the number of treatments) and there are n subjects, $\text{SS}_{\text{wit subjs}}$ is associated with $\text{DF}_{\text{wit subjs}} = n(m - 1)$ degrees of freedom.

The variation between subjects is quantified by computing the sum of squared deviations of the mean response of each subject about the grand mean

$$\text{SS}_{\text{bet subjs}} = m\sum_t (\bar{S}_s - \bar{X})^2$$

The sum is multiplied by m because each subject's mean is the mean response to the m treatments. (This situation is analogous to the computation of the between-groups sum of squares as the sum of squared deviations of the sample means about the grand mean in the analysis of variance developed in the last section.) This sum of squares has $\text{DF}_{\text{bet subjs}} = n - 1$ degrees of freedom.

It is possible to show that

$$\text{SS}_{\text{tot}} = \text{SS}_{\text{wit subjs}} + \text{SS}_{\text{bet subjs}}$$

that is, that the total sum of squares can be partitioned into the within- and between-subjects sums of squares.*

Next, we need to partition the within-subjects sum of squares into two components, variability in the observations due to the treatments and the *residual* variation due to random variation in how each individual responds to each treatment. The sum of squares due to the treatments is the sum of squared differences between the treatment means and the grand mean.

$$\text{SS}_{\text{treat}} = n\sum_t (\bar{T}_t - \bar{X})^2$$

*For a derivation of this equation, see B. J. Winer, D. R. Brown, and K. M. Michels, *Statistical Principles in Experimental Design*, 3d ed., McGraw-Hill, New York, 1991, chap. 4, "Single-Factor Experiments Having Repeated Measures on the Same Elements."

We multiply by n, the number of subjects used to compute each treatment mean, just as we did above when computing the between-subjects sum of squares. Since there are m different treatments, there are $DF_{treat} = m - 1$ degrees of freedom associated with SS_{treat}.

Since we are partitioning the within-subjects sum of squares into the treatment sum of squares and the residual sum of squares,

$$SS_{wit\ subjs} = SS_{treat} + SS_{res}$$

and so

$$SS_{res} = SS_{wit\ subjs} - SS_{treat}$$

The same partitioning for the degrees of freedom yields

$$\begin{aligned} DF_{res} &= DF_{wit\ subjs} - DF_{treat} \\ &= n(m - 1) - (m - 1) = (n - 1)(m - 1) \end{aligned}$$

Finally, our estimate of the population variance from the treatment sum of squares is

$$MS_{treat} = \frac{SS_{treat}}{DF_{treat}}$$

and the estimate of the population variance from the residual sum of squares is

$$MS_{res} = \frac{SS_{res}}{DF_{res}}$$

If the null hypothesis that the treatments have no effect is true, MS_{treat} and MS_{res} are both estimates of the same (unknown) population variance, so compute

$$F = \frac{MS_{treat}}{MS_{res}}$$

to test the null hypothesis that the treatments do not change the experimental subjects. If the hypothesis of no treatment effect is true, this F ratio will follow the F distribution with DF_{treat} numerator degrees of freedom and DF_{res} denominator degrees of freedom.

This development has been, by necessity, more mathematical than most of the explanations in this book. Let us apply it to a simple example to make the concepts more concrete.

Anti-Asthmatic Drugs and Endotoxin

Endotoxin is a component of gram-negative bacteria found in dust in both workplaces and homes. Inhaling endotoxin causes fever, chills, bronchoconstriction of airways in the lungs, and generalized bronchial hyperresponsiveness (wheezing). Prolonged endotoxin exposure is associated with chronic obstructive pulmonary disease and asthma. Olivier Michel and colleagues* thought that the anti-asthmatic drug, salbutamol, might protect against the endotoxin-induced inflammation that produces these symptoms. To test this hypothesis, they had four mildly asthmatic people breathe an aerosol containing a purified form of endotoxin and measured how many liters of air they could exhale in 1 second. This variable, known as forced expiratory volume in 1 second or FEV_1 is a measure of airway constriction. A decrease in FEV_1 indicates a higher degree of bronchoconstriction. They took three FEV_1 measurements in each person: baseline (before breathing the endotoxin), 1 hour later following endotoxin inhalation, and 2 hours later after each subject received an additional salbutamol treatment.

Figure 9–6 shows the results of this experiment. Simply looking at Fig. 9–6 suggests that salbutamol increases FEV_1, but there are only four people in the study. How confident can we be when asserting that the drug actually reduces bronchial constriction and makes it easier to breathe? To answer this question, we perform a repeated-measures analysis of variance.

Table 9–5 shows the same data as Fig. 9–6, together with the mean FEV_1 observed for each of the $n = 4$ experimental subjects (people) and

*O. Michel, J. Olbrecht, D. Moulard, R. Sergysels, "Effect of Anti-asthmatic Drugs on the Response to Inhaled Endotoxin." *Ann. Allergy Asthma Immunol.*, **85:**305–310, 2000.

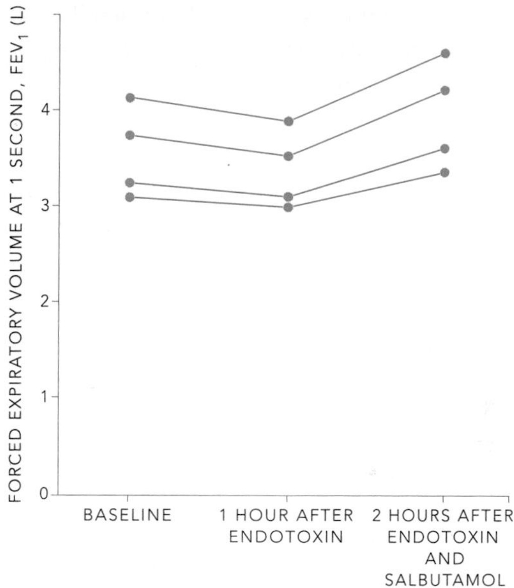

Figure 9–6 Forced expiratory volume at 1 second (FEV_1) in four people at baseline, 1 hour after inhaling endotoxin, and 2 hours following endotoxin and salbutamol exposure. Each individual's response is connected by straight lines. *(Adapted from table 2 and fig. 4 of O. Michel, J. Olbrecht, D. Moulard, R. Sergysels, "Effect of Anti-asthmatic Drugs on the Response to Inhaled Endotoxin,"* Ann. Allergy Asthma Immunol. ***85:****305–310, 2000.*

Table 9–5 Forced Expiratory Volume (L) at One Second before and after Bronchial Challenge with Endotoxin and Salbutamol Treatment

Person (subject)	No drug (baseline)	1 hour after endotoxin	2 hours after endotoxin and salbutamol	Subject	
				Mean	SS
1	3.7	3.4	4.0	3.70	0.1800
2	4.0	3.7	4.4	4.03	0.2467
3	3.0	2.8	3.2	3.00	0.0800
4	3.2	2.9	3.4	3.17	0.1267
Treatment mean	3.48	3.20	3.75		
Grand mean = 3.48				SS_{tot} = 2.6830 liters^2	

each of the $m = 3$ treatments (baseline, 1 hour, and 2 hours). For example, subject 2's mean response to all three treatments is

$$\bar{S}_2 = \frac{4.0 + 3.7 + 4.4}{3} = 4.03 \text{ liters}$$

and the mean response of all four subjects to treatment 1 (baseline) is

$$\bar{T}_1 = \frac{3.7 + 4.0 + 3.0 + 3.2}{4} = 3.48 \text{ liters}$$

The grand mean of all observations $\bar{X}$ is 3.48 liters and the total sum of squares is $SS_{tot} = 2.6830$ liters^2.

Table 9–5 also includes the sum of squares within each subject; for example, for subject 2

$$\begin{aligned} SS_{\text{wit subj}} &= (4 - 4.03)^2 + (3.7 - 4.03)^2 + (4.4 - 4.03)^2 \\ &= 0.2467 \text{ liters}^2 \end{aligned}$$

Adding the within-subjects sums of squares for the four subjects in the study yields

$$SS_{\text{wit subjs}} = 0.1800 + 0.2467 + 0.0800 + 0.1267 = 0.6333 \text{ liters}^2$$

We obtain sum of squares between subjects by adding up the squares of the deviations between the subjects' means and the grand mean and multiplying by the numbers of treatments ($m = 3$, the number of numbers used to compute each subject's mean response)

$$\begin{aligned} SS_{\text{bet subjs}} &= 3[(3.70 - 3.48)^2 + (4.03 - 3.48)^2 + (3.00 - 3.48)^2 \\ &\quad + (3.17 - 3.48)^2] = 2.0490 \text{ liters}^2 \end{aligned}$$

(Note that $SS_{\text{wit subjs}} + SS_{\text{bet subjs}} = 0.6333 + 2.0490 = 2.6830$ liters^2, the total sum of squares, as it should.)

We obtain the sum of squares for the treatments by multiplying the squares of the differences between the treatment means and the grand mean times the number of subjects (n = 4, the number of numbers used to compute each mean),

$$SS_{treat} = 4\,[(3.48 - 3.48)^2 + (3.20 - 3.48)^2 + (3.75 - 3.48)^2] = 0.6050 \text{ liters}^2$$

There are $DF_{treat} = m - 1 = 3 - 1 = 2$ degrees of freedom associated with the treatments. Therefore, the residual sum of squares is

$$SS_{res} = SS_{wit\ subjs} - SS_{treat} = 0.6333 - 0.6050 = 0.0283 \text{ liters}^2$$

and $DF_{res} = (n - 1)(m - 1) = (4 - 1)(3 - 1) = 6$ degrees of freedom.

Table 9–6, the analysis-of-variance table for this experiment, summarizes the results of all these calculations. Notice that we have partitioned the sums of squares into more components than we did in Table 9–3. We are able to do this because we made repeated measurements on the same experimental subjects.

From Table 9–6, our two estimates of the population variance are

$$MS_{treat} = \frac{SS_{treat}}{DF_{treat}} = \frac{0.6050}{2} = 0.3025 \text{ liters}^2$$

and

$$MS_{res} = \frac{SS_{res}}{DF_{res}} = \frac{0.0283}{6} = 0.0047 \text{ liters}^2$$

Table 9–6 Analysis-of-Variance Table for One-Way Repeated-Measures Analysis of FEV_1 in Endotoxin Response

Source of variation	SS	DF	MS
Between subjects	2.0490	3	
Within subjects	0.6333	8	
Treatments	0.6050	2	0.3025
Residual	0.0283	6	0.0047
Total	2.6830	11	

$$F = \frac{MS_{treat}}{MS_{res}} = \frac{0.3025}{0.0047} = 64.053$$

so our test statistic is

$$F = \frac{MS_{\text{treat}}}{MS_{\text{res}}} = \frac{0.3025}{0.0047} = 64.36$$

This value exceeds $F_{.01} = 10.92$, the critical value that defines the largest 1 percent of possible values of F with 2 and 6 degrees of freedom for the numerator and denominator. Therefore, these data permit concluding that endotoxin and salbutamol alter FEV_1 ($P < .01$).

So far we can conclude that at least one of the treatments produced a change. To isolate which one, we need to use a multiple-comparisons procedure analogous to the Holm t test (or Holm-Sidak test or other procedures) developed in Chapter 4.

How to Isolate Differences in Repeated-Measures Analysis of Variance

In Chapter 4, we made multiple pairwise comparisons between groups with the Holm t test.

$$t = \frac{\bar{X}_1 - \bar{X}_2}{\sqrt{2\, s_{\text{wit}}^2 / n}}$$

To use the Holm t-test to isolate differences following a repeated-measures analysis of variance, we simply replace s_{wit}^2 with our estimate of the variance computed from the residual sum of squares, MS_{res}:

$$t = \frac{\bar{T}_i - \bar{T}_j}{\sqrt{2\, \text{MS}_{\text{res}} / n}}$$

in which $\bar{T}_i$ and $\bar{T}_j$ represent the mean treatment responses of the pair of treatments (treatments i and j) you are comparing. The resulting value of t is compared with the critical value for DF_{res} degrees of freedom.

There are three comparisons ($k = 3$) for this experiment. To compare FEV_1 1 hour following endotoxin to FEV_1 2 hours following endotoxin and salbutamol exposure

$$t = \frac{3.20 - 3.75}{\sqrt{2(0.0047)/4}} = -11.346$$

To compare baseline FEV_1 to FEV_1 2 hours following endotoxin and salbutamol exposure

$$t = \frac{3.48 - 3.75}{\sqrt{2(0.0047)/4}} = -5.570$$

Finally, to compare baseline FEV_1 with FEV_1 1 hour following endotoxin exposure

$$t = \frac{3.48 - 3.20}{\sqrt{2(0.0047)/4}} = -5.776$$

There are 6 degrees of freedom for these comparisons. The uncorrected P values corresponding to these three comparisons are less than .0001, .001, and .001.

To keep the overall risk of erroneously reporting a difference for this family of three comparisons below 5 percent, we compare these P values to the Holm t test corrected P values based on $k = 3$: $.05/k = .05/3 = 0.017$, $.05/(k-1) = .05/2 = 0.025$, and $.05/(k-2) = .05/1 = .05$. All three of the uncorrected P values fall below the appropriate critical P. These results allow us to conclude that endotoxin decreases FEV_1, and subsequent administration of salbutamol appeared to reverse this effect, increasing FEV_1 to levels higher than baseline.

The Student-Newman-Keuls (SNK), Bonferroni, or Tukey test may also be used to compute all pairwise comparisons, and Dunnett's test to compute multiple comparison against a single control group. To do so, make the analogous changes in the computation: use MS_{res} in place of s^2_{wit} and use DF_{res} to determine the critical values of q or q'.

Power in Repeated-Measures Analysis of Variance

Power is computed exactly as in a simple analysis of variance, using the within-subjects variation (estimated by $\sqrt{MS_{res}}$) as the estimate of population standard deviation, σ, and the number of subjects in place of the sample size of each group, n.

EXPERIMENTS WHEN OUTCOMES ARE MEASURED ON A NOMINAL SCALE: McNEMAR'S TEST

The paired t test and repeated-measures analysis of variance can be used to analyze experiments in which the variable being studied can be measured on an interval scale (and satisfies the other assumptions required of parametric methods). What about experiments, analogous to the ones in Chapter 5, in which outcomes are measured on a *nominal* scale? This problem often arises when asking whether or not an individual responded to a treatment or when comparing the results of two different diagnostic tests that are classified as positive or negative in the same individuals. We will develop a procedure to analyze such experiments, *McNemar's test for changes,* in the context of one such study.

p7 Antigen Expression in Human Breast Cancer

The p7 antigen has been shown to be expressed in cell lines derived from ovarian cancers but not in cell lines derived from normal tissues. In addition, expression of this antigen has been increased in ovarian cancer cells after treatment with chemotherapeutic agents. Since there are similarities between ovarian and breast cancer, Xiaowei Yang and colleagues* wanted to study whether this antigen is present in tumor cells from women with breast cancer. They also wanted to investigate how treatment with radiation or chemotherapy affects appearance of p7, since presence of this antigen in a substantial fraction of breast cancer tumor cells has been associated with distant metastases and local recurrences. To investigate whether radiation and chemotherapy affected the expression of p7, the investigators took tissue samples from women with breast cancer before and after they were treated and used several molecular biology techniques to test for the presence of p7.

Table 9–7 shows the results of such an experiment. Four women had p7 both before and after treatment, none had p7 present before but not after treatment, 12 women who did not have p7 present before treatment had it afterwards, and 14 had p7 neither before nor after treatment.

*X. Yang, S. Groshen, S. C. Formenti, N. Davidson, and M. F. Press, "P7 Antigen Expression in Human Breast Cancer," *Clin. Cancer Res.* **9**:201–206, 2003.

Table 9–7 Presence of p7 Antigen in Breast Cancer Tumor Cells Before and After Women are Treated with Radiation and Chemotherapy

	After	
Before	Positive	Negative
Positive	4	0
Negative	12	14

This table looks very much like the 2 × 2 contingency tables analyzed in Chapter 5. In fact, most people simply compute a χ^2 statistic from these data and look the P value up in Table 5–7. The numbers in Table 9–7 are associated with a value of $\chi^2 = 2.165$ (computed including the Yates correction for continuity). This value is well below 3.841, the value of χ^2 that defines the largest 5 percent of possible values of χ^2 with 1 degree of freedom. As a result, one might report "no significant difference" in the expression of p7 before and after treatment of breast cancer and conclude that treatment has no effect on the likelihood of tumor recurrence or metastasis.

There is, however, a serious problem with this approach. The χ^2 test statistic developed for contingency tables in Chapter 5 was used to test the hypothesis that the *rows and columns of the tables are independent*. In Table 9–7, the rows and columns are *not* independent because they represent the p7 status of *the same individuals* before and after cancer treatment. (This situation is analogous to the difference between the unpaired t test presented in Chapter 4 and the paired t test presented earlier in this chapter.) In particular, the 4 women who were positive for p7 *both* before and after treatment and the 14 who were negative *both* before and after treatment do not tell you anything about whether or not breast cancer tumor cells change expression of p7 in response to radiation or chemotherapy. We need a statistical procedure that focuses on the 12 women who were negative before treatment and positive after treatment and the fact that there were no women positive before and negative after treatment.

If there is no effect of the treatment on p7 expression, we would expect half the 0 + 12 = 12 women whose p7 status condition before and after treatment was different to have been positive before treatment but not after and half to have been negative before but positive after treatment. Table 9–7 shows that the observed number of women who fell into each of these two categories was 0 and 12, respectively. To compare these observed and expected frequencies, we can use the χ^2 test statistic to compare these observed frequencies with the expected frequency of $12/2 = 6$.

$$\chi^2 = \sum \frac{\left(|0 - E| - \tfrac{1}{2})^2\right)}{E}$$

$$= \frac{\left(|0 - 6| - \tfrac{1}{2}\right)^2}{6} + \frac{\left(|12 - 6| - \tfrac{1}{2}\right)^2}{6} = 10.083$$

(Notice that this computation of χ^2 includes the Yates correction for continuity because it has only 1 degree of freedom.)

This value exceeds 7.879, the value of χ^2 that defines the biggest 0.5 percent of the possible values of χ^2 with 1 degree of freedom (from Table 5–7) if the differences in observed and expected are simply the effects of random sampling. This analysis leads to the conclusion that there *is* a difference in expression of p7 in breast cancer tumor cells after women are treated with radiation and chemotherapy ($P < .005$). This conclusion could have implications for the prognosis of these women as well as making p7 a potential target for antibody-based treatments or other types of target-based approaches.

This example illustrates that it is entirely possible to compute values of test statistics and look up P values in tables that are meaningless when the experimental design and underlying populations are not compatible with the assumptions used to derive the statistical procedure.

In sum, McNemar's test for changes consists of the following procedure:

- *Ignore individuals who responded the same way to both treatments.*
- *Compute the total number of individuals who responded differently to the two treatments.*

- *Compute the expected number of individuals who would have responded positively to each of the two treatments (but not the other) as half the total number of individuals who responded differently to the two treatments.*
- *Compare the observed and expected number of individuals that responded to one of the treatments by computing a χ^2 test statistic (including Yates correction for continuity).*
- *Compare this value of χ^2 with the critical values of the χ^2 distribution with 1 degree of freedom.*

This procedures yields a *P* value that quantifies the probability that the differences in treatment response are due to chance rather than actual differences in how the two treatments affect the same individuals.

PROBLEMS

9-1 In Prob. 8-8 you analyzed data from the study F. P. Ashley and colleagues completed on the effectiveness of an ammonium chloride-based mouthrinse. A group of people was randomly given either an inactive control rinse for 48 hours or the active rinse for 48 hours. When that period was over, those given the active rinse were given the inactive rinse, and vice versa. Ashley and coworkers measured a clinical score for the amount of plaque at 48 hours for each rinse and found:

Plaque Score

Active rinse	Control rinse
32	14
60	39
25	24
45	13
65	9
60	3
68	10
83	14
120	1
110	36

Do these rinses have different abilities to suppress plaque?

9-2 Secondhand tobacco smoke increases the risk of a heart attack. In order to investigate the mechanisms for this effect, C. Arden Pope III and his colleagues ("Acute Exposure to Environmental Tobacco Smoke and Heart Rate Variability," *Environ. Health Perspect.* **109:**711–716, 2001) studied whether breathing secondhand smoke affected autonomic (reflex) nervous system control of the heart. At rest the heart beats regularly, about once a second, but there are small beat-to-beat random fluctuations of the order of 100 msec (.1 sec) superimposed on the regular interval between heart beats. This random fluctuation in the length of time between heart beats is known as heart rate variability and quantified as the standard deviation of inter-beat intervals over many beats. For reasons that are not fully understood, reductions in this heart rate variability are associated with increased risk of an acute heart attack. Pope and his colleagues measured heart rate variability in eight healthy young adults before and after they spent 2 hours sitting in the smoking lounge at the Salt Lake City Airport. Did sitting in the smoking lounge reduce heart rate variability? Here are the observations on the standard deviation of the length of time between beats (in msec) measured over the 2 hours before and immediately after sitting in the smoking lounge:

	Standard Deviation in Beat-to-Beat Period (msec)	
Experimental Subject	Before	After
Tom	135	105
Dick	118	95
Harry	98	80
Lev	95	73
Joaquin	87	70
Stan	75	60
Aaron	69	68
Ben	59	40

9-3 What are the chances of detecting a halving of the heart rate variability in Prob. 9-2 with 95 percent confidence? Note that the power chart in Fig. 6–9 applies to the paired t test.

9-4 Rework Prob. 9-2 as a repeated-measures analysis of variance. What is the arithmetic relationship between F and t?

9-5 In addition to measuring FEV_1 (the experiment described in conjunction with Fig. 9–6), Michel and colleagues took measurements of immune response in their subjects, including measuring the amount of C-reactive protein (CRP mg/dL), a protein that is elevated when tissue is inflamed. Did endotoxin by itself or the combination of endotoxin and salbutamol affect CRP levels? If so, are the effects the same 1 and 2 hours after giving the bronchial challenge? Their results are:

	CRP (mg/dL)		
Person (subject)	No drug (baseline)	1 hour after endotoxin	2 hours after endotoxin and salbutamol
1	0.60	0.47	0.49
2	0.52	0.39	0.73
3	1.04	0.83	0.47
4	0.87	1.31	0.71

9-6 In general, levels of the hormone testosterone decrease during periods of stress. Because physical and psychological stressors are inevitable in the life of soldiers, the military is very interested in assessing stress response in soldiers. Many studies addressing this issue suffer from taking place in a laboratory setting, which may not accurately reflect the real world stresses on a soldier. To investigate the effects of stress on testosterone levels in a more realistic setting, Charles Morgan and colleagues ("Hormone Profiles in Humans Experiencing Military Survival Training," *Biol Psychiatry*, **47:**89–1901, 2000) measured salivary testosterone levels in 12 men before and during a military training exercise. The exercise included simulated capture and interrogation modeled on American prisoner of war experiences during the Vietnam and Korean wars. What conclusions can be drawn from these observations? Here are their data:

Testosterone (ng/dL)				
Soldier	Beginning of training exercise	Time of capture	12 hours post-capture	48 hours post-capture
1	17.4	11.2	12.8	5.9
2	13.6	6.9	9.8	7.4
3	17.3	12.8	13.7	9.0
4	20.1	16.6	15.5	15.7
5	21.1	13.5	15.4	11.0
6	12.4	2.9	3.7	3.4
7	13.8	7.9	10.5	7.8
8	17.7	12.5	14.9	13.1
9	8.1	2.6	2.3	1.3
10	16.3	9.2	9.3	7.3
11	9.2	2.9	5.8	5.5
12	22.1	17.5	15.3	9.3

9-7 Animal studies have demonstrated that compression and distension of the stomach trigger nerves that signal the brain to turn off the desire to eat. This fact has led some to propose surgery to reduce stomach size in clinically obese people as a way of reducing food intake and, ultimately, body weight. This surgery, however, has significant risks—including death—associated with it. Alan Geliebter and colleagues ("Extra-abdominal Pressure Alters Food Intake, Intragastric Pressure, and Gastric Emptying Rate," *Am. J. Physiol.*, **250:**R549–R552, 1986) sought to limit expansion of the stomach (and so increase pressure within the stomach) by placing a large inflatable cuff around the abdomen of experimental subjects, inflating the cuff to a specified pressure to limit abdominal (and, presumably, stomach) expansion, and then measuring the volume of food consumed at a meal following a control period during which diet was controlled. Subjects were told that the main purpose of the study was to detect expansion of the abdomen during eating by monitoring the air pressure in the cuff around their abdomen, with several pressure levels used to determine the one most sensitive to abdominal expansion. They were asked to drink a liquid lunch from a reservoir until they felt full. The subjects did not know that food intake was being measured. What do you conclude from this experiment? Why did Geliebter and his colleagues lie to the subjects about the purpose and design of the experiment? Here are the data:

	Food intake (milliliters) at abdominal pressure		
Subject	0 mmHg	10 mmHg	20 mmHg
1	448	470	292
2	472	424	390
3	631	538	508
4	634	496	560
5	734	547	602
6	820	578	508
7	643	711	724

9-8 What is the power of the test in Prob. 9-7 to find a 100 mL change in food intake with 95 percent confidence?

9-9 In the fetus, there is a connection between the aorta and the artery going to the lungs called the ductus arteriosus that permits the heart to bypass the nonfunctioning lungs and circulate blood to the placenta to obtain oxygen and nourishment and dispose of wastes. After the infant is born and begins breathing, these functions are served by the lungs and the ductus arteriosus closes. Occasionally, especially in premature infants, the ductus arteriosus remains open and shunts blood around the lungs. This shunting prevents the infant from getting rid of carbon dioxide and taking in oxygen. The drug indomethacin has been used to make the ductus arteriosus close. It is very likely that the outcome (with or without drugs) depends on gestational age, age after birth, fluid intake, other illnesses, and other drugs the infant is receiving. For these reasons, an investigator might decide to pair infants who are as alike as possible in each of these identified variables, and randomly treat one member of each pair with indomethacin or placebo, then judge the results as improved or not improved. Suppose the findings are:

		Indomethacin	
		Improved	Not improved
Placebo	Improved	65	13
	Not improved	27	40

Do these data support the hypothesis that indomethacin is no better than a placebo?

9-10 The data in Prob. 9-9 could also be presented in the following form:

	Improved	Not improved
Indomethacin	92	53
Placebo	78	67

How would these data be analyzed? If this result differs from the analysis in Prob. 9-9, explain why and decide which approach is correct.

9-11 Review all original articles published in the *New England Journal of Medicine* during the last 12 months. How many of these articles present the results of experiments that should be analyzed with a repeated-measures analysis of variance? What percentage of these articles actually did such an analysis? Of those that did not, how did the authors analyze their data? Comment on potential difficulties with the conclusions that are advanced in these papers.

Chapter 10

Alternatives to Analysis of Variance and the *t* Test Based on Ranks

Analysis of variance, including the *t* tests, is widely used to test the hypothesis that one or more treatments had no effect on the mean of some observed variable. All forms of analysis of variance, including the *t* tests, are based on the assumption that the observations are drawn from normally distributed populations in which the variances are the same even if the treatments change the mean responses. These assumptions are often satisfied well enough to make analysis of variance an extremely useful statistical procedure. On the other hand, experiments often yield data that are not compatible with these assumptions. In addition, there are often problems in which the observations are measured on an ordinal rather than an interval scale and may not be amenable to an analysis of variance. This chapter develops analogs to the *t* tests and analysis of variance based on *ranks* of the observations rather than the observations themselves. This approach uses information about the relative sizes of the observations without assuming anything about the specific nature of the population they were drawn from.* We will begin with the nonparametric analog to the unpaired and paired *t* tests, the *Mann-Whitney rank-sum test,* and *Wilcoxon's signed-rank test.* Then we will present the analogs of one-way analysis of variance, the *Kruskal-Wallis statistic,* and repeated-measures analysis-of-variance *Friedman statistic.*

HOW TO CHOOSE BETWEEN PARAMETRIC AND NONPARAMETRIC METHODS

As already noted, analysis of variance is called a *parametric* statistical method because it is based on estimates of the two population parameters, the mean and standard deviation (or variance), that completely define a normal distribution. Given the assumption that the samples are drawn from normally distributed populations, one can compute the distributions of the *F*- or *t*-test statistics that will occur in all possible experiments of a given size when the treatments have no effect. The critical values that define a value of *F* or *t* can then be obtained from that distribution. When the assumptions of parametric statistical methods are satisfied, they are the most powerful tests available.

If the populations the observations were drawn from are not normally distributed (or are not reasonably compatible with other assumptions of a parametric method, such as equal variances in all the treatment groups), parametric methods become quite unreliable because the mean and standard deviation, the key elements of parametric statistics, no longer completely describe the population. In fact, when the population substantially deviates from normality, interpreting the mean and standard deviation in terms of a normal distribution can produce a very misleading picture.

For example, recall our discussion of the distribution of heights of the entire population of Jupiter. The mean height of all Jovians is 37.6 cm in Fig. 2–3*A*, and the standard deviation is 4.5 cm. Rather than being equally distributed about the mean, the population is *skewed* toward taller heights. Specifically, the heights of Jovians range from 31 to 52 cm, with most heights around 35 cm. Figure 2–3*B* shows what the population of heights would have been if, instead of being skewed

*These methods do assume that the samples were drawn from populations with the same shape distributions, but there is no assumption about what that shape is.

toward taller heights, they had been normally distributed with the same mean and standard deviation as the actual population (in Fig. 2–3*A*). The heights would have ranged from 26 to 49 cm, with most heights around 37 to 38 cm. Simply looking at Fig. 2–3 should convince you that envisioning a population on the basis of the mean and standard deviation can be quite misleading if the population does not, at least approximately, follow the normal distribution.

The same thing is true of statistical tests that are based on the normal distribution. When the population the samples were drawn from does not at least approximately follow the normal distribution, these tests can be quite misleading. In such cases, it is possible to use the *ranks* of the observations rather than the observations themselves to compute statistics that can be used to test hypotheses. By using ranks rather than the actual measurements, it is possible to retain much of the information about the relative size of responses without making any assumptions about how the population the samples were drawn from is distributed. Since these tests are not based on the parameters of the underlying population, they are called *nonparametric* or *distribution-free* methods.* All the methods we will discuss require only that the distributions under the different treatments have similar shapes, but there is no restriction on what those shapes are.† When the observations are not drawn from normally distributed populations, the nonparametric methods in this chapter are about 95 percent as powerful as the analogous parametric methods. As a result, power for these tests can be estimated by computing the power of the analogous parametric test. When the observations are drawn from populations that are not normally distributed, nonparametric methods are not only more reliable but also more powerful than parametric methods.

Unfortunately, you can never observe the entire population. So how can you tell whether the assumptions such as normality are met, to permit using the parametric tests like analysis of variance? The simplest approach is to plot the observations and look at them. Do they seem

*The methods in this chapter are obviously not the first nonparametric methods we have encountered. The χ^2 for analysis of nominal data in contingency tables in Chapter 5, the Spearman rank correlation to analyze ordinal data in Chapter 8, and McNemar's test in Chapter 9 are three widely used nonparametric methods.

†They also require that the distributions be continuous (so that ties are impossible) to derive the mathematical forms of the sampling distributions used to define the critical values of the various test statistics. In practice, however, this restriction is not important, and the methods can be applied to observations with tied measurements.

compatible with the assumptions that they were drawn from normally distributed populations with roughly the same variances, that is, within a factor of 2 to 3 of each other? If so, you are probably safe in using parametric methods. If, on the other hand, the observations are heavily skewed (suggesting a population like the Jovians in Fig. 2–3*A*) or appear to have more than one peak, you probably will want to use a nonparametric method. When the standard deviation is about the same size or larger than the mean and the variable can take on only positive values, this is an indication that the distribution is skewed. (A normally distributed variable would have to take on negative values.) In practice, these simple rules of thumb are often all you will need.

There are two ways to make this procedure more objective. The first is to plot the observations on *normal-probability graph paper.* Normal-probability graph paper has a distorted scale that makes normally distributed observations plot as a straight line (just as exponential functions plot as a straight line on semilogarithmic graph paper). Examining how straight the line is will show how compatible the observations are with a normal distribution. One can also construct a χ^2 statistic to test how closely the observed data agree with those expected if the population is normally distributed with the same mean and standard deviation. Since in practice simply looking at the data is generally adequate, we will not discuss these approaches in detail.*

Unfortunately, none of these methods is especially convincing one way or the other for the small sample sizes common in biomedical research, and your choice of approach (i.e., parametric versus nonparametric) often has to be based more on judgment and preference than hard evidence.

Things basically come down to the following difference of opinion: Some people think that in the *absence* of evidence that the data were *not* drawn from a normally distributed population, one should use parametric tests because they are more powerful and more widely used. These people say that you should use a nonparametric test only when there is positive evidence that the populations under study are not normally

*For discussions and example of these procedures, see J. H. Zar, *Biostatistical Analysis,* 4th ed. Prentice-Hall, Upper Saddle River, N.J., 1999, chapter 7, "The Normal Distribution," or W. J. Dixon and F. J. Massey, Jr., *Introduction to Statistical Analysis,* 4th ed, McGraw-Hill, New York, 1983, chapter 5, "The Normal Distribution."

distributed. Others point out that the nonparametric methods discussed in this chapter are 95 percent as powerful as parametric methods when the data are from normally distributed populations and more reliable when the data are not from normally distributed populations. They also believe that investigators should assume as little as possible when analyzing their data; they therefore recommend that nonparametric methods be used *except* when there is *positive evidence* that parametric methods are suitable. At the moment there is no definitive answer stating which attitude is preferable. And there probably never will be such an answer.

TWO DIFFERENT SAMPLES: THE MANN-WHITNEY RANK-SUM TEST

When we developed the analysis of variance, t test, and Pearson product-moment correlation, we began with a specific (normally distributed) population and examined the values of the test statistic associated with all possible samples of a given size that could be selected from that population. The situation is different for methods based on ranks rather than the actual observations. We will replace the actual observations with their ranks, then focus on the population of all possible combinations of ranks. Since all samples have a finite number of members, we can simply list all the different possible ways to rank the members to obtain the distribution of possible values for the test statistic when the treatment has no effect.

To illustrate this process but keep this list relatively short, let us analyze a small experiment in which three people take a placebo and four people take a drug that is thought to be a diuretic. Table 10–1 shows the daily urine production observed in this experiment. Table 10–1 also shows the ranks of all the observations without regard to which experimental group they fall in; the smallest observed urine production is ranked 1 and the largest one is ranked 7. If the drug affected daily urine production, we would expect the rankings in the control group to be lower (or higher, if the drug decreased urine production) than the ranks for the treatment group. We will use the sum of ranks in the smaller group (in this case, the control group) as our test statistic T. The control-group ranks add up to 9.

Is the value of $T = 9$ sufficiently extreme to justify rejecting the hypothesis that the drug had no effect?

Table 10–1 Observations in Diuretic Experiment

Placebo (control)		Drug (treatment)	
Daily urine production, mL/day	Rank*	Daily urine production, mL/day	Rank*
1000	1	1400	6
1380	5	1600	7
1200	3	1180	2
		1220	4
	$T = 9$		

*1 = smallest; 7 = largest.

To answer this question, we examine the *population of all possible rankings* to see how likely we are to get a rank sum as extreme as that associated in Table 10–1. Notice that we are no longer discussing the actual observations but their ranks, so our results will apply to *any* experiment in which there are two samples, one containing three individuals and the other containing four individuals, regardless of the nature of the underlying populations.

We begin with the hypothesis that the drug did not affect urine production, so that the ranking pattern in Table 10–1 is just due to chance. To estimate the chances of getting this pattern when the two samples were drawn from a single population, we need not engage in any fancy mathematics, we just *list* all the possible rankings that could have occurred. Table 10–2 shows all 35 different ways the ranks could have been arranged with 3 people in one group and 4 in the other. The crosses indicate a person in the placebo group, and the

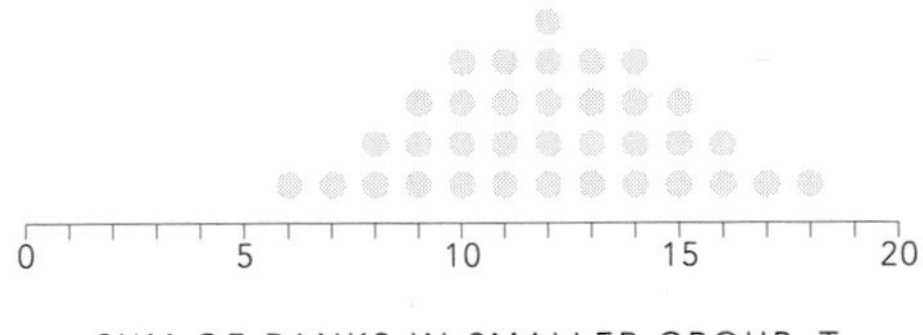

Figure 10–1 Sums of ranks in the smaller group for all possible rankings of seven individuals with three individuals in one sample and four in the other. Each circle represents one possible sum of ranks.

Table 10–2 Possible Ranks and Rank Sums for Three Individuals Out of Seven

Rank							
1	2	3	4	5	6	7	Rank sum T
X	X	X					6
X	X		X				7
X	X			X			8
X	X				X		9
X	X					X	10
X		X	X				8
X		X		X			9
X		X			X		10
X		X				X	11
X			X	X			10
X			X		X		11
X			X			X	12
X				X	X		12
X				X		X	13
X					X	X	14
	X	X	X				9
	X	X		X			10
	X	X			X		11
	X	X				X	12
	X		X	X			11
	X		X		X		12
	X		X			X	13
	X			X	X		13
	X			X		X	14
	X				X	X	15
		X	X	X			12
		X	X		X		13
		X	X			X	14
		X		X	X		14
		X		X		X	15
		X			X	X	16
			X	X	X		15
			X	X		X	16
			X		X	X	17
				X	X	X	18

blanks indicate a person in the treatment group. The right-hand column shows the sum of ranks for the people in the smaller (placebo) group for each possible combination of ranks. Figure 10–1 shows the distribution of possible values of our test statistic, the sum of ranks of the smaller group T that can occur when the treatment has no effect. This distribution looks a little like the t distribution in Fig. 4–5. Except that the distributions are not identical, there is another very important difference. Whereas the t distribution is continuous and, in theory, is based on an infinitely large collection of possible values of the t-test statistic, Fig. 10–1 shows *every possible* value of the sum-of-ranks test statistic T.

Since there are 35 possible ways to combine the ranks, there is 1 chance in 35 of getting rank sums of 6, 7, 17, or 18; 2 chances in 35 of getting 8 or 16; 3 chances in 35 of getting 9 or 15; 4 chances in 35 of getting 10, 11, 13, or 14; and 5 chances in 35 of getting 12. What are the chances of getting an extreme value of T? There is a $^2/_{35} = .057 = 5.7$ percent chance of obtaining $T = 6$ or $T = 18$ when the treatment has no effect. We use these numbers as the critical values to define extreme values of T and reject the hypothesis of no treatment effect. Hence, the value of $T = 9$ associated with the observations in Table 10–1 is not extreme enough to justify rejecting the hypothesis that the drug has no effect on urine production.

Notice that in this case $T = 6$ and $T = 18$ correspond to $P = .057$. Since T can take on only integer values, P can take on only discrete values. As a result, tables of critical values of T present pairs of values that define the proportion of possible values nearest traditional critical P values, for example, 5 and 1 percent, but the exact P values defined by these critical values generally do not equal 5 and 1 percent exactly. Table 10–3 presents these critical values. n_S and n_B are the number of members in the smaller and larger samples. The table gives the critical values of T that come nearest defining the most extreme 5 and 1 percent of all possible values of T that will occur if the treatment has no effect, as well as the exact proportion of possible T values defined by the critical values. For example, Table 10–3 shows that 7 and 23 define the 4.80 percent most extreme possible values of the rank sum of the smaller of two sample groups T when $n_S = 3$ and $n_B = 6$.

Table 10–3 Critical Values (Two-Tailed) of the Mann-Whitney Rank-Sum Statistic T

		Probability levels near			
		.05		.01	
n_S	n_B	Critical values	P	Critical values	P
3	4	6,18	.057		
	5	6,21	.036		
	5	7,20	.071		
	6	7,23	.048	6,24	.024
	7	7,26	.033	6,27	.017
	7	8,25	.067		
	8	8,28	.042	6,30	.012
4	4	11,25	.057	10,26	.026
	5	11,29	.032	10,30	.016
	5	12,28	.063		
	6	12,32	.038	10,34	.010
	7	13,35	.042	10,38	.012
	8	14,38	.048	11,41	.008
	8	....	....	12,40	.016
5	5	17,38	.032	15,40	.008
	5	18,37	.056	16,39	.016
	6	19,41	.052	16,44	.010
	7	20,45	.048	17,48	.010
	8	21,49	.045	18,52	.011
6	6	26,52	.041	23,55	.009
	6	....	....	24,54	.015
	7	28,56	.051	24,60	.008
	7	....	....	25,59	.014
	8	29,61	.043	25,65	.008
	8	30,60	.059	26,64	.013
7	7	37,68	.053	33,72	.011
	8	39,73	.054	34,78	.009
8	8	49,87	.050	44,92	.010

Source: Computed from F. Mosteller and R. Rourke, *Sturdy Statistics: Nonparametrics and Order Statistics,* Addison-Wesley, Reading, MA, 1973, Table A–9. Used by permission.

The procedure we just described is the *Mann-Whitney rank-sum test.** The procedure for testing the hypothesis that a treatment had no effect with this statistic is:

- *Rank all observations according to their magnitude, a rank of 1 being assigned to the smallest observation. Tied observations should be assigned the same rank, equal to the average of the ranks they would have been assigned had there been no tie (i.e., using the same procedure as in computing the Spearman rank correlation coefficient in Chapter 8).*
- *Compute* T, *the sum of the ranks in the smaller sample. (If both samples are the same size, you can compute* T *from either one.)*
- *Compare the resulting value of* T *with the distribution of all possible rank sums for experiments with samples of the same size to see whether the pattern of rankings is compatible with the hypothesis that the treatment had no effect.*

There are two ways to compare the observed value of T with the critical value defining the most extreme values that would occur if the treatment had no effect. The first approach is to compute the exact distribution of T by listing all the possibilities, as we just did, then tabulate the results in a table like Table 10–3. For experiments in which the samples are small enough to be included in Table 10–3, this approach gives the exact P value associated with a given set of experimental observations. For larger experiments, this exact approach becomes quite tedious because the number of possible rankings gets very large. For example, there are 184,756 different ways to rank two samples of 10 individuals each.

*There is an alternative formulation of this test that yields a statistic commonly denoted by U. U is related to T by the formula $U = T - n_S(n_S + 1)/2$, where n_s is the size of the smaller sample (or either sample if both contain the same number of individuals). For a presentation of the U statistic, see S. Siegel and N. J. Castellan, Jr., *Nonparametric Statistics for the Behavioral Sciences,* 2nd ed. McGraw-Hill, New York, 1988, Section 6.4, "The Wilcoxon-Mann-Whitney U Test." For a detailed derivation and discussion of the Mann-Whitney test as developed here, as well as its relationship to U, see F. Mosteller and R. Rourke, *Sturdy Statistics: Nonparametrics and Order Statistics,* Addison-Wesley, Reading, MA, 1973, chapter 3, "Ranking Methods for Two Independent Samples."

Second, when the large sample contains more than eight members, the distribution of T is very similar to the normal distribution with mean

$$\mu_T = \frac{n_S(n_S + n_B + 1)}{2}$$

and standard deviation

$$\sigma_T = \sqrt{\frac{n_S n_B(n_S + n_B + 1)}{12}}$$

in which n_S is the size of the smaller sample.* Hence, we can transform T into the test statistic

$$z_T = \frac{T - \mu_T}{\sigma_T}$$

and compare this statistic with the critical values of the normal distribution that define the, say 5 percent, most extreme possible values. z_T can also be compared with the t distribution with an infinite number of degrees of freedom (Table 4–1) because it equals the normal distribution.

This comparison can be made more accurate by including a *continuity correction* (analogous to the Yates correction for continuity in Chapter 5) to account for the fact that the normal distribution is continuous whereas the rank sum T must be an integer

$$z_T = \frac{|T - \mu_T| - \frac{1}{2}}{\sigma_T}$$

*When there are tied measurements, the standard deviation needs to be reduced according to the following formula, which depends on the number of ties.

$$\sigma_T \sqrt{\frac{n_S n_B(N + 1)}{12} - \frac{n_S n_B}{12N(N^2 - 1)} \sum(\tau_i - 1)\tau_i(\tau_i + 1)}$$

in which $N = n_S + n_B$, τ_i = number of tied ranks in ith set of ties, the sum indicated by Σ is computed over all sets of tied ranks.

The Leboyer Approach to Childbirth

Generally accepted methods of assisting low-risk women during childbirth have changed dramatically, with a general trend away from heavy sedation and increased emphasis on a role for the father during labor and delivery. The exact procedures to be used, however, are controversial. The French physician Leboyer heated up this debate with his book *Birth without Violence* in 1975. Leboyer suggested specific maneuvers to minimize the shock of the newborn child's first separation experience. He described the ideal birth as occurring in a dark, quiet room to minimize sensory overstimulation. He suggested placing the infant on his mother's abdomen and delaying cutting the umbilical cord until it stopped pulsating, calming the infant by gentle massaging, and placing the infant in a warm bath "to insure that this separation is not a shock but a joy." He claimed that children delivered this way were healthier and happier. Many medical practitioners objected to these procedures, saying that they interfered with accepted medical practice and increased risks to both the mother and child. Nevertheless, the Leboyer approach has gained popularity.

Like so many medical procedures, there is surprisingly little evidence to support or refute the claims Leboyer or his critics make. Until Nancy Nelson and colleagues* completed a randomized clinical trial of the methods, the only published evidence consisted of "clinical experience" and a single uncontrolled trial that supported Leboyer's position.

Nelson and her colleagues recruited low-risk pregnant women who were interested in the Leboyer method from an obstetrical practice at McMaster University, Ontario, Canada. The women had to have carried the infant for at least 36 weeks and be available for assessments of the child's development 3 days and 8 months after birth. After acceptance into the study, women were randomly allocated to be delivered by Leboyer techniques or by conventional (control) methods in a normally lit delivery room in which no particular attention was paid to sound levels, the umbilical cord was cut immediately after delivery, and the baby was wrapped in a blanket and given to the mother. In both groups the use of pain killers was minimized, and both parents participated actively in the labor and delivery. Thus, the study was designed to focus

*N. Nelson, M. Enkin, S. Saigal, K. Bennett, R. Milner, and D. Sackett, "A Randomized Clinical Trial of the Leboyer Approach to Childbirth," *N. Engl. J. Med.,* **302:** 655–660, 1980.

on the effects of the specific and controversial aspects of Leboyer's methods rather than the general principles of a gentle delivery.

Obviously the parents, physicians, and nurses who participated in the delivery knew which experimental group they were in. The researchers who were charged with evaluating the mothers and children before and after delivery and over the ensuing months, however, did not know how the children had been delivered. Thus, this is a *single-blind* protocol that minimizes the effects of observer biases but cannot control for the placebo effect.

Since the prime benefit of the Leboyer method is believed to be better development of the child, the investigators measured infant development on a specially constructed scale. They estimated that 30 percent of conventionally delivered infants would have "superior" scores on this scale. They reasoned that if the Leboyer method is really better, they would want to be able to detect a change that led to 90 percent of infants delivered by the Leboyer technique to rate "superior" in development. Computations using power revealed that the study had to include at least 20 infants in each treatment group to have a 90 percent chance of detecting such a difference with $P < .05$ (i.e., the power of the experiment is .90). Notice that they were, in effect, saying that they were not interested in detecting any smaller effect of the Leboyer treatment.

During the 1 year in which they recruited experimental subjects, they talked to 187 families and explained the trial to them; 34 did not meet the initial eligibility requirements, and 56 of the remaining 153 agreed to be randomized. Among the 97 who refused randomization, 70 insisted on a Leboyer delivery and 23 refused to participate in the study. One woman was delivered prematurely before randomization, and the remaining 55 were randomized. One of the women in the control group dropped out the study, leaving 26 women in the control group and 28 in the Leboyer (treatment) group. Six women in the control group and eight in the Leboyer group had complications that precluded delivery as planned, leaving the required 20 women in each group. This bit of bookkeeping illustrates how difficult it is to accumulate a sufficient number of cases in clinical studies, even ones as relatively simple and benign as this one.*

*The decision of whom to include and not include in a randomized trial, combined with the effects of people who drop out or are lost to follow-up, can have a profound effect on the outcome of the study. For a discussion of this problem, see D. Sackett and M. Gent, "Controversy in Counting and Attributing Events in Clinical Trials," *N. Engl. J. Med.*, **301:**1410–1412, 1979.

Although Nelson and colleagues examined a wide variety of variables before, during, immediately after, and several months after delivery, we will examine only one of the things they measured, the number of minutes the newborn child was alert during the first hour of life. If the Leboyer method leads to less traumatized newborns, we would expect them to be more alert immediately after delivery. Table 10–4 and Fig. 10–2 show the number of minutes of alertness during the first hour for the 20 infants in each of the two treatment groups.

The first thing that is evident from Fig. 10–2 is that the observations probably do not come from normally distributed populations. The length of time these infants were alert is skewed toward lower times, rather than being equally likely to be above the mean as below it. Since these data are *not* suitable for analysis with a parametric method such as the unpaired t test, we will use the Mann-Whitney rank-sum test.

Table 10–4 Minutes of Alert Activity during First Hour after Birth

Control delivery	Rank	Leboyer delivery	Rank
5.0	2	2.0	1
10.1	3	19.0	5
17.7	4	29.7	10
20.3	6	32.1	12
22.0	7	35.4	15
24.9	8	36.7	17
26.5	9	38.5	19
30.8	11	40.2	20
34.2	13	42.1	22
35.0	14	43.0	23
36.6	16	44.4	24
37.9	18	45.6	26
40.4	21	46.7	27
45.5	25	47.1	28
49.3	31	48.0	29
51.1	33	49.0	30
53.1	36	50.9	32
55.0	38	51.2	34
56.7	39	52.5	35
58.0	40	53.3	37
	$T = 374$		

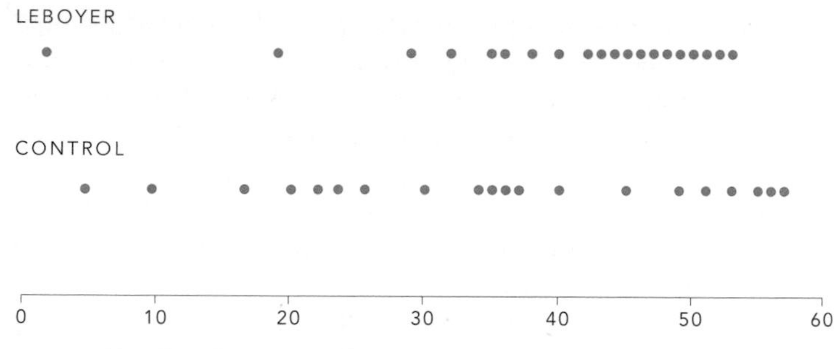

Figure 10–2 Number of minutes of alert behavior during first hour of life among infants delivered by conventional gentle techniques and the Leboyer method. Notice that the times are skewed toward higher values.

In addition to the observed number of minutes of alert behavior in the first hour, Table 10–4 shows the ranks of these observations, assigned without regard to which treatment group contains the individual infant being ranked. Since both samples are the same size, we can compute the rank sum T from either group. The rank sum for the control group is $T = 374$. Since there are 20 people in each group, we will compute the P value by computing z_T and comparing the resulting value with the normal distribution. The mean of all possible values of T for experiments of this size is

$$\mu_T = \frac{n_S(n_S + n_B + 1)}{2} = \frac{20(20 + 20 + 1)}{2} = 410$$

and the standard deviation is

$$\sigma_T = \sqrt{\frac{n_S n_B(n_S + n_B + 1)}{12}}$$

$$= \sqrt{\frac{20(20)(20 + 20 + 1)}{12}} = 36.97$$

So

$$z_T = \frac{|T - \mu_T| - \frac{1}{2}}{\sigma_T} = \frac{|374 - 410| - \frac{1}{2}}{36.9} = 0.962$$

This value is smaller than 1.960, the value of z that defines the biggest 5 percent of the normal distribution (from Table 4–1 with an infinite number of degrees of freedom). Hence, this study does not provide sufficient evidence to conclude that the Leboyer method is associated with more alert newborns.*

In fact, except for the feeling by mothers that the Leboyer method had influenced their child's behavior and the tendency of women using the Leboyer method to have shorter active labors, Nelson and colleagues could find no evidence that the Leboyer method led to outcomes different from those of a conventional gentle birth. These differences may actually be reflections of the placebo effect, since the mothers obviously knew the methods used for delivery and may have wanted better outcomes. The bottom line, for both the method's enthusiasts and critics, however, seems to be that nothing is gained or lost by choosing to use or not to use Leboyer's specific recommendations.

EACH SUBJECT OBSERVED BEFORE AND AFTER ONE TREATMENT: THE WILCOXON SIGNED-RANK TEST

Chapter 9 presented the paired *t* test to analyze experiments in which each experimental subject was observed before and after a single treatment. This test required that the changes accompanying treatment be normally distributed. We now develop an analogous test based on ranks that does not require this assumption. We compute the differences caused by the treatment in each experimental subject, rank these differences according to their magnitude (without regard for sign), then attach the sign of the difference to each rank, and finally sum the signed ranks to obtain the test statistic *W*.

This procedure uses information about the sizes of the differences the treatment produces in each experimental subject as well as its direction. Since it is based on ranks, it does not require making any assumptions about the nature of the population of the differences the treatment produces. As with the Mann-Whitney rank-sum test statistic, we can obtain the distribution of all possible values of the test statistic *W* by

*It is possible to compute a confidence interval for the median, but we will not discuss this procedure. For a discussion of confidence intervals for the median, see Mosteller and Rourke, *Sturdy Statistics: Nonparametrics and Order Statistics,* Addison-Wesley, Reading, MA, 1973, chapter 14, "Order Statistics: Distribution of Probabilities; Confidence Limits, Tolerance Limits."

simply listing all the possibilities of the signed-rank sum for experiments of a given size. We finally compare the value of W associated with our observations with the distribution of all possible values of W that can occur in experiments involving the number of individuals in our study. If the observed value of W is "big," the observations are not compatible with the assumption that treatment had no effect.

Remember that observations are ranked based on the *magnitude* of the changes *without regard for signs,* so that the differences that are equal in magnitude but opposite in sign, say −5.32 and +5.32, both have the same rank.

We begin with another hypothetical experiment in which we wish to test a potential diuretic on six people. In contrast to the experiments the last section described, we will observe daily urine production in each person *before* and *after* administering the drug. Table 10–5 shows the results of this experiment, together with the change in urine production that followed administering the drug in each person.

Daily urine production fell in five of the six people. Are these data sufficient to justify asserting that the drug was an effective diuretic?

To apply the signed-rank test, we first rank the magnitudes of each observed change, beginning with 1 for the smallest change and ending with 6 for largest change. Next, we attach the sign of the change to each rank (last column of Table 10–5) and compute the sum of the signed ranks W. For this experiment, $W = -13$.

If the drug has no effect, the ranks associated with positive changes should be similar to the ranks associated with the negative changes and W should be near zero. On the other hand, when the treatment alters the

Table 10–5 Effect of a Potential Diuretic on Six People

	Daily urine production mL/day				
Person	Before drug	After drug	Difference	Rank* of difference	Signed rank of difference
1	1600	1490	−110	5	−5
2	1850	1300	−550	6	−6
3	1300	1400	+100	4	+4
4	1500	1410	−90	3	−3
5	1400	1350	−50	2	−2
6	1010	1000	−10	1	−1
					$W = -13$

*1 = smallest magnitude; 6 = largest magnitude.

variable being studied, the changes with the larger or smaller ranks will tend to have the same sign and the signed rank sum W will be a big positive or big negative number.

As with all test statistics, we need only draw the line between "small" and "big." We do this by listing *all* 64 possible combinations of different ranking patterns, from all negative changes to all positive changes (Table 10–6). There is a 1 chance in 64 of getting any of these patterns by chance. Figure 10–3 shows all 64 of the signed-rank sums listed in Table 10–6.

Table 10–6 Possible Combinations of Signed Ranks for a Study of Six Individuals

Rank*						
1	2	3	4	5	6	Sum of signed ranks
−	−	−	−	−	−	−21
+	−	−	−	−	−	−19
−	+	−	−	−	−	−17
−	−	+	−	−	−	−15
−	−	−	+	−	−	−13
−	−	−	−	+	−	−11
−	−	−	−	−	+	−9
+	+	−	−	−	−	−15
+	−	+	−	−	−	−13
+	−	−	+	−	−	−11
+	−	−	−	+	−	−9
+	−	−	−	−	+	−7
−	+	+	−	−	−	−11
−	+	−	+	−	−	−9
−	+	−	−	+	−	−7
−	+	−	−	−	+	−5
−	−	+	+	−	−	−7
−	−	+	−	+	−	−5
−	−	+	−	−	+	−3
−	−	−	+	+	−	−3
−	−	−	+	−	+	−1
−	−	−	−	+	+	1
+	+	+	−	−	−	−9
+	+	−	+	−	−	−7
+	+	−	−	+	−	−5
+	+	−	−	−	+	−3

(continued)

Table 10–6 Possible Combinations of Signed Ranks for a Study of Six Individuals (*Continued*)

Rank*						
1	2	3	4	5	6	Sum of signed ranks
+	−	+	+	−	−	−5
+	−	+	−	+	−	−3
+	−	+	−	−	+	−1
+	−	−	+	+	−	−1
+	−	−	+	−	+	1
+	−	−	−	+	+	3
−	+	+	+	−	−	−3
−	+	+	−	+	−	−1
−	+	+	−	−	+	1
−	+	−	+	+	−	1
−	+	−	+	−	+	3
−	+	−	−	+	+	5
−	−	+	+	+	−	3
−	−	+	+	−	+	5
−	−	+	−	+	+	7
−	−	−	+	+	+	9
+	+	+	+	−	−	−1
+	+	+	−	+	−	1
+	+	+	−	−	+	3
+	+	−	+	+	−	3
+	+	−	+	−	+	5
+	+	−	−	+	+	7
+	−	+	+	+	−	5
+	−	+	+	−	+	7
+	−	+	−	+	+	9
+	−	−	+	+	+	11
−	+	+	+	+	−	7
−	+	+	+	−	+	9
−	+	+	−	+	+	11
−	+	−	+	+	+	13
−	−	+	+	+	+	15
+	+	+	+	+	−	9
+	+	+	+	−	+	11
+	+	+	−	+	+	13
+	+	−	+	+	+	15
+	−	+	+	+	+	17
−	+	+	+	+	+	19
+	+	+	+	+	+	21

*Signs denote whether rank is positive or negative.

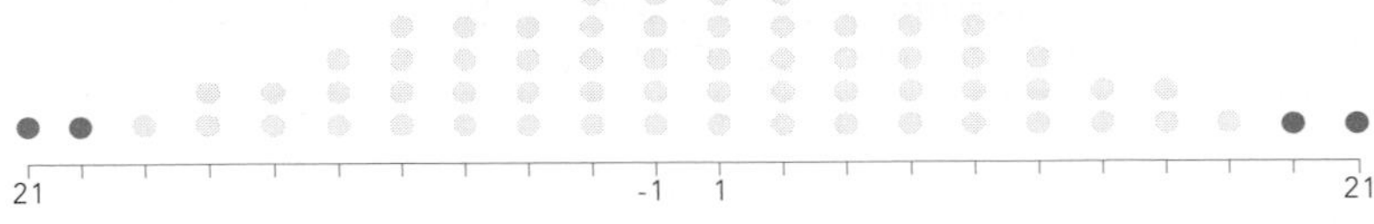

Figure 10–3 All 64 possible sums of signed ranks for observations before and after administering a treatment to six individuals. Table 10–6 lists all the possibilities. The colored circles show that 4 out of 64 have a magnitude of 19 or more, that is, fall at or below −19 or at or above +19.

To define a "big" value of *W*, we take the most extreme values of *W* that can occur when the treatment has no effect. Of the 64 possible rank sums, 4, or $^4/_{64} = .0625 = 6.25$ percent, fall at or beyond 19 (or −19), so we will reject the hypothesis that the treatment has no effect when the magnitude of *W* equals or exceeds 19 (i.e., *W* equals or is more negative than −19 or more positive than +19) with $P = .0625$.

Notice that, as with the Mann-Whitney rank-sum test, the discrete nature of the distribution of possible values of *W* means that we cannot always obtain *P* values precisely at traditional levels, like 5 percent. Since the value of *W* associated with the observations in Table 10–5 is only −13, these data are not sufficiently incompatible with the assumption that the treatment had no effect (that the drug is not an effective diuretic) to justify rejecting that hypothesis.

Table 10–7 presents the values of *W* that come closest to defining the most extreme 5 and 1 percent of all possible values for experiments with up to 20 subjects. For larger experiments, we use the fact that the distribution of *W* closely approximates a normal distribution with mean

$$\mu_W = 0$$

and standard deviation

$$\sigma_W = \sqrt{\frac{n(n+1)(2n+1)}{6}}$$

in which *n* equals the number of experimental subjects.

Table 10–7 Critical Values (Two-Tailed) of Wilcoxon *W*

n	Critical value	*P*	*n*	Critical value	*P*
5	15	.062	13	65	.022
6	21	.032		57	.048
	19	.062	14	73	.020
7	28	.016		63	.050
	24	.046	15	80	.022
8	32	.024		70	.048
	28	.054	16	88	.022
9	39	.020		76	.050
	33	.054	17	97	.020
10	45	.020		83	.050
	39	.048	18	105	.020
11	52	.018		91	.048
	44	.054	19	114	.020
12	58	.020		98	.050
	50	.052	20	124	.020
				106	.048

Source: Adapted from F. Mostelle; and R. Rourke, *Sturdy Statistics: Nonparametrics and Order Statistics,* Addison-Wesley, Reading, MA, 1973, Table A–11. Used by permission.

Therefore, we use

$$z_W = \frac{W - \mu_W}{\sigma_W} = \frac{W}{\sqrt{[n(n+1)(2n+1)]/6}}$$

as our test statistic. This approximation can be improved by including a continuity correction to obtain

$$z_W = \frac{|W| - \frac{1}{2}}{\sqrt{[n(n+1)(2n+1)]/6}}$$

There are two kinds of *ties* that can occur when computing *W*. First, there can be no change in the observed variable when the treatment is applied, so that the difference is zero. In this case, that individual provides no information about whether the treatment increases or decreases the response variable; so it is simply dropped from the analysis, and the sample size is reduced by 1. Second, the magnitudes of the change the treatment produces can be the same for two or more individuals. As with the Mann-Whitney test, all the individuals with that change are assigned the same rank as the average of the ranks that would be used for the same number of individuals if they were not tied.*

In summary, here is the procedure for comparing the observed effects of a treatment in a single group of experimental subjects before and after administering a treatment.

- *Compute the change in the variable of interest in each experimental subject.*
- *Rank all the differences according to their magnitude without regard for sign. (Zero differences should be dropped from the analysis with a corresponding reduction of sample size. Tied ranks should be assigned the average of the ranks that would be assigned to the tied ranks if they were not tied.)*
- *Apply the sign of each difference to its rank.*
- *Add all the signed ranks to obtain the test statistic W.*†
- *Compare the observed value of W with the distribution of possible values that would occur if the treatment had no effect, and reject this hypothesis if W is "big."*

To further illustrate this process, let us use the *Wilcoxon signed-rank test* to analyze the results of an experiment we discussed in Chapter 9.

*When there are tied ranks and you use the normal distribution to compute the P value, σ_W needs to be reduced by a factor that depends on the number of ties according to the formula

$$\sigma_W = \sqrt{\frac{n(n+1)(2n+1)}{6} - \sum \frac{(\tau_i - 1)\tau_i(\tau_i + 1)}{12}}$$

in which n is the number of experimental subjects, τ_i is the number of tied ranks in the ith set of ties, and Σ indicates summation over all the sets of tied ranks.

†Note that we have developed W as the sum of *all* the signed ranks of the differences. There are alternative deviations of the Wilcoxon signed-rank test that are based on the sum of only the positively or negatively signed ranks. These alternative forms are mathematically equivalent to the one developed here. You need to be careful when using tables of the critical value W to be sure which way the test statistic was computed when the table was constructed.

Cigarette Smoking and Platelet Function

Table 10–8 reproduces the results, shown in Fig. 9–2, of Levine's experiment measuring platelet aggregation of 11 people before and after each one smokes a cigarette. Recall that increased platelet aggregation indicates a greater propensity to form blood clots (capable of causing heart attacks, strokes, and other vascular disorders). The table's fourth column shows the change in platelet aggregation that accompanies smoking a cigarette.

Figure 10–4 shows these differences. While this figure may not present results that preclude using methods based on the normal distribution (like the paired t test), it does suggest that it would be more prudent to use a nonparametric method like the Wilcoxon signed-rank test because the differences do not appear to be symmetrically distributed about the mean and more likely to be near the mean as far from it. In particular, *outliers* like the point at 27 percent can bias methods based on a normal distribution.

To continue with our computation, which does not require the assumption of normally distributed changes, rank the magnitudes of each of these changes, the smallest change (1 percent) being ranked 1 and the largest change (27 percent) being ranked 11. The fifth column in Table 10–8 shows these ranks. The last column shows the same ranks

Table 10–8 Maximum Percentage Platelet Aggregation before and after Smoking One Cigarette

Person	Before smoking	After smoking	Difference	Rank of difference	Signed rank of difference
1	25	27	2	2	2
2	25	29	4	3.5	3.5
3	27	37	10	6	6
4	44	56	12	7	7
5	30	46	16	10	10
6	67	82	15	8.5	8.5
7	53	57	4	3.5	3.5
8	53	80	27	11	11
9	52	61	9	5	5
10	60	59	−1	1	−1
11	28	43	15	8.5	8.5
					$W = 64$

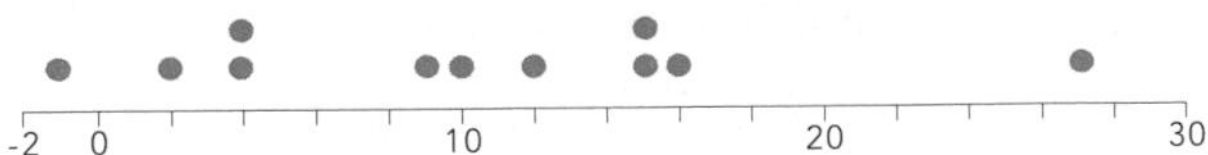

Figure 10–4 Change in platelet aggregation after smoking a cigarette. These changes do not seem to be normally distributed, especially because of the outlier at 27 percent. This plot suggests that a nonparametric method, such as the Wilcoxon signed-rank test, is preferable to a parametric method, such as the paired *t* test, to analyze the results of this experiment.

with the sign of the change attached. The sum of the signed ranks W is $2 + 3.5 + 6 + 7 + 10 + 8.5 + 3.5 + 11 + 5 + (-1) + 8.5 = 64$. This value exceeds 52, the value that defines the 1.8 percent most extreme values of W that can occur when the treatment has no effect (from Table 10–7), so we can report that these data support the assertion that smoking increases platelet aggregation ($P = .018$).

EXPERIMENTS WITH THREE OR MORE GROUPS WHEN EACH GROUP CONTAINS DIFFERENT INDIVIDUALS: THE KRUSKAL-WALLIS STATISTIC

Chapter 3 discussed experiments in which three or more different groups of experimental subjects are exposed to different treatments and the observations could be considered to come from normally distributed populations with similar variances. Now we shall develop an analogous procedure to the one-way analysis of variance (Chapter 3) based on ranks that does not require making these assumptions.

The *Kruskal-Wallis statistic* is a direct generalization of the Mann-Whitney rank-sum test. One first ranks all the observations *without regard for which treatment group they are in,* beginning with 1 for the smallest observation. (Ties are treated as before; i.e., they are assigned the average value that would be associated with the tied observations if they were not tied.) Next, compute the rank sum for each group. If the treatments have no effect, the *large and small ranks should be evenly distributed among the different groups,* so the average rank in each group should approximate the average of all the ranks computed without regard of the grouping. The more disparity there is between observed average ranks in each group and what you would expect if the hypothesis of no treatment effect was true, the less likely we will be to accept that hypothesis. Now, let us construct such a test statistic.

For simplicity, let us assume there are only three groups; then generalize the resulting equations to any number of groups when we are finished. The three different treatment groups contain n_1, n_2, and n_3 experimental subjects, and the rank sums for these three groups are R_1, R_2, R_3. Therefore, the mean ranks observed in the three groups are $\bar{R}_1 = R_1/n_1$, $\bar{R}_2 = R_2/n_2$, and $\bar{R}_3 = R_3/n_3$, respectively. The average rank of all the $n_1 + n_2 + n_3 = N$ observations is the average of the first N integers

$$\bar{R} = \frac{1 + 2 + 3 + \cdots + N}{N} = \frac{N + 1}{2}$$

We will use the sum of squared deviations between each sample group's average rank and the overall average rank, weighted by the sizes of each group, as a measure of variability between the observations and what you would expect if the hypothesis of no treatment effect was true. Call this sum D.

$$D = n_1(\bar{R}_1 - \bar{R})^2 + n_2(\bar{R}_2 - \bar{R})^2 + n_3(\bar{R}_3 - \bar{R})^2$$

This sum of squared deviations is exactly analogous to the weighted sum of squared deviations between the sample means and grand mean that define the between-groups sum of squares in the parametric one-way analysis of variance as developed in Chapter 9.

The distribution of possible values of D when the treatments have no effect depends on the size of the sample. It is possible to obtain a test statistic that does not depend on sample size by dividing D by $N(N + 1)/12$,

$$H = \frac{D}{N(N + 1)/12} = \frac{12}{N(N + 1)} \sum n_t(\bar{R}_t - \bar{R})^2$$

The summation denoted with Σ is over all the treatment groups, regardless of how many treatment groups there are. It is the *Kruskal-Wallis test statistic.*

The exact distribution of H can be computed by listing all the possibilities, as we did with Mann-Whitney and Wilcoxon tests, but there are so many different possibilities that the resulting table would be huge. Fortunately, if the sample sizes are not too small, the χ^2 distribution with $\nu = k - 1$ degrees of freedom, where k is the number of treatment groups, closely approximates the distribution of H. Hence, we can test the null hypothesis that the treatments had no effect by computing H for the observations and comparing the resulting value with the critical values for χ^2 in Table 5–7. This approximation works well in experiments with three treatment groups when each group contains at least 5 members and for experiments with four treatment groups when there are more than 10 individuals in the entire study. For smaller studies, consult a table of the exact distribution of the H to obtain the P value. (We do not include such a table because of its length and the relatively infrequent need for one; most intermediate statistics texts include one.)

In sum, the procedure for analyzing an experiment in which different groups of experimental subjects receive each treatment is as follows.

- *Rank each observation without regard for treatment group, beginning with a rank of 1 for the smallest observation. (Ties are treated in the same way as the other rank tests.*)*
- *Compute the Kruskal-Wallis test statistic* H *to obtain a normalized measure of how much the average ranks within each treatment group deviate from the average rank of all the observations.*
- *Compare* H *with* χ^2 *distribution with 1 less degree of freedom than the number of treatment groups, unless the sample size is small, in which case you must compare* H *with the exact distribution. If* H *exceeds the critical value that defines a "big"* H, *reject the hypothesis that the treatment has no effect.*

Now let us illustrate this procedure with an example.

*When there are ties, the approximation between the distributions of H and χ^2 can be improved by dividing H computed above by

$$1 - \frac{\sum(\tau_i - 1)\tau_i(\tau_i + 1)}{N(N^2 - 1)}$$

where τ_i is the number of ties in the ith set of tied ranks (as before). If there are only a few ties, this correction makes little difference and may be ignored.

Prenatal Marijuana Exposure and Child Behavior

Although most women stop using marijuana once they get pregnant, approximately 2.8 percent report using it during the first trimester of pregnancy and occasionally during the remainder of pregnancy. Exposure to marijuana is associated with attention deficits and impulsivity in young children whose mothers used marijuana while pregnant, but not as much is known about the long-term effects on cognitive function. Lidush Goldschmidt and colleagues* designed a prospective observational study to track children whose mothers used marijuana during pregnancy. They interviewed women who came to a prenatal clinic and attempted to recruit all women who used two or more joints of marijuana per month during the first trimester of pregnancy and a random selection of other women. They kept in touch with these women, then evaluated temperament and behavioral characteristics of the children when they were 10 years old. One of the assessments used to address attentional deficit disorder and hyperactivity was the Swanson, Noland, and Pelham (SNAP) checklist, which is a questionnaire completed by mothers.

Table 10–9 gives the SNAP scores for the 31 children in this study. It shows the ranks of each observation together with the sum of ranks and mean ranks for each of the three exposure groups. The mean rank of all 31 observations is

$$\bar{R} = \frac{1 + 2 + 3 + \cdots + 31}{31} = \frac{N + 1}{2} = \frac{31 + 1}{2} = 16$$

Therefore, the weighted sum of squared deviations between the average ranks observed in each treatment group and the average of all ranks is

$$D = 13(11.23 - 16)^2 + 9(16.89 - 16)^2 + 9(22.00 - 16)^2$$

$$= 13(-4.77)^2 + 9(0.89)^2 + 9(6.00)^2 = 626.92$$

$$H = \frac{D}{N(N + 1)/12} = \frac{626.92}{31(31 + 1)/12} = 7.58$$

*L. Goldschmidt, N. L. Day, and G. A. Richardson, "Effects of Prenatal Marijuana Exposure on Child Behavior Problems at Age 10," *Neurotoxicol. and Tetratol.* **22:**325–336, 2000.

Table 10–9 Average Number of Joints per day (ADJ)

	ADJ = 0 $n_1 = 13$		$0 < \text{ADJ} \leq 0.89$ $n_1 = 9$		ADJ > 0.89 $n_1 = 9$	
	SNAP score	Rank	SNAP score	Rank	SNAP score	Rank
	7.79	4	8.84	12	8.65	11
	9.16	17	9.92	24	10.70	31
	7.34	2	7.20	1	10.24	28
	10.28	29	9.25	20	8.62	10
	9.12	15	9.45	21	9.94	25
	9.24	19	9.14	16	10.55	30
	8.40	7	9.99	26	10.13	27
	8.60	9	9.21	18	9.78	23
	8.04	5	9.06	14	9.01	13
	8.45	8				
	9.51	22				
	8.15	6				
	7.69	3				
Sum of ranks, R_t		146		152		198
Mean rank, $\bar{R}_t = R_t/n_t$		11.23		16.89		22.00

This value exceeds 5.991, the value that defines the largest 5 percent of the χ^2 distribution with $\nu = k - 1 = 3 - 1 = 2$ degrees of freedom (from Tables 5–7). Therefore, we conclude that at least one of these three groups differed in hyperactivity and attention deficit ($P < .05$).

Nonparametric Multiple Comparisons

Just as with parametric analysis of variance, there are multiple comparison procedures to identify subgroups among the different treatment groups and to conduct multiple comparisons against a single control group. When there are equal numbers of observations in each treatment group, these multiple comparisons can be done with variants of the Student-Newman-Keuls (SNK) and Dunnett's tests, for all pairwise comparisons and multiple comparisons against a single control, respectively. There is not an equivalent of the Bonferroni or Holm t test. When the sample sizes are not equal, multiple comparisons are conducted with *Dunn's test.* Because the SNK and Dunnett's procedures differ only in the way the test statistics q and q' are defined, we briefly summarize them, then concentrate on Dunn's test, because it is applicable when the sample sizes are not equal.

When the sample sizes are equal, the nonparametric *SNK test* statistic is computed as

$$q = \frac{R_A - R_B}{\sqrt{\dfrac{n(np)(np + 1)}{12}}}$$

where R_A and R_B are the rank sums of the two treatments to be compared, n is the sample size of each group, and p is the number of groups spanned by the comparison, after ranking the rank sums in descending (or ascending) order. The resulting values of q are compared to the table of critical values in Table 4–3 with an infinite number of degrees of freedom.

Likewise, the nonparametric *Dunnett's test* statistic is computed as

$$q' = \frac{R_{\text{con}} - R_A}{\sqrt{\dfrac{n(np)(np + 1)}{6}}}$$

where R_{con} is the rank sum associated with the control group and the other variables are defined as before. The resulting values of q' are compared to the table of critical values in Table 4–4 with an infinite number of degrees of freedom, and p is the number of groups being compared.

When there are unequal sample sizes, one should use Dunn's test. (Dunn's test can also be used for equal sample sizes.) For all pairwise comparisons, compute the test statistic

$$Q = \frac{\bar{R}_A - \bar{R}_B}{\sqrt{\dfrac{N(N + 1)}{12}\left(\dfrac{1}{n_A} + \dfrac{1}{n_B}\right)}}$$

where $\bar{R}_A$ and $\bar{R}_B$ are the average ranks for the two groups being compared, N is the total sample size, and n_A and n_B are the number of observations in samples *A* and *B*, respectively.* The critical values for Q depend on the number of treatment groups, k, and appear in Table 10–10. The computations are organized as with the SNK test; order the mean rank sums from smallest to largest, and test from the largest difference to the smallest. When the test fails to detect a significant difference, do not test the smaller differences.

Dunn's test may also be used for multiple comparisons against a single control group. The test statistic is computed in the same way just described, but the value is compared with the table of critical values of Q' in Table 10–11.

More on Marijuana

Now that we have a procedure that is suitable for nonparametric multiple comparison testing following the Kruskal-Wallis test, let us complete our study of the data on the effects of marijuana during pregnancy on SNAP scores in children presented in Table 10–9. The largest difference in mean ranks is between the mothers who smoked an average of 0 joints per day and those who smoked greater than 0.89. The associated value of Dunn's Q is

$$Q = \frac{\bar{R}_{ADJ>.89} - \bar{R}_0}{\sqrt{\dfrac{N(N+1)}{12}\left(\dfrac{1}{n_{ADJ>0.89}} + \dfrac{1}{n_0}\right)}}$$

$$= \frac{22 - 11.23}{\sqrt{\dfrac{31(31+1)}{12}\left(\dfrac{1}{9} + \dfrac{1}{13}\right)}} = 2.73$$

This value exceeds the critical value of Q for $k = 3$ treatment groups, 2.394 for $\alpha = .05$, so we conclude that SNAP scores for

*If there are ties, Q should be corrected for the ties according to

$$Q = \frac{\bar{R}_A - \bar{R}_B}{\sqrt{\left(\dfrac{N(N+1)}{12} - \dfrac{\Sigma(\tau_i^3 - \tau_i)}{12(N-1)}\right)\left(\dfrac{1}{n_A} + \dfrac{1}{n_B}\right)}}$$

where τ_i is the number of ties in the *i*th set of tied ranks (as before). If there are only a few ties, this correction makes little difference and can be ignored.

Table 10–10 Critical Values of Q for Nonparametric Multiple Comparison Testing

	α_T	
k	**0.05**	**0.01**
2	1.960	2.576
3	2.394	2.936
4	2.639	3.144
5	2.807	3.291
6	2.936	3.403
7	3.038	3.494
8	3.124	3.570
9	3.197	3.635
10	3.261	3.692
11	3.317	3.743
12	3.368	3.789
13	3.414	3.830
14	3.456	3.868
15	3.494	3.902
16	3.529	3.935
17	3.562	3.965
18	3.593	3.993
19	3.622	4.019
20	3.649	4.044
21	3.675	4.067
22	3.699	4.089
23	3.722	4.110
24	3.744	4.130
25	3.765	4.149

Adapted from Table B. 14 of J. H. Zar, *Biostatistical Analysis,* 2nd ed., Prentice-Hall, Englewood Cliffs, N.J., 1984, p. 569.

children exposed to none or more than 0.89 joints per day during gestation differ. Next, we compare the children exposed to more than 0.89 joints per day to those exposed to more than 0, but less than or equal to 0.89.

$$Q = \frac{\bar{R}_{0<ADJ\leq 0.89} - \bar{R}_0}{\sqrt{\dfrac{N(N+1)}{12}\left(\dfrac{1}{n_{0<ADJ\leq 0.89}} + \dfrac{1}{n_0}\right)}}$$

Table 10–11 Critical Values of Q' for Nonparametric Multiple Comparison Testing Against a Control Group

	α_T	
k	0.05	0.01
2	1.960	2.576
3	2.242	2.807
4	2.394	2.936
5	2.498	3.024
6	2.576	3.091
7	2.639	3.144
8	2.690	3.189
9	2.735	3.227
10	2.773	3.261
11	2.807	3.291
12	2.838	3.317
13	2.866	3.342
14	2.891	3.364
15	2.914	3.384
16	2.936	3.403
17	2.955	3.421
18	2.974	3.437
19	2.992	3.453
20	3.008	3.467
21	3.024	3.481
22	3.038	3.494
23	3.052	3.506
24	3.066	3.518
25	3.078	3.529

Adapted from Table B. 15 of J. H. Zar, *Biostatistical Analysis,* 2nd ed., Prentice-Hall, Englewood Cliffs, N.J., 1984, p. 569.

$$Q = \frac{16.89 - 11.23}{\sqrt{\dfrac{31(31+1)}{12}\left(\dfrac{1}{9} + \dfrac{1}{13}\right)}} = 1.435$$

which does not exceed the critical value of 2.394, so we cannot conclude that there is a difference in SNAP scores of children between the children in the ADJ $= 0$ and $0 <$ ADJ ≤ 0.89 groups. Since this difference is not significant, we do not need to test the smaller, spanned difference between no marijuana and less than 0.89 joints per day.

Therefore, we conclude that marijuana smoking while pregnant affects the hyperactivity and attention deficit of the child if the woman smokes more than 0.89 joints per day while pregnant.

EXPERIMENTS IN WHICH EACH SUBJECT RECEIVES MORE THAN ONE TREATMENT: THE FRIEDMAN TEST

Often it is possible to complete experiments in which each individual is exposed to a number of different treatments. This experimental design reduces the uncertainty due to variability in the responses between individuals and provides a more sensitive test of what the treatments do in a given person. When the assumptions required for parametric methods can be reasonably satisfied, such experiments can be analyzed with the repeated-measures analysis of variance in Chapter 9. Now we will derive an analogous test based on ranks that does not require that the observations be drawn from normally distributed populations. The resulting test statistic is called *Friedman's statistic.*

The logic of this test is quite simple. Each experimental subject receives each treatment, so we rank *each subject's* responses to the treatments without regard for the other subjects. If the hypothesis that the treatment has no effect is true, then, for each subject, the ranks will be randomly distributed, and the sums of the ranks for each *treatment* will be similar. Table 10–12 illustrates such a case, in which 5 different subjects receive 4 treatments. Instead of the measured responses, this table contains the *ranks* of each experimental subject's responses. Hence, the treatments are ranked 1, 2, 3, and 4 separately for each subject. The bottom line in the table gives the sums of the ranks for all people receiving each treatment. These rank sums are all similar and also roughly equal to 12.5, which is the average rank, $(1 + 2 + 3 + 4)/4 = 2.5$, times the number of subjects, 5. This table does not suggest that any of the treatments had any systematic effect on the experimental subjects.

Now consider Table 10–13. The first treatment *always* produces the greatest response in all experimental subjects, the second treatment always produces the smallest response, and the third and fourth treatments always produce intermediate responses, the third treatment

Table 10–12 Ranks of Outcomes for Experiment When Five Subjects Each Receive Four Treatments

Experimental subject	Treatment 1	2	3	4
1	1	2	3	4
2	4	1	2	3
3	3	4	1	2
4	2	3	4	1
5	1	4	3	2
Rank sum R_t	11	14	13	12

producing a greater response than the fourth treatment. The bottom line shows the column rank sums. In this case there is a great deal of variability in the rank sums, some being much larger or smaller than 5 times the average rank, or 12.5. Table 10–13 strongly suggests that the treatments affect the variable being studied.

All we have left to do is to reduce this objective impression of a difference to a single number. In a way similar to that used in deriving the Kruskal-Wallis statistic, let us compute the sum of squared deviations between the rank sums observed for each treatment and the rank sum that we would expect if each treatment were as likely to have any of the possible rankings. This latter number is the average of the possible ranks.

For the examples in Tables 10–12 and 10–13, there are four possible treatments, so there are four possible ranks. Therefore, the average

Table 10–13 Ranks of Outcomes for Another Experiment When Five Subjects Each Receive Four Treatments

Experimental subject	Treatment 1	2	3	4
1	4	1	3	2
2	4	1	3	2
3	4	1	3	2
4	4	1	3	2
5	4	1	3	2
Rank sum R_t	20	5	15	10

rank is $(1 + 2 + 3 + 4)/4 = 2.5$. In general, if there are k treatments, the average rank will be

$$\frac{1 + 2 + 3 + \cdots + k}{k} = \frac{k + 1}{2}$$

In our example there are five experimental subjects, so we would expect each of the rank sums to be around 5 times the average rank for each person, or $5(2.5) = 12.5$. In Table 10–12 this is the case whereas in Table 10–13 it is not. If there are n experimental subjects and the ranks are randomly distributed between the treatments, each of the rank sums should be about n times the average rank, or $n(k + 1)/2$. Hence, we can collapse all this information into a single number by computing the sum of squared differences between the observed rank sums and rank sums that would be expected if the treatments had no effect.

$$S = \Sigma[R_t - n(k + 1)/2]^2$$

in which Σ denotes the sum over all the treatments and R_t denotes the sum of ranks for treatment t.

For example, for the observations in Table 10–12, $k = 4$ treatments and $n = 5$ experimental subjects, so

$$\begin{aligned} S &= (11 - 12.5)^2 + (14 - 12.5)^2 + (13 - 12.5)^2 + (12 - 12.5)^2 \\ &= (-1.5)^2 + (1.5)^2 + (.5)^2 + (-.5)^2 = 5 \end{aligned}$$

and for Table 10–13

$$\begin{aligned} S &= (20 - 12.5)^2 + (5 - 12.5)^2 + (15 - 12.5)^2 + (10 - 12.5)^2 \\ &= (7.5)^2 + (-7.5)^2 + (2.5)^2 + (-2.5)^2 = 125 \end{aligned}$$

In the former case, S is a small number; in the latter S is a big number. The more of a pattern there is relating the ranks within each subject to the treatments, the greater the value of our test statistic S.

We could stop here and formulate a test based on S, but statisticians have shown that we can simplify the problem by dividing this sum of squared differences between the observed and expected rank sums by $nk(k + 1)/12$ to obtain

$$\chi_r^2 = \frac{S}{nk(k+1)/12} = \frac{12\Sigma[R_t - n(k+1)/2]^2}{nk(k+1)}$$

$$= \frac{12}{nk(k+1)}\Sigma R_t^2 - 3n(k+1)$$

The test statistic χ_r^2, is called *Friedman's statistic* and has the desirable property that, for large enough samples, it follows the χ^2 distribution with $\nu + k - 1$ degrees of freedom, regardless of sample size.* When there are three treatments and nine or fewer experimental subjects or four treatments with four or fewer experimental subjects each, the χ^2 approximation is not adequate, so one needs to compare χ_r^2 to the exact distribution of possible values obtained by listing all the possibilities in Table 10–14.

In sum, the procedure for using the Friedman statistic to analyze experiments in which the same individuals receive several treatments is as follows:

- *Rank each observation within each experimental subject, assigning 1 to the smallest response. (Treat ties as before.)*
- *Compute the sum of the ranks observed in all subjects for each treatment.*
- *Compute the Friedman test statistic χ_r^2 as a measure of how much the observed rank sums differ from those that would be expected if the treatments had no effect.*
- *Compare the resulting value of the Friedman statistic with the χ^2 distribution if the experiment involves large enough samples or with the exact distribution of χ_r^2 in Table 10–14 if the sample is small.*

Now, let us apply this test to two experiments, one old and one new.

*When there are tied measurements, χ_r^2 needs to be increased by dividing it by

$$1 - \frac{\displaystyle\sum_{\text{subjects, } i} \sum_{\substack{\text{ties} \\ \text{within} \\ \text{subject, } j}} (\tau_{ij} - 1)\tau_{ij}(\tau_{ij} + 1)}{Nk(k^2 - 1)}$$

in which τ_{ij} = number of tied ranks in the ith set of ties within the ranks for subject j, and the double sum $\Sigma\Sigma$ is computed over all ties within each subject. If there are only a few ties, this correction makes little difference and can be ignored.

Table 10–14 Critical Values for Friedman χ_r^2

k = 3 treatments			k = 4 treatments		
n	χ_r^2	P	n	χ_r^2	P
3	6.00	.028	2	6.00	.042
4	6.50	.042	3	7.00	.054
	8.00	.005		8.20	.017
5	5.20	.093	4	7.50	.054
	6.40	.039		9.30	.011
	8.40	.008	5	7.80	.049
6	5.33	.072		9.96	.009
	6.33	.052	6	7.60	.043
	9.00	.008		10.20	.010
7	6.00	.051	7	7.63	.051
	8.86	.008		10.37	.009
8	6.25	.047	8	7.65	.049
	9.00	.010		10.35	.010
9	6.22	.048			
	8.67	.010			
10	6.20	.046			
	8.60	.012			
11	6.54	.043			
	8.91	.011			
12	6.17	.050			
	8.67	.011			
13	6.00	.050			
	8.67	.012			
14	6.14	.049			
	9.00	.010			
15	6.40	.047			
	8.93	.010			

Source: Adapted from Owen, *Handbook of Statistical Tables,* U.S. Department of Energy, Addison-Wesley, Reading, MA., 1962. Used by permission.

Anti-Asthmatic Drugs and Endotoxin

Table 10–15 reproduces the observed forced expiratory volume 1 (FEV_1) at one second in Table 9–5 that Berenson and colleagues used to study whether or not salbutamol had a protective effect on endotoxin

Table 10–15 Forced Expiratory Volume at 1 Second before and after Bronchial Challenge with Endotoxin and Salbutamol

	FEV_1 (L)					
	No drug (baseline)		1 hour after endotoxin		2 hours after endotoxin and salbutamol	
Person	Units	Rank	Units	Rank	Person (subject)	No drug (baseline)
1	3.7	2	3.4	1	4.0	3
2	4.0	2	3.7	1	4.4	3
3	3.0	2	2.8	1	3.2	3
4	3.2	2	2.9	1	3.4	3
Rank sums for each group		8		4		12

induced bronchoconstriction. In Chapter 9, we analyzed these data with a repeated-measures one-way analysis of variance. Now, let us reexamine them using ranks to avoid having to make any assumptions about the population these patients represent.

Table 10–15 shows how the three treatments rank in terms of FEV_1 for each of the four people in the study. The last row gives the sums of the ranks for each treatment. Since the possible ranks are 1, 2, and 3, the average rank is $(1 + 2 + 3)/3 = 2$. Since there are 4 people, if the treatments had no effect, these rank sums should all be about $4(2) = 8$. Hence, our measure of the difference between this expectation and the observed data is

$$S = (8 - 8)^2 + (4 - 8)^2 + (12 - 8)^2$$

$$= (0)^2 + (4)^2 + (4)^2 = 32$$

We convert S into χ_r^2 by dividing by $nk(k + 1)/12 = 4(3)(3 + 1)/12 = 4$ to obtain $\chi_r^2 = 32/4 = 8.0$. Table 10–14 shows that for an experiment with $k = 3$ treatments and $n = 4$ experimental subjects there is only a $P = .042$ chance of obtaining a value of χ_r^2 as big or bigger than 8 by chance if the treatments have no effect. Therefore, we can report that endotoxin and salbutamol alter FEV_1 ($P = .042$).

Multiple Comparisons after Friedman's Test

Because Friedman's test is a repeated-measures design in which all subjects receive all treatments, and the number of observations under each experimental condition are the same, it is possible to adapt the Student-Newman-Keuls and Dunnett's tests for use in multiple comparisons following Friedman's test for all pairwise comparisons and multiple comparisons against a single control group. These two test statistics are used just as in the parametric versions of these tests.

To compute all pairwise comparisons, compute the SNK test statistic

$$q = \frac{R_A - R_B}{\sqrt{\dfrac{pn(p+1)}{12}}}$$

where R_A and R_B are the rank sums for the two groups being compared, p is the number of groups spanned by the comparison, and n is the number of experimental subjects. The resulting value of q is compared with the critical value of q for p comparisons with an infinite number of degrees of freedom in Table 4–3.

Likewise, the Dunnett's test statistic is

$$q' = \frac{R_{\text{con}} - R_A}{\sqrt{\dfrac{pn(p+1)}{6}}}$$

The resulting value of q' is compared to the critical value of Dunnett's test statistic for p comparisons with an infinite number of degrees of freedom in Table 4–4.

Effect of Secondhand Smoke on Angina Pectoris

Cigarette smoking aggravates the conditions of people with coronary artery disease for several reasons. First, the arteries that supply blood to the heart muscle to deliver oxygen and nutrients and remove metabolic wastes are narrowed and are less able to maintain the needed flow of blood. Second, cigarette smoke includes carbon monoxide; it binds to the hemoglobin in blood and displaces oxygen that would otherwise be delivered to the heart muscle. In addition, chemicals in tobacco smoke act directly on the heart muscle to depress its ability to pump and deliver the blood containing oxygen and nutrients to the entire body, including the heart muscle. When the heart muscle is not adequately supplied with oxygen, a person with coronary artery disease experiences a well-defined chest pain called *angina pectoris.* People with coronary artery disease often feel fine when resting but develop pain when they exercise and increase the heart muscle's need for oxygen. It is well established that smoking can precipitate angina pectoris in people with severe coronary artery disease and decrease the ability of other people with milder disease to exercise. Wilbur Aronow* wondered whether exposing people with coronary artery disease to someone else's cigarette smoke would produce similar effects on people with coronary artery disease, even though they were not smoking the cigarette themselves.

To answer this question, he measured how long 10 men with well-documented coronary artery disease could exercise on a bicycle. Aronow tested each subject to see how long he could exercise before developing chest pain. After obtaining these control measurements, he sent each subject to a waiting room for 2 h, where three other volunteers were waiting who either (1) did not smoke, (2) smoked five cigarettes with the room ventilator turned on, or (3) smoked five cigarettes with the room ventilator turned off. After this exposure, Aronow again measured each subject's exercise tolerance.

The experimental subjects were exposed to these different environments on different days in random order. The investigator knew whether or not they had been exposed to the secondhand smoke, but the subjects themselves did not know that the purpose of the study was to assess their response to secondhand smoke. Therefore, this is a single-blind experiment that minimizes placebo effects but not observer biases.

Table 10–16 shows the results of this experiment together with the ranks of exercise duration in each experimental subject, 1 being assigned to the shortest duration and 6 being assigned to the longest. Since there are 6 possible ranks, the average rank for each subject is $(1 + 2 + 3 + 4 + 5 + 6)/6 = 3.5$; since there are 10 people in the study, we

*W. S. Aronow, "Effect of Passive Smoking on Angina Pectoris," *N. Engl. J. Med.*, **299:**21–24, 1978.

Table 10–16 Duration of Exercise until Angina in the Control Periods and after Exposure to Clean Air, Smoking in a Well-Ventilated Room, and Smoking in an Unventilated Room

	Clean air				Well-ventilated room				Unventilated room			
	Control		Placebo		Control		Smoke		Control		Smoke	
Person	Time, s	Rank	Time, s	Rank	Time, s	Rank	Time, s	Rank	Time, s	Rank	Time, s	Rank
1	193	4	217	6	191	3	149	2	202	5	127	1
2	206	5	214	6	203	4	169	2	189	3	130	1
3	188	4	197	6	181	3	145	2	192	5	128	1
4	375	3	412	6	400	5	306	2	387	4	230	1
5	204	5	199	4	211	6	170	2	196	3	132	1
6	287	3	310	5	304	4	243	2	312	6	198	1
7	221	5	215	4	213	3	158	2	232	6	135	1
8	216	5	223	6	207	3	155	2	209	4	124	1
9	195	4	208	6	186	3	144	2	200	5	129	1
10	231	6	224	4	227	5	172	2	218	3	125	1
Rank sum		44		53		39		20		44		10
Mean	231.6		241.9		232.3		181.1		233.7		145.8	

Source: W. S. Aronow, "Effect of Passive Smoking on Angina Pectoris," *N. Engl. J. Med.* **299:**21–24, 1978, table 1.

would expect the rank sums to all be around 10(3.5) = 35 if the different treatments all had no effect on how long a person could exercise. The rank sums at the bottom of the table appear to differ from this value.

To convert this impression to a single number, compute

$$\chi_r^2 = \frac{12}{10(6)(6+1)}(44^2 + 53^2 + 39^2 + 20^2 + 44^2 + 10^2) - 3(10)(6+1) = 38.629$$

This value exceeds 20.515, the critical value that defines the .1 percent of largest values of the χ^2 distribution with $\nu = k - 1 = 6 - 1 = 5$ degrees of freedom (from Table 5–7), so we can report that there are differences in the amount of exercise a person with coronary artery disease can do in this experiment ($P < .001$).

To determine whether this difference is due to exposure to the secondhand smoke, we do all pairwise comparisons for the data in Table 10–16 with the Student-Newman-Keuls test. To do this, we first order the groups in descending order of the rank sums, then compute q using the formula above. For example, for the comparison of the clean air control (C,C) condition with the unventilated room smoke (U,S) condition (the greatest difference), there are $p = 6$ included treatments, so

$$q = \frac{R_{C,C} - R_{U,S}}{\sqrt{\dfrac{pn(p+1)}{12}}} = \frac{53 - 10}{\sqrt{\dfrac{6(10)(6+1)}{12}}} = 7.268$$

7.268 exceeds 4.030, the critical value of q for $\alpha_T = .05$ with $p = 6$ and infinite degrees of freedom (from Table 4–3), so we conclude that people can do significantly less exercise in an unventilated smoky room than in a room with clean air and no smoking. All the pairwise comparisons are shown in Table 10–17. These comparisons clearly define three subgroups: All cases when there is smoke-free air (the three controls and the clean-air placebo) form the subgroup with the greatest ability to exercise, the second subgroup consists of a well-ventilated room where smoke is present, and the third subgroup consists of the unventilated smoky room. Thus, we conclude that exposure to secondhand smoke

Table 10–17 All Pairwise Multiple Comparisons of the Data on Passive Smoking and Exercise Tolerance in Table 10–16

Comparison*	$R_A - R_B$	p	D	q	q_{crit}	$P < .05$?
C,P vs. U,S	53 − 10 = 43	6	5.916	7.268	4.030	Yes
C,P vs. W,S	53 − 20 = 33	5	5.000	6.600	3.858	Yes
C,P vs. W,C	53 − 39 = 14	4	4.082	3.430	3.633	No
C,P vs. U,C	53 − 44 = 9	3	3.162			Do not test
C,P vs. C,C	53 − 44 = 9	2	2.236			Do not test
C,C vs. U,S	44 − 10 = 34	5	5.000	6.800	3.828	Yes
C,C vs. W,S	44 − 20 = 24	4	4.082	5.879	3.633	Yes
C,C vs. W,C	44 − 39 = 5	3	3.162	1.581	3.314	No
C,C vs. U,C	44 − 44 = 0	2	2.236			Do not test
U,C vs. U,S	44 − 10 = 34	4	4.082	8.329	3.633	Yes
U,C vs. W,S	44 − 20 = 24	3	3.162	7.590	3.314	Yes
U,C vs. W,C	44 − 39 = 5	2	2.236	2.236	2.772	No
W,C vs. U,S	39 − 10 = 29	3	3.162	9.171	3.314	Yes
W,C vs. W,S	39 − 20 = 19	2	2.236	8.497	2.772	Yes
W,S vs. U,S	20 − 10 = 10	2	2.236	4.472	2.772	Yes

*Abbreviations: First letter: C = clean air, W = well-ventilated room, U = Unventilated room. Second letter: C = control, P = placebo, S = smoke. $D = \sqrt{pn(p + 1)/12}$.

significantly reduces the ability of people with heart disease to exercise, with a greater effect as the room becomes smokier ($P < .05$).

SUMMARY

The methods in this chapter permit testing hypotheses similar to those we tested with analysis-of-variance and t tests but do not require us to assume that the underlying populations follow normal distributions. We avoid having to make such an assumption by replacing the observations with their ranks before computing the test statistic (T, W, H, or χ_r^2). By dealing with ranks we preserve most of the information about the relative sizes (and signs) of the observations. More important, by dealing with ranks, we do not use information about the population or populations the samples were drawn from to compute the distribution of possible values of the test statistic. Instead we consider the population of all possible ranking patterns (often by simply listing all the possibilities) to compute the P value associated with the observations.

It is important to note that the procedures we used in this chapter to compute the P value from the ranks of the observations is essentially the same as the methods we have used everywhere else in this book.

- *Assume that the treatment(s) had no effect, so that any differences observed between the samples are due to the effects of random sampling.*
- *Define a test statistic that summarizes the observed differences between the treatment groups.*
- *Compute all possible values this test statistic can take on when the assumption that the treatments had no effect is true. These values define the distribution of the test statistic we would expect if the hypothesis of no effect was true.*
- *Compute the value of the test statistic associated with the actual observations in the experiment.*
- *Compare this value with the distribution of all possible values; if it is "big," it is unlikely that the observations came from the same populations (i.e., that the treatment had no effect), so conclude that the treatment had an effect.*

The specific procedure you should use to analyze the results from a given experiment depends on the design of the experiment and the nature of the data. When the data are measured on an ordinal scale or you cannot or do not wish to assume that the underlying populations follow normal distributions, the procedures developed in this chapter are appropriate.

PROBLEMS

10-1 A person who has decided to enter the medical care system as a patient has relatively little control over the medical services (laboratory tests, x-rays, drugs) purchased. These decisions are made by the physician and other medical care providers, who are often unaware of how much of the patient's money they are spending. To improve awareness of the financial impacts of their decisions regarding how they use medical resources in making a diagnosis and treatment, there is an accelerating trend toward auditing how individual physicians choose to diagnose and treat their patients. Do such audits affect practice? To answer this question, Steven Schroeder and colleagues ("Use of Laboratory Tests and Pharmaceuticals: Variation among Physicians and Effect of Cost Audit on Subsequent Use," *JAMA*, **225**:969–973, 1973, copyright 1970–1973, American Medical Association) measured the total of money a sample of physicians practicing in the George Washington University outpatient clinic spent on laboratory tests (including x-rays) and drugs for comparable patients for 3 months. The physicians were either salaried or volunteers. None received any direct compensation for the tests or drugs ordered. To be included, a patient must have been seen in the clinic for at least 6 months and have at least 1 of the 15 most common diagnoses among patients seen at the clinic. In addition, they excluded patients who were receiving a therapy that required laboratory tests as part of routine management, for example, anticoagulant therapy. They selected 10 to 15 patients at random from the people being seen by each physician and added up the total amount of money spent over a 3-month period, then computed the average annual cost for laboratory tests and drug costs for each physician. They then assigned each physician a number (unknown to the other participants in the study) and gave the physicians the results of the audit. In this way, the physicians could see how their costs compared with those of the other physicians, but they could not identify specific costs with any other individual physician. Then, unknown to the physicians, Schroeder and his colleagues repeated their audit using the same patients. Here is what they found:

	Mean annual lab charges per patient		Mean annual drug charges per patient	
Physician	Before audit	After audit	Before audit	After audit
1	$20	$20	$32	$42
2	17	26	41	90
3	14	1	51	71
4	42	24	29	47
5	50	1	76	56
6	62	47	47	43
7	8	15	60	137
8	49	7	58	63
9	81	65	40	28
10	54	9	64	60
11	48	21	73	87
12	55	36	66	69
13	56	30	73	50

Did knowledge of the audit affect the before the audit amount of money physicians spent for laboratory tests? For drugs before the audit? Is there any relationship between expenditures for laboratory tests and drugs? What are some possible explanations for these results? (Raw data supplied by Steven Schroeder.)

Grade	Definition
0	No adhesions
1	One band between organs or between one organ and the peritoneum
2	Two bands between organs or between one organ and the peritoneum
3	More than two bands between organs or mass formed by intestines not adhering to the peritoneum
4	Organs adhering to peritoneum or extensive adhesions

10-2 Despite progress in technique, adhesions (the abnormal connection between tissues inside the body formed during healing following surgery) continues to be a problem in abdominal surgery, such as when operating on the uterus. To see if it would be possible to reduce adhesions following uterine surgery by placing a membrane around the area of incision in the uterus, Nurullah Bülbüller and colleagues ("Effect of a Bioresorbable Membrane on Postoperative Adhesions and Wound Healing," *J. Reprod. Med.* **48:** 547–550, 2003) operated on the uteruses of two groups of rats, a control group that simply received the surgery and a test group that had the membrane applied over the uterus. This bioresorbable membrane prevented the tissue of the uterus from connecting to other internal organs of

Control	Bioresorbable membrane
3	1
4	1
4	2
4	0
2	0
1	0
3	2
2	0
1	1
0	3

the peritoneum (the inside lining of the abdomen), then was slowly absorbed by the surrounding tissue after healing was complete. They allowed the rats to heal, then sacrificed them and measured the amount of adhesions, according to the scale shown at the top of p. 408. The scores for the two groups of rats are shown at the bottom of p. 408. Does use of the membrane affect the extent of adhesions?

10-3 The inappropriate and overuse of antibiotics is a well-recognized problem in medicine. To test whether it was possible to encourage more appropriate use of antibiotics in elderly hospitalized patients, Monika Lutters and her colleagues monitored the number of patients receiving antibiotics in a 304-bed geriatric unit at her hospital before any intervention, after providing information to the physicians taking care of patients in the unit, after providing pocket cards with specific therapeutic guidelines for the use of antibiotics to treat the most common need for antibiotics in these patients (urinary and respiratory tract infections) combined with weekly lectures on appropriate use of antibiotics, then while the pocket cards were continued but the lectures stopped. The number of patients in the unit receiving antibiotics was recorded on each of 12 days under each experimental condition.

Number of Patients Receiving Antibiotics (out of 304 in the Geriatric Unit)

Baseline	Information	Pocket cards plus weekly lectures	Pocket cards only
55	51	50	45
54	53	51	59
57	67	52	58
54	55	50	45
59	51	53	49
57	50	52	55
67	52	64	46
80	56	52	52
55	84	53	50
55	54	51	53
56	54	52	45
65	67	45	56

Did the educational interventions have any effect on the number of patients receiving antibiotics? If so, how?

10-4 Rework Probs. 9-5 and 9-6 using methods based on ranks.

10-5 Chapter 3 discussed a study of whether or not offspring of parents with type II diabetes have abnormal glucose levels compared to offspring without a parental history of type II diabetes. Gerald Berenson and colleagues ("Abnormal Characteristics in Young Offspring of Parents with Non-Insulin-Dependent Diabetes Mellitus." *Am. J. Epidemiol.*, **144:** 962–967, 1996) also collected data on whether these offspring had different cholesterol levels. Here are the data for 30 subjects:

Offspring with a diabetic parent					Offspring without a diabetic parent				
181	183	170	173	174	168	165	163	175	176
179	172	175	178	176	166	163	174	175	173
158	179	180	172	177	179	180	176	167	176

Are these data consistent with the hypothesis that these offspring differ in cholesterol levels?

10-6 People with problem gambling habits are often substance abusers; these behaviors may be connected by an underlying personality trait such as impulsivity. Nancy Petry ("Gambling Problems in Substance Abusers are Associated with Increased Sexual Risk Behaviors," *Addiction*, **95:** 1089–1100, 2000) investigated whether problem gamblers would also be at higher risk for contracting HIV, since the underlying impulsivity might make problem gamblers more likely to engage in riskier sexual behavior. They administered a questionnaire known as the HIV Risk Behavior Scale (HRBS) to assess sexual risk behavior in two groups of substance abusers, those with and without problem gambling. The HRBS is an 11-item questionnaire with questions addressing drug and sex behavior and responses are coded on a 6-point scale from 0 to 5, with higher values associated with riskier behavior. The results of the HRBS sex composite score are given below. What do these data indicate?

HRBS Sex Composite Score

Non-problem gambling substance abusers	Problem gambling substance abusers
12	14
10	15
11	15
10	16
13	17
10	15
14	15
11	14
9	13
9	13
9	14
12	13
13	12
11	

10-7 Many studies show that women are less satisfied with their bodies than men and that the main source of this dissatisfaction is body weight. A negative body image is found not only in girls and women with eating disorders, but also in those who do not have an eating disorder. Salvatore Cullari and colleagues ("Body-image Perceptions across Sex and Age Groups," *Percept. Mot. Skills.,* **87:** 839–847, 1988) investigated whether these gender differences in body image are present in elementary and middle school boys and girls. Cullari and colleagues administered the kids' Eating Disorder Survey to a group of 98 students. This survey includes a Weight Dissatisfaction subscale with questions like "Do you want to lose weight now?" and "Have you ever been afraid to eat because you thought you would gain weight?" A higher score indicates more weight dissatisfaction. Here are their data:

Weight Dissatisfaction Score

Grade 5 boys	Grade 5 girls	Grade 8 boys	Grade 8 girls
1.0 1.2	1.5 2.4	1.2 1.1	2.9 2.8
0.8 1.0	2.3 0.8	0.9 1.3	2.7 3.1
0.9 0.7	0.1 0.3	1.5 1.4	2.6 2.2
1.1 0.6	2.1 0.9	0.5 0.8	2.5
	1.8 1.5	0.7 1.6	
	1.1		

Are there differences in weight dissatisfaction in any of these groups? If so, in which groups?

10-8 In his continuing effort to become famous, the author of an introductory biostatistics text invented a new way to test if some treatment changes an individual's response. Each experimental subject is observed before and after treatment, and the change in the variable of interest is computed. If this change is positive, we assign a value of +1 to that subject; if it is negative, we assign a value of zero (assume that there are never cases that remain unchanged). The soon-to-be famous G test statistic is computed by summing up the values associated with the individual subjects. For example:

Subject	Before treatment	After treatment	Change	Contribution
1	100	110	+10	+1
2	95	96	+ 1	+1
3	120	100	−20	0
4	111	123	+12	+1

In this case, $G = 1 + 1 + 0 + 1 = 3$. Is G a legitimate test statistic? Explain briefly. If so, what is the sampling distribution for G when $n = 4$? $n = 6$? Can you use G to conclude that the treatment had an effect in the data given above with $P < .05$? How confident can you be about this conclusion? Construct a table of critical values for G when $n = 4$ and $n = 6$.

Chapter 11

How to Analyze Survival Data

All the methods that we have discussed so far require "complete" observations, in the sense that we know the outcome of the treatment or intervention we are studying. For example, in Chapter 5, we considered a study in which we compared the rate of blood clot (thrombus) formation in people receiving aspirin versus people taking a placebo (Table 5–1). We compared these two groups of people by computing the expected pattern of thrombus formation in each of the two comparison groups under the null hypothesis that there was no difference in the rate of thrombus formation in the two treatment groups, then used the chi-square test statistic to examine how closely the observed pattern in the data matched the expected pattern under the null hypothesis of no treatment effect. The resulting value of χ^2 was "big," so we rejected the null hypothesis of no treatment effect and concluded that aspirin reduced the risk of thrombus formation. In this study we knew the outcome in *all* the people in the study. Indeed, in all the methods we have considered in this book so far, we knew the outcome of the variable under study for all the individuals in the study being analyzed. There are, however, situations, in which we do not know the ultimate outcome for all the individuals in the study because the study ended before the final outcome had been observed in all the study subjects or because the outcome in some of the individuals is not known.* We now turn our attention to developing procedures for such data.

The most common type of study in which we have incomplete knowledge of the outcome are clinical trials or survival studies in which individuals enter the study and are followed up over time until some event—typically death or development of a disease—occurs. Since such studies do not go on forever, it is possible that the study will end before the event of interest has occurred in all the study subjects. In such cases, we have incomplete information about the outcomes in these individuals. In clinical trials it is also common to lose track of patients who are being observed over time. Thus, we would know that the patient was free of disease up until the last time that we observed them, but we do not know what happened later. In both cases, we know that the individuals in the study were event free for some length of time, but not the actual time to an event. These people are *lost to follow-up;* such data are known as *censored data.* Censored data are most common in clinical trials or survival studies.

CENSORING ON PLUTO

The tobacco industry, having been driven farther and farther from Earth by protectors of the public health, invades Pluto and starts to promote smoking. Since it is very cold on Pluto, Plutonians spend most of their time indoors and begin dropping dead from the secondhand tobacco smoke. Since it would be unethical to purposely expose Plutonians to secondhand smoke, we will simply observe how long it takes Plutonians to drop dead after they begin to be exposed to secondhand smoke in bars.

Figure 11–1*A* shows the observations for 10 nonsmoking Plutonians selected at random and observed over the course of a study

*Another reason for not having all the data would be the case of *missing data,* in which samples are lost because of experimental problems or errors. Missing data are analyzed using the same statistical techniques as complete data sets, with appropriate adjustments in the calculations to account for the missing data. For a complete discussion of the analysis of studies with missing data, see S. Glantz and B. Slinker, *Primer of Applied Regression and Analysis of Variance* (2nd ed), McGraw-Hill, New York, 2001.

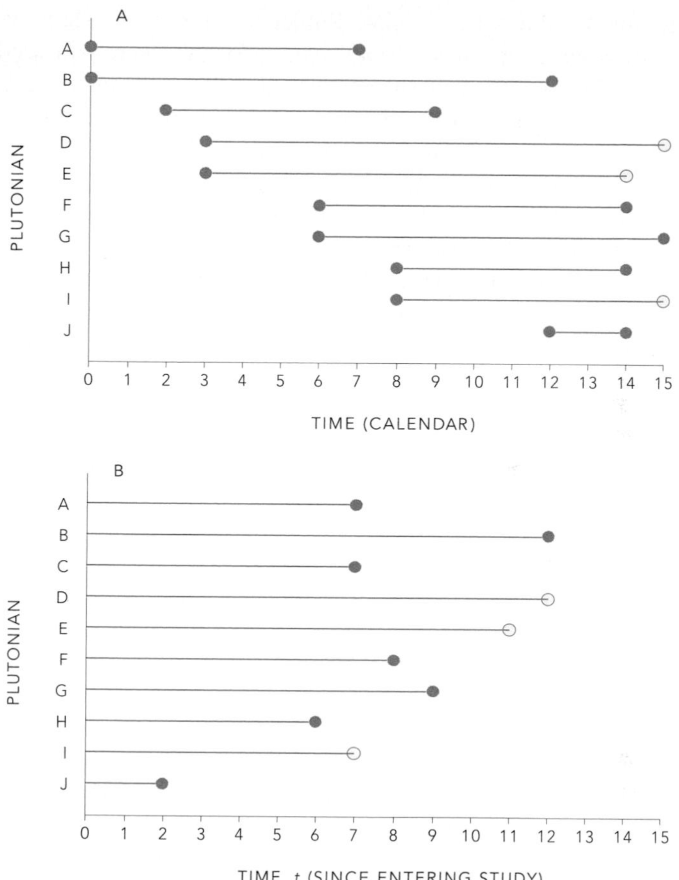

Figure 11–1 ***(A)*** This graph shows the observations in our study of the effect of hanging out in a smoky bar on Plutonians. The horizontal axis represents calendar time, with Plutonians entering the study at various times, when tobacco smoke invades their bars. Solid points indicate known times. Open points indicate the time at which observations are censored. Seven of the Plutonians die during the study (A, B, F, G, H, and J), so we know how long they were breathing secondhand smoke when they expired. Two of the Plutonians were still alive when the study ended at time 15 (D and I), and one (E) was lost to observation during the study, so we know that they lived at least as long as we were able to observe them, but do not know their actual time of death. ***(B)*** This graph shows the same data as panel ***A***, except that the horizontal axis is the length of time each subject was observed after they entered the study, rather than calendar time.

lasting for 15 Pluto time units. Subjects entered the study when they started hanging out at smoky bars, and they were followed-up until they dropped dead or the study ended. As with many survival studies, individuals were recruited into the study at various times as the study progressed. Of the 10 subjects, 7 died during the period of the study (A, B, C, F, G, H, and J). As a result, we know the exact length of time that they lived after their exposure to secondhand smoke in bars. These observations are *uncensored.* In contrast, two of the Plutonians were still alive at the end of the study (D and I); we know that they lived at least until the end of the study, but do not know how long they lived after being exposed to secondhand smoke. In addition, Plutonian E was vaporized in a freak accident while on vacation before the study was completed, so was lost to follow-up. We do know, however, that these individuals lived *at least as long* as we observed them. These observations are *censored.**

Figure 11 − 1*B* shows the data in another format, where the horizontal axis is the length of time that each subject is observed after starting exposure to secondhand smoke, as opposed to calendar time. The Plutonians who died by the end of the study have a solid point at the end of the line; those that were still alive at the end of the observation period are indicated with an open circle. Thus, we know that Plutonian A lived exactly 7 time units after starting to go to a smoky bar (an uncensored observation), whereas Plutonian J lived *at least* two time units after hanging out in a smoky bar (a censored observation).

*More precisely, these observations are *right censored* because we know the time the subjects entered the study, but not when they died (or experienced the event we are monitoring). It is also possible to have *left censored* data, when the actual survival time is less than that observed, such as when patients are studied following surgery, and the precise dates at which some patients had surgery before the beginning of the study are not known. Other types of censoring can occur when studies are designed to observe subjects until some specified fraction (say, half) die. We will concentrate on right censored data; for a discussion of other forms of censoring, see D. Collett, *Modelling Survival Data in Medical Research,* Chapman and Hall, London, 1994, chapter 1, "Survival Analysis," or E. T. Lee, *Statistical Methods for Survival Data Analysis* Wiley, 2d ed., New York, 1992, chapter 1, "Introduction."

This study has the necessary features of a clinical follow-up study.

- *There is a well-defined starting point for each subject (date smoking at work started in this example or date of diagnosis or medical intervention in a clinical study).*
- *There is a well-defined endpoint (death in this example or relapse in many clinical studies) or the end of the study period.*
- *The subjects in the study are selected at random from a larger population of interest.*

If all subjects were studied for the same length of time or until they reached a common endpoint (such as death), we could use the methods of Chapters 5 or 10 to analyze the results. Unfortunately, in clinical studies these situations often do not exist. The fact that the study period often ends before all the subjects have reached the end point makes it impossible to know the actual time that all the subjects reach the common end point. In addition, because subjects are recruited throughout the length of the study, the follow-up time often varies for different subjects. These two facts require that we develop new approaches to analyzing these data. The first step is to characterize the pattern of the occurrence of endpoints (such as death). This pattern is quantified with a *survival curve.* We will now examine how to characterize survival curves and test hypotheses about them.

ESTIMATING THE SURVIVAL CURVE

When discussing survival curves, one often considers death the end point—hence, the name *survival* curves—but any well-defined end point can be used. Other common end points include relapse of a disease, need for additional treatment, and failure of a mechanical component of a machine. Survival curves can also be used to study the length of time to desirable events as well, such as time to pregnancy in couples having fertility problems. We will generally talk in terms of the death end point, recognizing that these other end points are also possible.

The parameter of the underlying population we seek to estimate is the *survival function,* which is the fraction of individuals who are alive at time 0 who are surviving at any given time. Specifically,

The survival function, S(t), *is the probability of an individual in the population surviving beyond time* t.

In mathematical terms, the survival function is

$$S(t) = \frac{\text{Number of individuals surviving longer than time } t}{\text{Total number of individuals in population}}$$

Figure 11–2 shows a hypothetical survival function for a population. Note that it starts at 1 (or 100 percent alive) at time $t = 0$ and falls to 0 percent over time, as members of the population die off. The time at which half the population is alive and half is dead is called the *median survival time.*

Our goal is to estimate the survival function from a sample. Note that it is only possible to estimate the entire survival curve if the study lasts long enough for all members of the sample to die. When we are able to follow the sample until all members die, estimating the survival curve is easy: Simply compute the fraction of surviving individuals at each time someone dies. In this case, the estimate of the survival function from the data would simply be

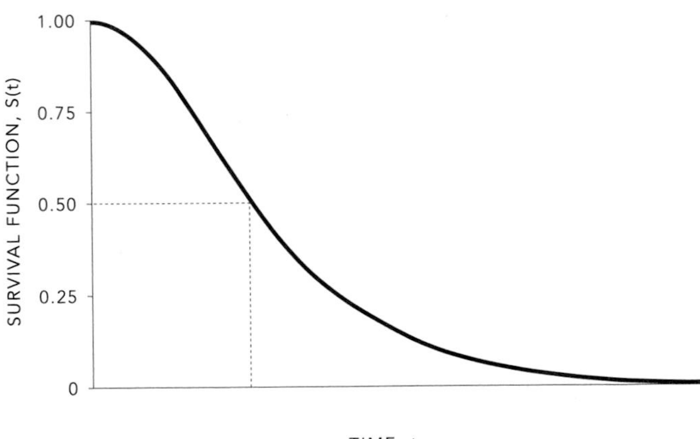

Figure 11–2 All population survival curves begin at 1 (100%) at time 0, when all the individuals in the study are alive, and falls to 0 as individuals die over time. The time at which 50 percent of the population has died is the *median survival time.*

$$\hat{S}(t) = \frac{\text{Number of individuals surviving longer than time } t}{\text{Total number of individuals in sample}}$$

where $\hat{S}(t)$ is the estimate of the population survival function computed from the observations in the sample.

Unfortunately, as we have already seen on Pluto, we often do not know the length of time every individual in the sample lives, so we cannot use this approach. In particular, we need a method to estimate the survival curve from real data, in the presence of censoring, when we do not know the precise times of death of all the individuals in the sample. To estimate the survival function from censored data, we need to compute the probability of surviving at each time we observe a death, based on the number of individuals *known* to be surviving immediately before that death.

The first step in estimating the survival function is to list all the observations in the order of the time of death or the last available observation. Table 11–1 shows these results for the data in Fig. 11–1, in the order that death occurred. Uncensored observations (where the actual time of death is known) are listed before censored observations. Censored observations are indicated with a "+," indicating that the time of death is some unknown time after the last time at which

Table 11–1 Pattern of Deaths over Time for Plutonians after Starting to Go to Smoky Bars

Plutonian	Survival time, t_i	No. alive at beginning of interval, n_i	No. of deaths at end of interval, d_i
J	2	10	1
H	6	9	1
A and C	7	8	2
I	7+	—	—
F	8	5	1
G	9	4	1
E	11+	—	—
B	12	2	1
D	12+	—	—

the subject was observed. For example, the first death took place (Plutonian J) at time 2, and the second death (Plutonian H) took place at time 6. Two Plutonians (A and C) died at time period 7, and one more observation (Plutonian I) *after* time 7. Thus, we know that Plutonian I lived longer than J, H, A, and C, *but we do not know how much longer.*

The second step is to estimate the probability of death within any time period, based on the number of subjects that survive to the beginning of the time period. Thus, just before the first Plutonian (J) dies at time 2, there are 10 Plutonians alive. Since one dies at time 2, there are $10 - 1 = 9$ survivors. Thus, our best estimate of the probability of surviving *past* time 2 *if alive just before time 2* is

$$\text{Fraction alive just before time 2 surviving past time 2} = \frac{n_2 - d_2}{n_2} = \frac{10 - 1}{10} = \frac{9}{10} = 0.900$$

where n_2 is the number of individuals alive *just before* time 2 and d_2 is the number of deaths *at* time 2. At the beginning of the time interval ending at time 2, 100 percent of the Plutonians are alive, so the estimate of the cumulative survival rate at time 2, $\hat{S}(2)$, is $1.000 \times 0.900 = 0.900$.

Next, we move on to the time of the next death, at time 6. One Plutonian dies at time 6 and there are 9 Plutonians alive immediately before time 6. The estimate of the probability of surviving past time 6 if one is alive just before time 6 is

$$\text{Fraction alive just before time 6 surviving past time 6} = \frac{n_6 - d_6}{n_6} = \frac{9 - 1}{9} = \frac{8}{9} = 0.889$$

At the beginning of the time interval ending at time 6, 90 percent of the Plutonians are alive, so the estimate of the cumulative survival rate at time 6, $\hat{S}(6)$, is $0.900 \times 0.889 = 0.800$. (Table 11–2 summarizes these calculations.)

Table 11–2 Estimation of Survival Curve for Plutonians after Starting to Go to Smoky Bars

Plutonian	Survival time, t_i	No. alive at beginning of interval, n_i	No. of deaths at end of interval, d_i	Fraction surviving interval, $(n_i - d_i)/n_i$	Cumulative survival rate, $\hat{S}(t)$
J	2	10	1	0.900	0.900
H	6	9	1	0.889	0.800
A and C	7	8	2	0.750	0.600
I	7+				
F	8	5	1	0.800	0.480
G	9	4	1	0.750	0.360
E	11+				
B	12	2	1	0.500	0.180
D	12+				

Likewise, just before time 7 there are 8 Plutonians alive and 2 die at time 7. Thus,

$$\text{Fraction alive just before time 7 surviving past time 7} = \frac{n_7 - d_7}{n_7} = \frac{8 - 2}{8} = \frac{6}{8} = 0.750$$

At the beginning of the time interval ending at time 7, 80 percent of the Plutonians are alive, so the estimate of the cumulative survival rate at time 7, $\hat{S}(7)$, is $0.800 \times 0.750 = 0.600$.

Up to this point, the calculations probably seem unnecessarily complex. After all, at time 7 there are 6 survivors out of 10 original individuals in the study, so why not simply compute the survival estimate as $6/10 = 0.600$? The answer to this question becomes clear after time 7, when we encounter our first censored observation. Because of censoring, we know that Plutonian I died sometime *after* time 7, but we do not know exactly when.

The next known death occurs at time 8, when Plutonian F dies. Because of the censoring of Plutonian I, who was last observed at time 7, we do not know whether this individual is alive or dead at time 8. As a result, we must drop Plutonian I from the calculation of the survival function. Just before time 8, there are 5 Plutonians *known* to be alive and one dies at time 8, so, following the procedure outlined previously

$$\text{Fraction alive just before time 8 surviving past time 8}$$
$$= \frac{n_8 + d_8}{n_8} = \frac{5 - 1}{5} = \frac{4}{5} = 0.800$$

At the beginning of the time interval ending at time 8, 60 percent of the Plutonians are alive, so the estimate of the cumulative survival rate at time 8, $\hat{S}(8)$, is $0.600 \times 0.800 = 0.480$. Because of the censoring, it would be impossible to estimate the survival function based on all the Plutonians who initially entered the study.

Table 11–2 presents the remainder of the computations to estimate the survival curve. This approach is known as the *Kaplan-Meier product-limit estimate* of the survival curve. The general formula for the Kaplan-Meier product-limit estimate of the survival curve is

$$\hat{S}(t_j) = \Pi\left(\frac{n_i - d_i}{n_i}\right)$$

where there are n_i individuals alive just before time t_i and d_i deaths occur at time t_i. The Π symbol indicates the product* taken over all the times, t_i, at which deaths occurred up to and including time t_j. (Note that the survival curve is *not* estimated at the times of censored observations because no known deaths occur at those times.) For example,

$$\hat{S}(7) = \left(\frac{10 - 1}{10}\right)\left(\frac{9 - 1}{9}\right)\left(\frac{8 - 2}{8}\right) = 0.600$$

Figure 11–3 shows a plot of the results. By convention, the survival function is drawn as a series of step changes, with the steps occurring at the times of known deaths. The curve ends at the time of the last observation, whether censored or not. Note that the curve, as all survival curves, begins at 1.0 and falls toward 0 as individuals die. Because

*The Π symbol for multiplication is used similarly to the symbol Σ for sums.

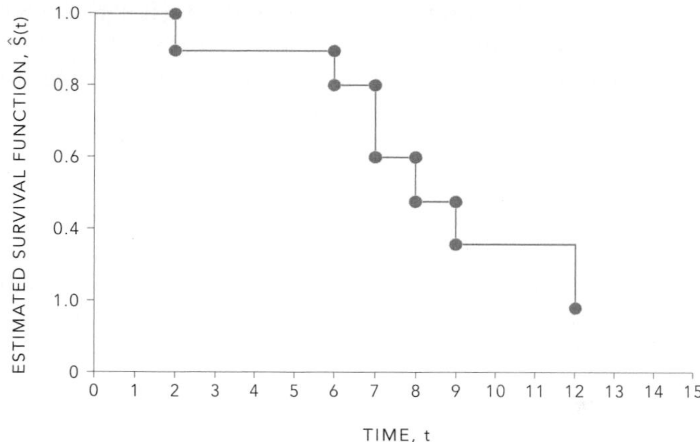

Figure 11-3 The survival curve for Plutonians hanging out in smoky bars, computed from the data in Table 11-1 as outlined in Table 11-2. Note that the curve is a series of horizontal lines, with the drops in survival at the times of known deaths. The curve ends at 12 time units because that is the survival time of the last known observation.

some individuals are still alive at the end of the study period, the data are censored and the estimated survival curve does not reach 0 during the time observations were available.

Median Survival Time

It is often desirable to provide a single statistic that summarizes a survival curve with a single number. Because the survival times tend to be positively skewed, the *median survival time* is generally used. After the survival curve has been estimated, it is simple to estimate the median survival time.

> *The median survival time is defined to be the smallest observed survival time for which the estimated survival function is less than .5.**

For example, in our study of the effect of secondhand smoke on Plutonians, the median survival time is 8 time units, because that is the first

*An alternative approach is to connect the two observed values above and below .5 with a straight line and read the time that corresponds to $\hat{S}(t) = .5$ off the resulting line.

time at which the survival function drops below .5. (It equals .480.) If fewer than half the individuals in the study die before the end of the study, it is not possible to estimate the median survival time. Other percentiles of the survival time are estimated analogously.

Standard Errors and Confidence Limits for the Survival Curve

Like all statistics, which are based on random samples drawn from underlying populations, there is a sampling distribution of the statistic around the population parameter, in this case, the true survival function, $S(t)$. The standard deviation of the sampling distribution is estimated by the standard error of the survival function. The standard error of the estimate of the survival curve can be estimated with the following equation, known as *Greenwood's formula.**

$$s_{\hat{S}(t_j)} = \hat{S}(t_j)\sqrt{\sum \frac{d_i}{n_i(n_i - d_i)}}$$

where the summation (indicated by Σ) extends over all times, t_i, at which deaths occurred up to and including time t_j. As with estimates of the survival curve itself, the standard error is only computed using times at which actual deaths occur. For example, the standard error for the estimated value of the survival function for the Plutonians going to smoky bars for time 7 is (using the results from Table 11–2)

$$s_{\hat{S}(7)} = .600\sqrt{\frac{1}{10(10-1)} + \frac{1}{9(9-1)} + \frac{2}{8(8-2)}} = .155$$

Table 11–3 shows all the computations for the standard errors of the survival curve using the data in Table 11–2.

The standard error can be used to compute a confidence interval for the survival function, just as we used the standard error to compute a confidence interval for rates and proportions in Chapter 7. Recall

*For a derivation of Greenwood's formula, see D. Collett, *Modelling Survival Data in Medical Research* Chapman and Hall, London, 1994, pages 22–26.

Table 11–3 Estimation of Standard Error of Survival Curve and 95% Confidence Interval (CI) for Survival Curve for Plutonians after Starting to Go to Smoky Bars

Plutonian	Survival time, t_i	No. alive at beginning of interval, n_i	No. of deaths at end of interval, d_i	Fraction surviving interval, $(n_i - d_i)/n_i$	Cumulative survival rate, $\hat{S}(t)$	$\frac{d_i}{n_i(n_i - d_i)}$	Standard error, $s_{\hat{S}(t)}$	Lower 95% CI	Upper 95% CI
J	2	10	1	0.900	0.900	0.011	0.095	0.714	1.000*
H	6	9	1	0.889	0.800	0.014	0.126	0.552	1.000*
A and C	7	8	2	0.750	0.600	0.042	0.155	0.296	0.904
I	7+								
F	8	5	1	0.800	0.480	0.050	0.164	0.159	0.801
G	9	4	1	0.750	0.360	0.083	0.161	0.044	0.676
E	11+								
B	12	2	1	0.500	0.180	0.500	0.151	0.000*	0.475
D	12+								

*The computed values were truncated at 1 and 0 because the survival function cannot go above 1 or below 0.

that we defined the 100(1 − α) percent confidence interval for a proportion to be

$$\hat{p} - z_\alpha s_{\hat{p}} < p < \hat{p} + z_\alpha s_{\hat{p}}$$

where z_α is the two-tail critical value of the standard normal distribution that defines the most α extreme values, $\hat{p}$ is the observed proportion with the characteristic of interest, and $s_{\hat{p}}$ is its standard error. Analogously, we define the 100(1 − α) percent confidence interval for the survival curve at time t_j to be

$$\hat{S}(t_j) - z_\alpha s_{\hat{S}(t_j)} < S(t_j) < \hat{S}(t_j) + z_\alpha s_{\hat{S}(t_j)}$$

To obtain the 95 percent confidence intervals, α = 0.05, and z_α = 1.960. Table 11–3 and Fig. 11–4 show the estimated survival curve for Plutonians exposed to secondhand smoke in bars. Note the confidence interval widens as time progresses because the number of individuals remaining in the study that form the basis for the estimate of $S(t)$ falls as people die.

As with computation of the confidence intervals for rates and proportions, this normal approximation works well when the observed values of the survival function are not near 1 or 0, in which case the confidence interval is no longer symmetric. (See Fig. 7–4 and the associated discussion.) As a result, applying the previous formula for values of $\hat{S}(t)$ near 1 or zero will yield confidence intervals that extend above 1 or below 0, which cannot be correct. From a pragmatic point of view, one can often simply truncate the intervals at 1 and 0 without introducing serious errors.*

*A better way to deal with this problem is to transform the observed survival curve according to ln [−ln $\hat{S}(t)$], which is not bounded by 0 and 1, compute the standard error of the transformed variable, then transform the result back into the survival function. The standard error of the transformed survival function is

$$s_{\ln[-\ln \hat{S}(y)]} = \sqrt{\frac{1}{[\ln \hat{S}(t)]^2} \sum \frac{d_i}{n_i(n_i - d_i)}}$$

The 100 (1 − α) percent confidence interval for $S(t)$ is

$$\hat{S}(t)^{\exp(-z_\alpha s_{\ln[-\ln \hat{S}(t)]})} < S(t) < \hat{S}(t)^{\exp(+z_\alpha s_{\ln[-\ln \hat{S}(t)]})}$$

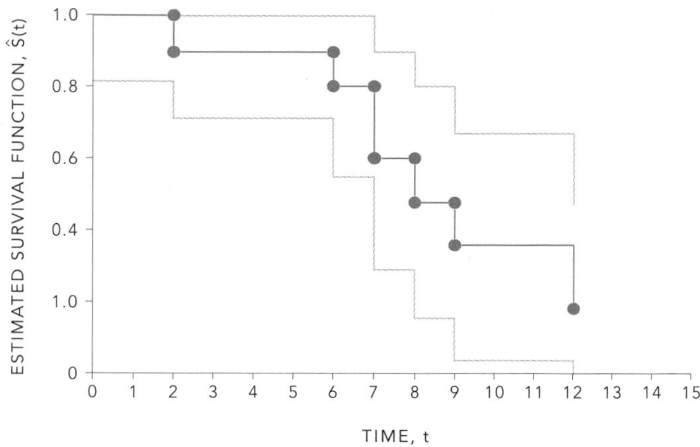

Figure 11–4 Survival curve for Plutonians hanging out in smoky bars, together with the 95 percent confidence interval (computed in Table 11–3). The upper and lower bounds of the 95 percent confidence interval are shown as dashed lines.

COMPARING TWO SURVIVAL CURVES*

The end goal of much of medical practice is to prolong life, so the need to compare survival curves for groups of people receiving different treatments naturally arises in many clinical studies. We discuss how to compare the survival curves for two groups of different patients receiving different treatments. The null hypothesis we will test is that the treatments have the same effect on the pattern of survival, that is, that the two groups of people are drawn from the same population. If all individuals in the study are followed up for the same length of time and there are no censored observations, we could simply analyze the data using contingency tables as described in Chapter 5. If all individuals are followed up until death (or whatever the defining event is), we could compare the time to deaths observed in the different groups using nonparametric methods, such as the Mann-Whitney rank sum test or Kruskal-Wallis analysis of variance

*There are methods for comparing more than two survival curves that are direct generalizations of the methods discussed in this book. The computations, however, require a computer and the use of more advanced mathematical notation (in particular, matrix notation), which is beyond the scope of this text.

based on ranks, described in Chapter 10. Unfortunately, in clinical studies of different treatments, these situations rarely hold. People are often lost to follow-up and the study often ends while many of the people in the study are still alive. As a result, some of the observations are censored and we need to develop appropriate statistical hypothesis testing procedures that will account for the censored data. We will use the *log-rank test.*

There are three assumptions that underlie the log-rank test.

- *The two samples are independent random samples.*
- *The censoring patterns for the observations are the same in both samples.*
- *The two population survival curves exhibit proportional hazards, so that they are related to each other according to* $S_2(t) = [S_1(t)]^{\Psi}$ *where* Ψ *is a constant called the hazard ratio.*

Note that if the two survival curves are identical, $\Psi = 1$. If $\Psi < 1$, people in group 2 die more slowly than people in group 1, and if $\Psi > 1$, people in group 2 die more quickly than people in group 1. The *hazard function* is the probability that an individual who has survived until time t dies at time t.* Hence, the assumption of proportional hazards means that the probability of dying at time t for individuals who have lived up to that point is a constant proportion between the two test groups.

*The mathematical definition of the hazard function is

$$h(t) = \lim_{\Delta t \to 0} \frac{\text{Probability an individual alive at time } t \text{ dies between } t \text{ and } t + \Delta t}{\Delta t}$$

The hazard function is related to the survival function according to

$$h(t) = \frac{f(t)}{S(t)}$$

where $f(t)$ is the probability density function corresponding to the failure function, $F(t) = 1 - S(t)$. The failure function begins at 0 and increases to 1, as all the members of the population die. For a discussion of these representations of the survival curve and their use, see E. T. Lee, *Statistical Methods for Survival Data Analysis,* 2nd ed., Wiley, New York, 1992.

Bone Marrow Transplantation to Treat Adult Leukemia

Acute lymphoblastic leukemia is a form of cancer in which a cancerous mutation of a lymph cell leads to greatly increased numbers of white blood cells (leukocytes). These leukemic white blood cells, however, are usually not functional in terms of the usual protections that white blood cells provide the body. At the same time, the cancerous tissue usually spreads to the bone marrow, where it interferes with the normal production of red blood cells, together with other adverse effects. The destruction of the bone marrow's ability to produce blood cells often leads to severe anemia (lack of red blood cells), which is one of the most common reasons people with this disease die.

This form of leukemia is treated through a combination of radiation and chemotherapy, which is effective in preventing recurrence in children. In adults, however, the chances of recurrence of the disease are high, even after the disease has been put into remission through chemotherapy and radiation. The chemotherapy and radiation are toxic not only to the cancer cells but also to many normal cells. In particular, at the doses used in adults, these treatments often destroy the normal bone marrow's ability to produce red blood cells. This side effect of the cancer treatment is treated by giving the person with leukemia a bone marrow transplant to reestablish function of the bone after the end of the chemotherapy and radiation. This bone marrow transplant ideally comes from a sibling who has the same type of bone marrow, a so-called *allogenic transplant.* Unfortunately, not everyone has an available sibling with matching tissue type to serve as a donor. Another option is to remove bone marrow from the person with cancer, treat the marrow with drugs in an effort to kill any residual cancer cells, preserve the "cleaned" marrow, and then inject it back into the person after the end of chemotherapy and radiation, a so-called *autologous transplant.** N. Vey

*Note that, because of ethical considerations and the fact that many of the people simply did not have appropriate siblings to serve as bone marrow donors, the investigators could not randomize the people in the study. They did, however, demonstrate that the two groups of people were similar in important clinical respects. This procedure is a common and reasonable way to deal with the fact the sometimes randomization is simply not possible. (See further discussion of these issues in Chapter 12.)

and colleagues* asked the question: Is there a difference in the survival patterns of the people who receive allogenic bone marrow transplants compared to those who receive autologous transplants?

To be included in the study, patients had to have a clear diagnosis of acute lymphoblastic leukemia that involved at least 30 percent of their bone marrow and had to have achieved a first complete remission before receiving their bone marrow transplant. Everyone was treated using the same treatment protocols. Patients who had a willing sibling with compatible bone marrow received an allogenic transplant and the remaining people received autologous transplants. Vey and colleagues observed the two groups of people for 11 years.

Table 11–4 shows the data we seek to analyze, Table 11–5 shows the computation of the survival curves for the two groups of people, and Figure 11–5 shows the survival curves. Examining this figure suggests that an allogenic transplant from a sibling leads to better survival than an autologous transplant from the cancer patient to himself or herself. The question remains, however, whether this difference is simply due to random sampling variation. Our null hypothesis is that there is no difference in the underlying populations represented by the two treatment groups.

The first step in constructing the test statistic used in the log-rank test is to consider the patterns of death in the two groups at each time a death occurs in either group. Table 11–6 summarizes all the deaths actually observed in the study. (Censored observations are not listed in this table.) One month following the bone marrow transplantation, 3 of the 33 people who had autologous transplants died, compared to 1 of 21 of the people who had allogenic transplants. How does this pattern compare with what would be expected by chance?

There are a total of $3 + 1 = 4$ deaths out of a total of $33 + 21 = 54$ people alive before the end of month 1 in the study. Thus, $4/54 = 0.074 = 7.4\%$ of all the people died, regardless of the kind of bone marrow transplant that was received. Thus, if the type of bone marrow transplantation did not matter, we would expect that 7.4 percent of the 33 people who received autologous transplants, $0.074 \times 33 = 2.444$

*N. Vey, D. Blaise, A. M. Stoppa, R. Bouaballah, M. Lafage, D. Sainty, D. Cowan, P. Viens, G. Lepeu, A. P. Blanc, D. Jaubert, C. Gaud, P. Mannoni, J. Camerlo, M. Resbeut, J. A. Gastaut, D. Maraninchi, "Bone Marrow Transplantation in 63 Adult Patients with Acute Lymphoblastic Leukemia in First Complete Remission," *Bone Marrow Transplant.* **14:**383–388, 1994.

Table 11–4 Time to Death (or Lost to Follow-Up) for People Receiving Autologous and Allogenic Bone Marrow Transplants

Autologous transplant ($n = 33$)		Allogenic transplant ($n = 21$)	
Month	Deaths or lost to follow-up	Month	Deaths or lost to follow-up
1	3	1	1
2	2	2	1
3	1	3	1
4	1	4	1
5	1	6	1
6	1	7	1
7	1	12	1
8	2	15+	1
10	1	20+	1
12	2	21+	1
14	1	24	1
17	1	30+	1
20+	1	60+	1
27	2	85+	2
28	1	86+	1
30	2	87+	1
36	1	90+	1
38+	1	100+	1
40+	1	119+	1
45+	1	132+	1
50	3		
63+	1		
132+	2		

people, to die at the end of month 1. This expected number of deaths compares to the observed 3 autologous transplant patients who died at month 1. If there is no difference between the patterns of survival between the two treatments, the observed and expected number of deaths at each time of a death should be similar for the autologous transplant patients.

To quantify the overall difference between the observed and expected number of deaths in the autologous group, we first compute the expected number of deaths at the time each death is observed in *either* group, then

Table 11–5 Computation of Survival Curves for Data in Table 11–4

Autologous bone marrow transplant					Allogenic bone marrow transplant				
Month, t_i	No. of deaths at end of interval d_i or lost to follow-up	No. alive at beginning of interval, n_i	Fraction surviving interval, $(n_i - d_i)/n_i$	Cumulative survival rate, $\hat{S}_{\text{autologous}}(t)$	Month, t_i	No. of deaths at end of interval d_i or lost to follow-up	No. alive at beginning of interval, n_i	Fraction surviving interval, $(n_i - d_i)/n_i$	Cumulative survival rate, $\hat{S}_{\text{allogenic}}(t)$
1	3	33	0.909	0.909	1	1	21	0.952	0.952
2	2	30	0.933	0.848	2	1	20	0.950	0.904
3	1	28	0.964	0.817	3	1	19	0.947	0.857
4	1	27	0.963	0.787	4	1	18	0.944	0.809
5	1	26	0.962	0.757	6	1	17	0.941	0.762
6	1	25	0.960	0.727	7	1	16	0.938	0.714
7	1	24	0.958	0.697	12	1	15	0.933	0.666
8	2	23	0.913	0.636	15+	1	14		
10	1	21	0.952	0.605	20+	1	13		
12	2	20	0.900	0.545	21+	1	12		
14	1	18	0.944	0.514	24	1	11	0.909	0.605
17	1	17	0.941	0.484	30+	1	10		
20+	1	16			60+	1	9		
27	2	15	0.867	0.420	85+	2	8		
28	1	13	0.923	0.388	86+	1	6		
30	2	12	0.833	0.323	87+	1	5		
36	1	10	0.900	0.291	90+	1	4		
38+	1	9			100+	1	3		
40+	1	8			119+	1	2		
45+	1	7			132+	1	1		
50	3	6	0.500	0.145					
63+	1	3							
132+	2	2							

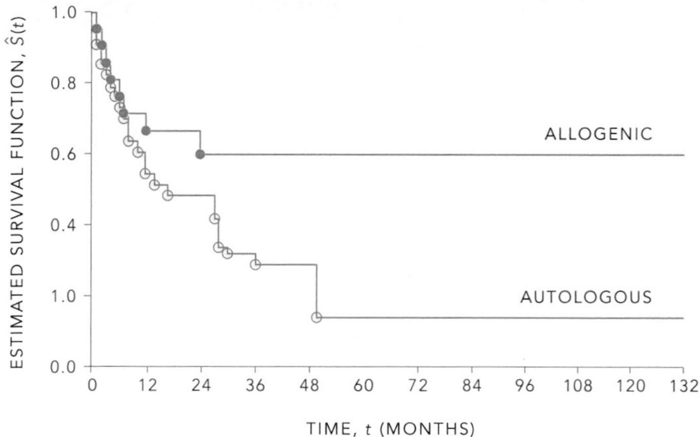

Figure 11–5 Survival curves for adults with leukemia who received autologous or allogenic bone marrow transplants (according to data in Table 11–4; survival curve computations are in Table 11–5). The curves extend to 132 months because that is the survival time of the last observation (even though the subsequent observations are censored at that time).

sum these differences up. In terms of equations, the expected number of deaths in the autologous group at time t_i is

$$e_{\text{autologous},i} = \frac{n_{\text{autologous},i}\, d_{\text{total}}}{n_{\text{total}}}$$

where $n_{\text{autologous},i}$ is the number of people who are known to be alive in the autologous transplant group immediately before time t_i, d_{total} is the total number of deaths in both groups at time t_i, and n_{total} is the total number of people who are known to be alive at immediately before time t_i.

Note that, while we do not explicitly include the censored observations in our summation, the censored observations do affect the results because they are included in the n's before the time at which they are censored. For example, the number of people in the allogenic transplant group known to be alive at the beginning at month 17 drops from 15 to 14 even though there were no known deaths in this group at this time

Table 11–6 Computation of Log-Rank Test to Compare Survival Curves for Autologous and Allogenic Bone Marrow Transplants

	Autologous		Allogenic		Total					
Month, t_i	Deaths at end of interval, $d_{autologous,i}$	No. alive at beginning of interval, $n_{autologous,i}$	Deaths at end of interval, $d_{allogenic,i}$	No. alive at beginning of interval, $n_{allogenic,i}$	Deaths at end of interval, $d_{total,i}$	No. alive at beginning of interval, $n_{total,i}$	Fraction of all people who die, $d_{total,i}/n_{total,i} = f_i$	Expected no. of autologous deaths, $n_{autologous,i}$ $f_i = e_i$	Observed minus expected autologous deaths, $d_{autologus,i} - e_i$	Contribution to standard error of U_L (see text)
1	3	33	1	21	4	54	0.074	2.444	0.556	0.897
2	2	30	1	20	3	50	0.060	1.800	0.200	0.691
3	1	28	1	19	2	47	0.043	1.191	−0.191	0.471
4	1	27	1	18	2	45	0.044	1.200	−0.200	0.469
5	1	26	0	17	1	43	0.023	0.605	0.395	0.239
6	1	25	1	17	2	42	0.048	1.190	−0.190	0.470
7	1	24	1	16	2	40	0.050	1.200	−0.200	0.468
8	2	23	0	15	2	38	0.053	1.211	0.789	0.465
10	1	21	0	15	1	36	0.028	0.583	0.417	0.243
12	2	20	1	15	3	35	0.086	1.714	0.286	0.691
14	1	18	0	14	1	32	0.031	0.563	0.438	0.246
17	1	17	0	14	1	31	0.032	0.548	0.452	0.248
24	0	16	1	11	1	27	0.037	0.593	−0.593	0.241
27	2	15	0	10	2	25	0.080	1.200	0.800	0.460
28	1	13	0	10	1	23	0.044	0.572	0.435	0.246
30	2	12	0	10	2	22	0.091	1.091	0.909	0.472
36	1	10	0	9	1	19	0.053	0.526	0.474	0.249
50	3	6	0	9	3	15	0.200	1.200	1.800	0.617
								Total	$U_L = 6.575$	$s^2_{UL} = 7.884$

because one of the patients in this group was lost to observation (censored) after month 15. In computing the log-rank test, it is important that the censored observations be carefully taken into account even though they do not explicitly appear in the calculations.

The first part of our test statistic is the sum of the differences between the observed and expected number of deaths in the autologous transplant group.

$$U_L = \sum(d_{\text{autologous},i} - e_{\text{autologous},i})$$

where the summation is over all the times at which anyone died in either group. For the study we are analyzing, $U_L = 6.575$ (Table 11–6). If this number is "small," it would indicate that there is not much difference between the two survival curves; if it is "big," we would reject the null hypothesis of no difference and report a difference in the survival associated with the two treatments.

As in earlier tests, we need to estimate the uncertainty associated with this sum to assess whether it is large. As in earlier tests, U_L follows a sampling distribution which is approximately normally distributed, with standard deviation*

$$s_{U_L} = \sqrt{\sum \frac{n_{\text{autologous},i}\, n_{\text{allogenic},i}\, d_{\text{total},i}(n_{\text{total},i} - d_{\text{total},i})}{n^2_{\text{total},i}(n_{\text{total},i} - 1)}}$$

where the summation is over all times at which deaths occurred. The last column in Table 11–6 includes these computations; $s^2_{U_L} = 7.884$ and $s_{U_L} = 2.808$. Finally, our test statistic is obtained by dividing the observed value of the test statistic by its standard error (the standard deviation of its sampling distribution).

$$z = \frac{U_L}{s_{U_L}} = \frac{6.575}{2.808} = 2.342$$

*For a derivation of this result, see D. Collett, *Modelling Survival Data in Medical Research,* Chapman & Hall, London, 1994, pages 40–42.

The test statistic is approximately normally distributed, so we compare its value with the critical values for the normal distribution (the last row in Table 4–1).* The critical value for the most extreme 2 percent of the normal distribution is 2.326, so we reject the null hypothesis of no difference in survival, $P < .02$. The allogenic bone marrow transplants are associated with better survival than the autologous bone marrow transplants. Bone marrow transplants from healthy siblings work better than autologous transplants from someone with leukemia to himself or herself.

This analysis could be done using either group; we simply use autologous transplants because it is the first group. Using the allogenic group as the reference group would have led to identical results.

The Yates Correction for the Log-Rank Test

When we used the normal approximation to test for differences between two proportions in Chapters 5 and 10, we noted that, while the normal distribution is continuous, the actual sampling distribution of the test statistic will be discrete because we were analyzing counts. The Yates correction was applied to correct for the fact that simply using the normal approximation will yield P values that are slightly too small. The situation is exactly the same for the log-rank test, so many statisticians apply the Yates correction to the computation of the log-rank statistic. The resulting test statistic (using the data in Table 11–6) is

$$z = \frac{|U_L| - \frac{1}{2}}{s_{U_L}} = \frac{6.575 - .500}{2.808} = 2.163$$

The value of the test statistic has been reduced from 2.342 to 2.163, and the associated P value increased to $P < .05$. The conclusion that the two types of bone marrow transplants have different effects on survival, however, remains unchanged.

*Some people compute the test statistic as U_L^2/s_U^2. This test statistic follows the chi-square distribution with 1 degree of freedom. The results are identical to those as described in the main text. The Yates correction, discussed in the following subsection, may also be applied to the log-rank test when computed in this manner.

GEHAN'S TEST

The log-rank test is not the only procedure available to compare two survival curves. Another procedure, known as *Gehan's test* is a generalization of the Wilcoxon signed rank test. As discussed below, however, the log-rank test is generally considered to be a superior method because Gehan's test can be dominated by a small number of early deaths. Gehan's test is computed by comparing every observation in the first treatment with every observation in the second treatment. For each comparison, score +1 if the second treatment *definitely* has a longer survival time than the first treatment, −1 if the first treatment *definitely* has a longer survival time than the second treatment, and 0 if censoring makes it impossible to say which treatment has a longer survival time for a given pair. Finally, sum up all the scores, to get U_W. A simpler way to compute U_W is to rank all the observations in time, and for each observation compute R_1 as the total number of observations whose survival time is *definitely* less than the current observation. Likewise, let R_2 be the number of cases whose survival time is *definitely* longer than the current observation. (If the observation is censored, you do not know the actual survival time, so $R_2 = 0$.) Let $h = R_1 - R_2$. U_W equals the sum of all the h's associated with the first treatment group. The standard error of U_W equals

$$s_{U_W} = \sqrt{\frac{n_1 n_2 \sum h^2}{(n_1 + n_2)(n_1 + n_2 - 1)}}$$

Finally, the test statistic

$$z = \frac{U_W}{s_{U_W}}$$

is compared to the standard normal distribution to obtain a P value. (The Yates correction can also be applied to this test, just as with the log-rank test.)

The log-rank test is also superior to Gehan's test if the assumption of *proportional hazards* is reasonably satisfied. If two survival functions exhibit proportional hazards, they will not cross.* Note that, because of random sampling variation, it is possible for the observed survival curves to cross, even if the underlying population survival functions exhibit proportional hazards.

POWER AND SAMPLE SIZE

As with all the other statistical hypothesis tests that we have considered, the power, $1 - \beta$, of a log-rank test to detect a real difference in the survival functions for two treatments depends on the size of the difference to be detected, the false-positive risk one is willing to accept (Type I error, α), and the sample size. Conversely, the sample size required to detect a given difference depends on the power one is seeking and the false-positive risk one is willing to accept. For a given risk of Type I error and power, larger studies are required to detect smaller differences in survival.

In the interest of simplicity, we limit ourselves to estimating the sample size for the log-rank test and assume that there are the same number of individuals in each of the test groups.† As with other statistical tests, making the sample sizes equal yields the minimum total sample size to detect a given difference or, alternatively, yields the maximum power to detect a given difference.

To compute the sample size needed to achieve a given power, we must first estimate the total number of deaths (or other events we are treating as the outcome variable) that must be observed. The total number of deaths, d, required is

$$d = (z_{\alpha(2)} - z_{1-\beta(\text{upper})})^2 \left(\frac{1 + \psi}{1 - \psi} \right)^2$$

where $z_{\alpha(2)}$ is the critical value of the normal distribution for a 2 tail test with $p = \alpha$ and $z_{1-\beta(\text{upper})}$ is the value of z that defines the upper

*A quick test for proportional hazards is to plot $\ln[-\ln \hat{S}_1(t)]$ and $\ln[-\ln \hat{S}_2(t)]$ against t. If the two lines are parallel, the assumption of proportional hazards is met.

†For a derivation of these results, see L. S. Freedman, "Tables of Number of Patients Required in Clinical Trials Using the Log-rank Test," *Stat. Med.* **1**:121–129, 1982.

(one tail) value of the normal distribution corresponding to $1 - \beta$, the desired power. Note that since $S_2(t) = [S_1(t)]^{\Psi}$,

$$\psi = \frac{\ln S_2(\infty)}{\ln S_1(\infty)}$$

where $S_1(\infty)$ and $S_2(\infty)$ are the expected survival rates of the two groups at the end of the experiment. Once we have the required number of deaths, d, we can compute the required sample size, n, for *each* experimental group, given

$$n = \frac{d}{2 - S_1(\infty) - S_2(\infty)}$$

Therefore, we can estimate the sample size based on the expected survival in the two treatment groups at the end of the study.

For example, suppose we want to design a study in which we wish to detect a difference in survival from 30 percent to 60 percent at the end of the study, with $\alpha = 0.05$ and power, $1 - \beta = .8$. From Table 4–2 $z_{\alpha(2)} = z_{.05(2)} = 1.960$ from Table 6–2, $z_{1-\beta(\text{upper})} = z_{.80(\text{upper})} = -.842$, and

$$\psi = \frac{\ln S_2(\infty)}{\ln S_1(\infty)} = \frac{\ln .6}{\ln .3} = \frac{-.511}{-1.203} = .425$$

Substituting into the formula for the number of deaths above,

$$d = (z_{\alpha(2)} - z_{1-\beta(\text{upper})})^2 \left(\frac{1 + \psi}{1 - \psi}\right)^2$$

$$= (1.960 + .842)^2 \left(\frac{1 + .425}{1 - .425}\right)^2 = 48.1$$

So, we need a total of 49 deaths. To obtain this number of deaths, the number of individuals required in each of the two samples would be

$$n = \frac{d}{2 - S_1(\infty) - S_2(\infty)} = \frac{49}{2 - .3 - .6} = 44.5$$

Thus, we need 45 individuals in each group, for a total sample size of 90 individuals.

These same equations can be used to compute power, by solving for $z_{1-\beta(\text{upper})}$ in terms of the other variables in the equations.

SUMMARY

This chapter developed procedures to describe outcome patterns in clinical trials where people are observed over time until a discrete event, such as death, occurs. Such trials are gaining in importance as cost pressures demand that medical treatment be demonstrated to be effective. Analysis of such data is complicated by the fact that because of the very nature of survival studies, some of the individuals in the study live beyond the end of the study and others are lost to observation because they move or die for reasons unrelated to the disease or treatment being studied. In order to construct descriptive statistics and test hypotheses about these kind of data, we used all the available information at each time an event occurred. The procedures we describe in this chapter can be generalized to include more complicated experimental designs in which several different treatments are being studied.* The final chapter places all the tests we have discussed in this book in context, together with some general comments on how to assess what you read and write.

PROBLEMS

11-1 Surgery is an accepted therapeutic approach for treating cancer patients with metastases in their lungs. Philippe Girard and colleagues ("Surgery for Pulmonary Metastases: Who Are the 10-year Survivors?" *Cancer* **74:**2791–2797, 1994) collected data on 35 people who had metastases removed from their lungs. Estimate the survival curve and associated 95% confidence interval.

*The methods we discuss in this chapter are *nonparametric* methods because they do not make any assumptions about the shape of the survival function. There are also a variety of parametric procedures that one can use when you know that the survival function follows a known functional form.

Month	Death or loss to follow-up during month
1	1
2	1
3	3
3+	1
4	1
5	1
6	1
7	2
8	1
9	1
10+	1
11+	2
12	2
13	1
15	1
16	3
20	3
21	1
25+	1
28	1
34	1
36+	1
48+	1
56	1
62	1
84	1

11-2 Taking care of old people on an outpatient basis is less costly than caring for them in nursing homes or hospitals, but health professionals have expressed concern about how well it is possible to predict clinical outcomes among people cared for on an outpatient basis. As part of an investigation of predictors of death in geriatric patients, Brenda Keller and Jane Potter ("Predictors of Mortality in Outpatient Geriatric Evaluation and Management Clinic Patients," *J. Gerontol.* **49:**M246–M251, 1994) compared survival in people aged 78.4 +/= 7.2 (SD) years who scored high on the Instrumental Activities of Daily Living (IADL) scale and those who scored low. Based on the following survival data, is there a difference in the survival patterns of these two groups of people?

High IADL scores		Low IADL scores	
Month	Death or lost to follow-up	Month	Death or lost to follow-up
14	1	6	2
20	2	12	2
24	3	18	4
25+	1	24	1
28	1	26+	1
30	2	28	4
36+	1	32	4
37+	1	34+	2
38	2	36	3
42+	1	38+	3
43+	1	42	3
48	2	46+	2
48+	62	47	3
		48	2
		48+	23

11-3 In Japan, cancer is the leading cause of death from disease in children under the age of 15. Wakiko Ajiki and colleagues ("Survival Rates of Childhood Cancer Patients in Osaka, Japan, 1975–1984," *Jpn. J. Cancer Res.* **86:**13–20, 1995) compared the survival rates for children with several cancers, including neuroblastoma, a malignant tumor of the peripheral nervous system, for children diagnosed between 1975 and 1979 and 1980 and 1984. The data appear on the next page.

Children diagnosed 1975–1979		Children diagnosed 1980–1984	
Month	Death or lost to follow-up	Month	Death or lost to follow-up
2	3	2	4
4	4	4	1
6	3	6	3
8	4	8	10
10+	1	12	4
12	2	14	3
14	3	18+	1
16+	1	20+	1
18	2	22	2
22+	1	24	1
24	1	30	2
30	2	36	3
36	1	48	2
52+	1	54+	1
54	1	56	2
56	1	60	1
60	1	60+	9
60+	18		

(a) Estimate the survival curves and 95 percent confidence intervals for the two survival curves. (b) Estimate the median survival times for the two groups of children. (c) Compare the two survival curves; are they significantly different? (d) What is the power of the log-rank test to detect a significant difference (with $\alpha = 0.05$) where the steady state survival rates, S_∞, are equal to the observed estimates of the survival observed at 60 months. (e) Calculate the total number of deaths and total sample size needed to obtain a power of .80 if there are changes in steady state survival rate from 0.40 from the 1975–1979 period to 0.20 for the 1980–1984 period.

Chapter 12

What Do the Data Really Show?

The statistical methods we have been discussing permit you to estimate the certainty of statements and precision of measurements that are common in the biomedical sciences and clinical practice about a population after observing a random sample of its members. To use statistical procedures correctly, one needs to use a procedure that is appropriate for the experiment (or survey) and the scale (i.e., interval, nominal, or ordinal) used to record the data. All these procedures have, at their base, the assumption that the samples were selected at random from the populations of interest. If the real experiment does not satisfy this randomization assumption, the resulting P values and confidence intervals are meaningless. In addition to seeing that the individuals in the sample are selected at random, there is often a question of exactly what actual populations the people in any given study represent. This question is especially important and often difficult to answer when the experimental subjects are patients in academic medical centers, a group of people hardly typical of the population as a whole. Even so, identifying the population in question is the crucial step in deciding the broader applicability of the findings of any study.

WHEN TO USE WHICH TEST

We have reached the end of our discussion of different statistical tests and procedures. It is by no means exhaustive, for there are many other approaches to problems and many kinds of experiments we have not even discussed. (For example, *two-factor* experiments in which the investigator administers two different treatments to each experimental subject and observes the response. Such an experiment yields information about the effect of each treatment alone as well as the joint effect of the two treatments acting together.) Nevertheless, we have developed a powerful set of tools and laid the groundwork for the statistical methods needed to analyze more complex experiments. Table 12–1 shows that it is easy to place all these statistical hypothesis-testing procedures this book presents into context by considering two things: the *type of experiment* used to collect the data and the *scale of measurement.*

To determine which test to use, one needs to consider the experimental design. Were the treatments applied to the same or different individuals? How many treatments were there? Were all treatments applied to the same or different individuals? Was the experiment designed to define a tendency for two variables to increase or decrease together?

How the response is measured is also important. Were the data measured on an interval scale? If so, are you satisfied that the underlying population is normally distributed? Do the variances within the treatment groups or about a regression line appear equal? When the observations do not appear to satisfy these requirements—or if you do not wish to assume that they do—you lose little power by using nonparametric methods based on ranks. Finally, if the response is measured on a nominal scale in which the observations are simply categorized, one can analyze the results using contingency tables.

Table 12–1 comes close to summarizing the lessons of this book, but there are three important things that it excludes. First, as Chapter 6 discussed, it is important to consider the power of a test when determining whether or not the failure to reject the null hypothesis of no treatment effect is likely to be because the treatment really has no effect or because the sample size was too small for the test to detect the treatment effect. Second, Chapters 7 and 8 discussed the importance of quantifying the size of the treatment effect (with confidence intervals) in addition to the

Table 12–1 Summary of Some Statistical Methods to Test Hypotheses

	Type of experiment				
Scale of measurement	Two treatment groups consisting of different individuals	Three or more treatment groups consisting of different individuals	Before and after a single treatment in the same individuals	Multiple treatments in the same individuals	Association between two variables
Interval (and drawn from normally distributed populations*)	Unpaired *t* test (Chapter 4)	Analysis of variance (Chapter 3)	Paired *t* test (Chapter 9)	Repeated-measures analysis of variance (Chapter 9)	Linear regression, Pearson product-moment correlation, or Bland-Altman analysis (Chapter 8)
Nominal	Chi-square analysis-of-contingency table (Chapter 5)	Chi-square analysis-of-contingency table (Chapter 5)	McNemar's test (Chapter 9)	Cochrane Q†	Relative risk or odds ratio (Chapter 5)
Ordinal†	Mann-Whitney rank-sum test (Chapter 10)	Kruskal-Wallis statistic (Chapter 10)	Wilcoxon signed-rank test (Chapter 10)	Friedman statistic (Chapter 10)	Spearman rank correlation (Chapter 8)
Survival time	Log-rank test or Gehan's test (Chapter 11)				

*If the assumption of normally distributed populations is not met, rank the observations and use the methods for data measured on an ordinal scale.

†Or interval data that are not necessarily normally distributed.

certainty with which you can reject the hypothesis that the treatment had no effect (the P value). Third, one must consider how the samples were selected and whether or not there are biases that invalidate the results of any statistical procedure, however elegant or sophisticated. This important subject has been discussed throughout this book; we will finish with a few more comments and examples relating to it.

RANDOMIZE AND CONTROL

As already noted, all the statistical procedures assume that the observations represent a sample *drawn at random* from a larger population. What, precisely, does "drawn at random" mean? It means that any specific member of the population is as likely as any other member to be selected for study, and further that any given individual is as likely to be selected for one sample group as the other (i.e., control or treatment). The only way to achieve randomization is to use an objective procedure, such as a table of random numbers, to select subjects for a sample or treatment group. When other criteria are used that permit the investigator (or participant) to influence which treatment a given individual receives, one can no longer conclude that observed differences are due to the treatment rather than *biases* introduced by the process of assigning different individuals to different groups. When the randomization assumption is not satisfied, the logic underlying the distributions of the test statistics (F, t, q, q', χ^2, z, r, r_s, T, W, H, Q, Q', or χ^2_r) used to estimate that the observed differences between the different treatment groups are due to chance as opposed to the treatment fails and the resulting P values (i.e., estimates that the observed differences are due to chance) are meaningless.

To reach meaningful conclusions about the efficacy of some treatment, one must compare the results obtained in the individuals who receive the treatment with an appropriate *control* group that is identical to the treatment group in all respects except the treatment. Clinical studies often fail to include adequate controls. *This omission generally biases the study in favor of the treatment.*

Despite the fact that questions of proper randomization and control are really distinct statistical questions, in practice these two areas are so closely related that we will discuss them together by considering two classic examples.

Internal Mammary Artery Ligation to Treat Angina Pectoris

People with coronary artery disease develop chest pain (angina pectoris) when they exercise because the narrowed arteries cannot deliver enough blood to carry oxygen and nutrients to the heart muscle and remove waste products fast enough. Relying on some anatomical studies and clinical reports during the 1930s, some surgeons suggested that tying off (ligating) the mammary arteries would force blood into the arteries that supplied the heart and increase the amount of blood available to it. By comparison with major operations that require splitting the chest open, the procedure to ligate the internal mammary arteries is quite simple. The arteries are near the skin, and the entire procedure can be done under local anesthesia.

In 1958, J. Roderick Kitchell and colleagues* published the results of a study in which they ligated the internal mammary arteries of 50 people who had angina before the operation, then observed them for 2 to 6 months; 34 of the patients (68 percent) improved clinically in that they had no more chest pain (36 percent) or fewer and less severe attacks (32 percent); 11 patients (22 percent) showed no improvement, and 5 (10 percent) died. On its face, this operation seems an effective treatment for angina pectoris.

In fact, even before this study was published, *Reader's Digest* carried an enthusiastic description of the procedure in an article entitled "New Surgery for Ailing Hearts."† (This article probably did more to promote the operation than the technical medical publications.)

Yet, despite the observed symptomatic relief and popular appeal of the operation, no one uses it today. Why not?

In 1959, Leonard Cobb and colleagues†† published the results of a double-blind randomized controlled trial of this operation. Neither the patients nor the physicians who evaluated them knew whether or not a given patient had the internal mammary arteries ligated. When the patient reached the operating room, the surgeon made the incisions

*J. R. Kitchell, R. Glover, and R. Kyle, "Bilateral Internal Mammary Artery Ligation for Angina Pectoris: Preliminary Clinical Considerations," *Am. J. Cardiol.*, **1**:46–50, 1958.

†J. Ratcliff, "New Surgery for Ailing Hearts," *Reader's Dig.*, **71**:70–73, 1957.

††L. Cobb, G. Thomas, D. Dillard, K. Merendino, and R. Bruce, "An Evaluation of Internal-Mammary-Artery Ligation by a Double-Blind Technic," *N. Engl. J. Med.*, **260**:1115–1118, 1959.

necessary to reach the internal mammary arteries and isolated them. At that time, the surgeon was handed an envelope instructing whether or not actually to ligate the arteries. The treated patients had their arteries ligated, and the control patients had the wound closed without touching the artery.

When evaluated in terms of subjective improvement as well as more quantitative measures, for example, how much they could exercise before developing chest pain or the appearance of their electrocardiogram, there was little difference between the two groups of people, although there was a suggestion that the control group did better.

In other words, the improvement that Kitchell and colleagues reported was a combination of observer biases and, probably more important, the placebo effect.

The Portacaval Shunt to Treat Cirrhosis of the Liver

Alcoholics often develop cirrhosis of the liver when the liver's internal structure breaks down and increases the resistance to the flow of blood through the liver. As a result, blood pressure increases and often affects other parts of the circulation, such as the veins around the esophagus. If the pressure reaches a high enough level, these vessels can rupture, causing internal bleeding and even death. To relieve this pressure, many surgeons performed a major operation to redirect blood flow away from the liver by constructing a connection between the portal artery (which goes to the liver) and the vena cava (the large veins on the other side of the liver). This connection is called a *portacaval shunt.*

Like many medical procedures, the early studies that supported this operation were completed without controls. The investigators completed the operation on people, then watched to see how well they recovered. If their clinical condition improved, the operation was considered a success. This approach has the serious flaw of not allowing for the fact that some of the people would have been fine (or died) regardless of whether or not they had the operation.

In 1966, more than 20 years after the operation was introduced, Norman Grace and colleagues* examined 51 papers that sought to evaluate this procedure. They examined the nature of the control group,

*N. Grace, H. Muench, and T. Chalmers, "The Present Status of Shunts for Portal Hypertension in Cirrhosis," *Gastroenterology,* **50:**684–691, 1966.

if one was present, whether or not patients were assigned to treatment or control at random, and how enthusiastic the authors were about the operation after they finished their study. Table 12–2 shows that the overwhelming majority of investigators who were enthusiastic about the procedure did studies failing to include a control group or including a control group that was not the result of a random assignment of patients between control and the operation. The few investigators who included controls and adequate randomization were not enthusiastic about the operation.

The reasons for biases on behalf of the operation in the studies that did not include controls—the placebo effect and observer biases—are the same as in the study of internal mammary artery ligation we just discussed.

The situation for the 15 studies with nonrandomized controls contains some of these same difficulties, but the situation is more subtle. Specifically, there *is* a control group that provides some basis of comparison; the members of the control were not selected at random, however, but assigned on the basis of the investigators' judgment. In such cases, there is often a bias to treat only patients who are well enough to respond (or occasionally, hopeless cases). This selection procedure biases the study in behalf of (or occasionally against) the treatment under study. This bias can slip into studies in quite subtle ways. For example, suppose that you are studying some treatment and decide to assign patients who are admitted to the control and

Table 12–2 Value of Portacaval Shunt According to 51 Different Studies

	Degree of enthusiasm		
Design	Marked	Moderate	None
No controls	24	7	1
Controls			
Not randomized	10	3	2
Randomized	0	1	3

Source: Adapted from N. D. Grace, H. Muench, and T. C. Chambers, "The Present Status of Shunts for Portal Hypertension in Cirrhosis," *Gastroenterology,* **50:**684–691, 1966, table 2.

treatment groups alternately in the order in which they are admitted or on alternate days of the month. It then makes it easy for the investigators to decide which group a given person will be a member of by manipulating the day or time of admission to the hospital. The investigators may not even realize they are introducing such a bias.

A similar problem can arise in laboratory experiments. For example, suppose that you are doing a study of a potential carcinogen with rats. Simply taking rats out of a cage and assigning the first 10 rats to the control group and the next 10 rats to the treatment group (or alternate rats to the two groups) will not produce a random sample because more aggressive, or bigger, or healthier rats may, as a group, stay in the front or back of the cage.

The only way to obtain a random sample that avoids these problems is *consciously to assign the experimental subjects at random* using a table of random numbers, dice, or other procedure.

Table 12–2 illustrates that the four randomized trials done of the portacaval shunt showed the operation to be of little or no value. This example illustrates a common pattern.

The better the study, the less likely it is to be biased in favor of the treatment.

The biases introduced by failure to randomize the treatments in clinical trials can be substantial. For example, Kenneth Schulz and coworkers* examined 250 controlled trials and assessed how the subjects in the studies had been allocated to the different treatment groups. A well-randomized trial was one in which subjects were assigned to treatments based on a random number generator or some similar process. A study was deemed to have an inadequate treatment allocation procedure if the subjects were treated based on the date they entered the study (including alternating one treatment or the other), which could be subject to manipulation by the investigators or others participating in the study. The authors found that the treatments appeared 41 percent better in the poorly randomized studies than in the ones with careful application of strict randomization procedures.

*K. F. Schulz, I. Chalmers, R. J. Hayes, D. G. Altman, "Empirical Evidence of Bias: Dimensions of Methodological Quality Associated with Estimates of Treatment effects in Controlled Trials," *JAMA* **273:**408–412, 1995.

Thus, it is very important that the randomization be conducted using a random number generator, table of random digits, or other similarly objective procedure to avoid the introduction of serious upward biases in the estimate of how well the treatment under study works.

Is Randomization of People Ethical?

Having concluded that the randomized clinical trial is the definitive way to assess the value of a potential therapy, we need to pause to discuss the ethical dilemma that some people feel when deciding whether or not to commit someone's treatment to a table of random numbers. The short answer to this problem is that *if no one knows* which therapy is better, there is no ethical imperative to use one therapy or another.

In reality, all therapies have their proponents and detractors, so one can rarely find a potential therapy that everyone feels neutral about at the start of a trial. (If there were no enthusiasts, no one would be interested in trying it.) As a result, it is not uncommon to hear physicians, nurses, and others protesting that some patient is being deprived of effective treatment (i.e., a therapy that the individual physician or nurse believes in) simply to answer a scientific question. Sometimes these objections are well-founded, but when considering them it is important to ask: *What evidence of being right does the proponent have*? Remember that uncontrolled and nonrandomized studies tend to be biased in favor of the treatment. At the time, Cobb and colleagues' randomized controlled trial of internal mammary artery ligation may have seemed unethical to enthusiasts for the surgery on the grounds that it required depriving some people of the potential benefits of the surgery. In hindsight, however, they spared the public the pain and expense of a worthless therapy.

These genuine anxieties, as well as the possible vested interests of the proponent of the procedure, must be balanced against the possible damage and costs of subjecting the patient to a useless or harmful therapy or procedure. The same holds for the randomized controlled trials of the portacaval shunt. To complete a randomized trial it is necessary to assess carefully just *why* you believe some treatment to have an effect.

This situation is complicated by the fact that once something becomes accepted practice, it is almost impossible to evaluate it, even though it is as much as a result of tradition and belief as scientific evidence, for example, the use of leeches. To return to the theme we opened this book with, a great deal of inconvenience, pain, and money is wasted pursuing diagnostic tests and therapies that are of no demonstrated value. For example, despite the fact that the provision of coronary artery bypass graft surgery has become a major American industry, there is continuing debate over precisely who the operation helps.

Another seemingly more difficult issue is what to do when the study suggests that the therapy is or is not effective but enough cases have not yet been accumulated to reach conventional statistical significance, that is, $P = .05$. Recall (from Chapter 6) that the power of a test to detect a difference of a specified size increases with the sample size and as the risk of erroneously concluding that there is a difference between the treatment groups (the Type I error α) increases. Recall also that α is simply the largest value of P that one is willing to accept and still conclude that there is a difference between the sample groups (in this case, that the treatment had an effect). Thus, if people object to continuing a clinical trial until the trial accumulates enough patients (and sufficient power) to reject the hypothesis of no difference between the treatment groups with $P < .05$ (or $\alpha = 5$ percent), all they are really saying is that they are willing to conclude that there is a difference when P is greater than .05.* In other words, they are willing to accept a higher risk of being wrong in the assertion that the treatment was effective when, in fact, it is not, because they believe the potential benefits of the treatment make it worth pursuing despite the increased uncertainty about whether or not it is really effective. Viewed in this light, the often diffuse debates over continuing a clinical trial can be focused on the real question underlying the disagreements: How confident does one need to be that the observed difference is not due to chance before concluding that the treatment really did cause the observed differences?

*When one examines the data as they accumulate in a clinical trial, one can encounter the same multiple-comparisons problem discussed in Chapters 3 and 4. Therefore, it is important to use techniques (such as a Bonferroni correction to the P values) that account for the fact that you are looking at the data more than once. See K. McPherson, "Statistics: The Problem of Examining Accumulating Data More than Once," *N. Engl. J. Med.*, **290:**501–502, 1974, and the comments on sequential analysis in the footnote at the end of Chapter 6.

The answer to this question depends on personal judgment and values, not statistical methodology.

Is a Randomized Controlled Trial Always Necessary?

No. There are rare occasions, such as the introduction of penicillin, when the therapy produces such a dramatic improvement that one need not use statistical tools to estimate the probability that the observed effects are due to chance.

In addition, sometimes medical realities make it impossible to do a randomized trial. For example, in Chapter 11 we considered a study of the effects of bone marrow transplants on survival among adults with leukemia. One group of people received bone marrow transplants from a tissue-matched sibling (allogenic transplants), and the other group received bone marrow removed from themselves before beginning treatment with chemotherapy and radiation for the cancer (autologous transplants). Since everyone does not have a tissue-matched sibling that could serve as a transplant donor, it was impossible to randomize the treatments. To minimize bias in this study, however, the investigators treated all the people in the study the same and carefully matched people in the two treatment groups on other characteristics that could have affected the outcome. This situation often exists in clinical studies; it is particularly important to see that the subjects in different experimental groups are as similar as possible when a strict randomization is not possible.

There are also often accidents of nature that force attentive practitioners to reassess the value of accepted therapy. For example, Ambroise Paré, a French military surgeon, followed the accepted therapy of treating gunshot wounds with boiling oil. During a battle in Italy in 1536 he ran out of oil and simply had to dress the untreated wounds. After spending a sleepless night worrying about his patients who had been deprived of the accepted therapy, he was surprised to find them "free from vehemencie of paine to have had good rest" while the conventionally treated soldiers were feverish and tormented with pain.*

*This example is taken from H. R. Wulff, *Rational Diagnosis and Treatment,* Blackwell, Oxford, 1976. This excellent short book builds many bridges between the ideas we have been discussing and the diagnostic therapeutic thought processes.

History does not record whether Paré then prepared a proposal to do a randomized clinical trial to study the value of boiling oil to treat gunshot wounds. Should and would it be necessary if he had made his discovery today?

DOES RANDOMIZATION ENSURE CORRECT CONCLUSIONS?

The randomized controlled trial is the most convincing way to demonstrate the value of a therapy. Can you assume that it will always lead to correct conclusions? No.

First, as Chapter 6 discussed, the trial may involve too few patients to have sufficient power to detect a true difference.

Second, if the investigators require $P < .05$ to conclude that the data are incompatible with the hypothesis that the treatment had no effect, in the long run 5 percent of the "statistically significant" effects they find will be due to chance in the random-sampling process when, in actuality, the treatment had no effect, that is, the null hypothesis is correct. (Since investigators are more likely to publish positive findings than negative findings, more than 5 percent of the published results are probably due to chance rather than the treatments.) This means that as you do more and more tests, you will accumulate more and more incorrect statements. When one collects a set of data and repeatedly subdivides the data into smaller and smaller subgroups for comparison, it is not uncommon to "find" a difference that is due to random variation rather than a real treatment effect.

Most clinical trials, especially those of chronic disease like coronary artery disease or diabetes, are designed to answer a single broad question dealing with the effect on survival of competing treatments. These trials involve considerable work and expense and yield a great many data, and the investigators are generally interested in gleaning as much information (and as many publications) as possible from their efforts. As a result, the sample is often divided into subgroups based on various potential prognostic variables, and the subgroups are compared for the outcome variable of interest (usually survival). This procedure inevitably yields one or more subgroups of patients in whom the therapy is effective. For example, the Veterans Administration's prospective randomized controlled trial[*] of coronary artery bypass surgery did not detect a difference between the operation and medical therapy for the study group taken as a whole but did suggest that surgery improved survival in patients with left main coronary artery disease (disease of a specific artery, the left main coronary artery). This conclusion has had a major impact on the treatment physicians now recommend to their patients.

One needs to be extremely cautious when interpreting such findings, especially when they are associated with relatively large *P* values (of the order of five percent as opposed to less than one percent).

To demonstrate the difficulties that can arise when one begins examining subgroups of patients in a randomized controlled trial, Kerry Lee and colleagues[†] took 1073 patients who had coronary artery disease and were being treated with medical therapy at Duke University and randomly divided them into two groups. *The "treatment" was randomization.* Therefore, if the samples are representative, one would not expect any systematic differences between the two groups. Indeed, when they compared the two groups with respect to age, sex, medical history, electrocardiographic findings, number of blocked coronary arteries, or whether or not the heart exhibited a normal contraction pattern, using the methods this book describes, they found no significant differences between the two groups, except in the left ventricular contraction pattern. This result is not surprising, given that the two groups were created by randomly dividing a single group into two samples. Most important, there was virtually no difference in the pattern of survival in the two groups (Figure 12–1*A*). So far, this situation is analogous to a randomized clinical trial designed to compare two groups receiving different therapies.

As already noted, after going to all the trouble of collecting such data, investigators are usually interested in examining various subgroups to see whether any finer distinctions can be made that will help the individual clinician deal with each individual patient according to the particular circumstances to the case. To simulate this procedure, Lee and

*M. Murphy, H. Hultgren, K. Detre, J. Thomsen, and T. Takaro, "Treatment of Chronic Stable Angina: A Preliminary Report of Survival Data of the Randomized Veterans Administration Cooperative Study," *N. Engl. J. Med.*, **297:**621–627, 1977.

†K. Lee, F. McNeer, F. Starmer, P. Harris, and R. Rosati, "Clinical Judgment and Statistics: Lessons from a Simulated Randomized Trial in Coronary Artery Disease," *Circulation,* **61:**508–515, 1980.

colleagues subdivided (the technical statistical term is *stratified*) the 1073 patients into six subgroups depending on whether one, two, or three coronary arteries were blocked and whether or not the patient's left ventricle was contracting normally. They also further subdivided these six groups into subgroups based on whether or not the patient had a history of heart failure. They analyzed the resulting survival data for the 18 subgroups (6 + 12) using the techniques discussed in Chapter 11. This analysis revealed, among others, a statistically significant ($P < .025$) difference in survival between the two groups of patients who had three diseases vessels and an abnormal contraction pattern (Fig. 12–1*B*). How could this be? After all, *randomization was the treatment.*

This result is another aspect of the multiple-comparisons problem discussed at length in Chapters 3 and 4. Without counting the initial test of the global hypothesis that the survival in the two original sample groups is not different, Lee and colleagues completed 18 different comparisons on the data. Thus, according to the Bonferroni inequality, the chances of obtaining a statistically significant result with $P < .05$, by chance is not above 18(.05) = .90.* The result in Fig. 12–1*B* is an example of this fact. When the total patient sample in a clinical trial is subdivided into many subgroups and the treatment compared within these subgroups, the results of these comparisons need to be interpreted very cautiously, especially when the P values are relatively large (say, around .05, as opposed to being around .001).

One approach to this problem would be to use the Bonferroni inequality (much as we used it in earlier chapters) and require that the value of the test statistic exceed the critical value for $P = \alpha_T/k$; however, this approach is too conservative when there are a large number of comparisons.

*When there are so many tests, the Bonferroni inequality overestimates the true probability of making a Type I error. It also increases the probability of making a Type II error. If you complete k comparisons each at the α level of significance, the total risk of making a Type I error is

$$\alpha_T = 1 - (1 - \alpha)^k$$

In the case of 18 comparisons with $\alpha = 0.05$, the total chance of obtaining $P < .05$ at least once by chance is

$$\alpha_T = 1 - (1 - .05)^{18} = .60$$

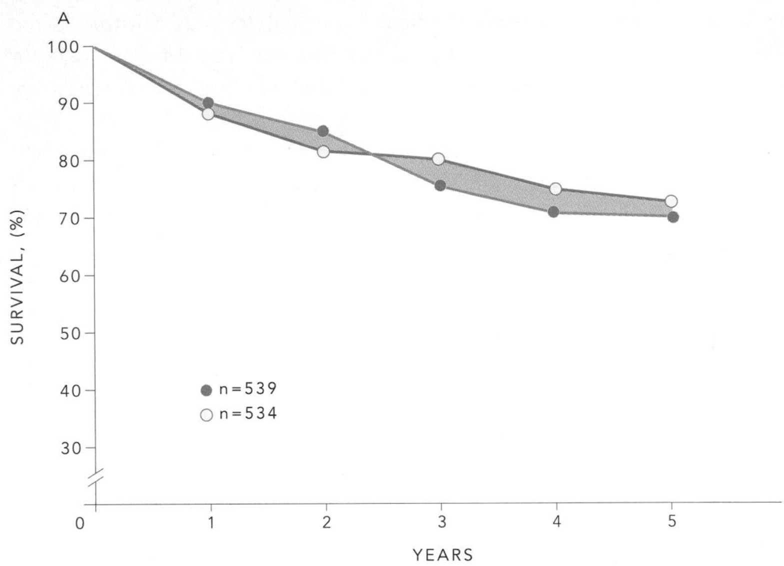

Figure 12–1 ***(A)*** Survival over time of 1073 people with medically treated coronary artery disease who were randomly divided into two groups. As expected, there is no detectable difference. ***(B)*** Survival in two subgroups of the patients shown in panel ***A*** who have three-vessel disease and abnormal left ventricular function. The two different groups were selected at random and received the same medical treatment. The difference is statistically significant ($P < .025$) if one does not include a Bonferroni correction for the fact that many hypotheses were tested even though the only treatment was randomization into two groups. *(Data for panel* ***A*** *from the text of K. Lee, J. McNeer, C. Starmer, P. Harris, and R. Rosati, "Clinical Judgment and Statistics: Lessons from a Simulated Randomized Trial in Coronary Artery Disease,"* Circulation, ***61:****508–515, 1980, and personal communication with Dr. Lee. Panel* ***B*** *is reproduced from fig. 1 of the same paper. By permission of the American Heart Association, Inc. Survival curves appear smooth because of the large number of deaths in all cases.).*

Another approach is to use more advanced statistical techniques that permit looking at all the variables together rather than just one at a time. (These methods, called *multivariate analysis,* are generalizations of linear regression, and are beyond the scope of this book.[†]) In fact, although the patients in the two randomized

[†]For a discussion of multivariate methods, see S. A. Glantz and B. K. Slinker, *Primer of Applied Regression and Analysis of Variance* (2nd ed), McGraw-Hill, New York, 2001.

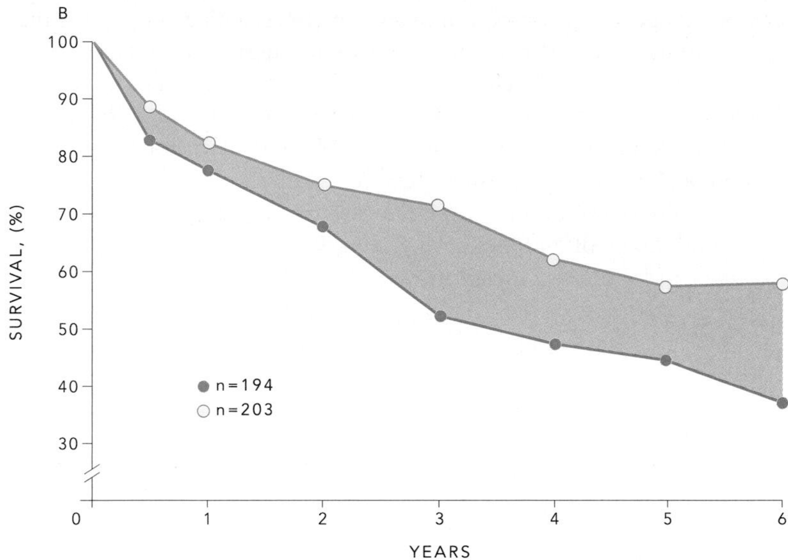

Figure 12–1 *(continued)*

groups were not detectably different when their baseline characteristics were examined one at a time, when Lee and colleagues looked at all of them together, the statistical analysis showed that one of the treatment groups with three-vessel disease and abnormal contraction was slightly sicker than the other; and when these differences were taken into account, there no longer appeared to be a difference in survival between the two groups.

This exercise illustrates an important general rule for all statistical analysis: design the experiment to *minimize the total number of statistical tests of hypotheses that need to be computed.*

Another way that perfectly correct application of statistical tests of hypotheses (from an arithmetical point of view) can lead to unreliable conclusions is when they are used *after the fact.* All the procedures to test hypotheses begin with the assumption that the samples are all drawn from the same population (the null hypothesis). It is not uncommon to conduct a clinical trial—or, for that matter, any experiment—to answer a question, then notice an interesting pattern in the data that may have been totally unrelated to the original reason for the study. This pattern certainly can suggest further research. It might even be striking enough to lead you to conclude that there is actually a relationship present. *But,* it is not fair to turn around and apply a statistical test to obtain a *P* value after you have already observed that a difference probably exists. The temptation to do this is often quite strong and, while it produces impressive *P* values, they are quite meaningless.

PROBLEMS WITH THE POPULATION

In most laboratory experiments and survey research, including marketing research and political polling, it is possible to define and locate the population of interest clearly, and then arrange for an appropriate random sample. In contrast, in clinical research, the sample generally has to be drawn from patients and volunteers at medical centers who are willing to participate in the project. This fact can make the interpretation of the study in terms of the population as a whole quite difficult.

Most medical research involving human subjects is carried out on people who either attend clinics or are hospitalized at university medical centers. Yet, these groups of people are not really typical of the population as a whole or even the population of sick people. Figure 12–2 shows that, of 1000 people in the United States, only eight are admitted to a hospital in any given month, and *less than one* is referred to an academic medical center. It is often that one person who is available to participate in a clinical research protocol. Often the population of interest consists of people with the arcane or complex problems that lead to referral to an academic medical center; in such cases, a sample consisting of such people can be considered to represent the relevant population. However, as Fig. 12–2 makes clear, a sample of people drawn (even at random) from the patients at a university medical center can hardly be considered to be representative of the population as a whole. This fact must be carefully considered when evaluating a research report

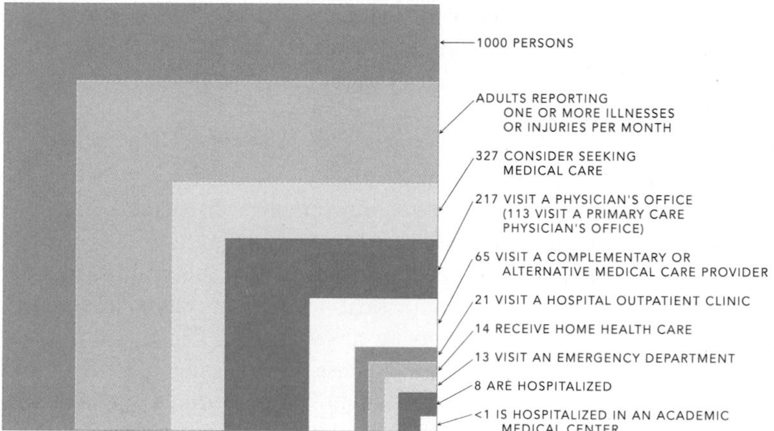

Figure 12–2 Estimates of the number of people in the United States who report illnesses and receive various forms of health care. Less than 1 in 1000 is hospitalized in an academic medical center. (*Redrawn from Fig. 2 of L. A. Green, et al., "The Ecology of Medical Care Revisited,"* N. Engl. J. Med. ***344:****2021–2025, 2001. Used by permission.*)

to decide just what population (that is, whom) the results can be generalized to.

In addition to the fact that people treated at academic medical centers do not really represent the true spectrum of illness in the community, there is an additional difficulty due to the fact that hospitalized patients do not represent a random sample of the population as a whole. It is not uncommon for investigators to complete studies of the association between different diseases based on hospitalized patients (or patients who seek medical help as outpatients). In general, different diseases lead to different rates of hospitalization (or physician consultation). Unless extreme care is taken in analyzing the results of such studies to ensure that there are comparable rates of including all classes of disease, any apparent association (or lack of association) between various diseases and symptoms is as likely to be due to the differential rates at which patients seek help (or die, if it is an autopsy study) as to a true association between the diseases. This problem is called *Berkson's fallacy,* after the statistician who first identified the problem.*

HOW YOU CAN IMPROVE THINGS

Using statistical thinking to reach conclusions in clinical practice and the biomedical sciences amounts to much more than memorizing a few formulas and looking up P values in tables. Like all human endeavors, applying statistical procedures and interpreting the results requires insight—not only into the statistical techniques but also into the clinical or scientific question to be answered. As Chap. 1 discussed, these methods will continue to increase in importance as economic pressures grow for evidence that diagnostic procedures and therapies actually are worth the cost both to the individual patient and to society at large. Statistical arguments play a central role in many of these discussions.

Even so, the statistical aspects of most medical research are supervised by investigators who only have heard of t tests (and, perhaps, contingency tables) regardless of the nature of the experimental design and the data. Since the investigators themselves best know what they are trying to establish and are responsible for drawing the conclusions, they should take the lead in the analysis of the data. Unfortunately, this task often falls to a laboratory technician or statistical consultant who does not really understand the question at hand or the data collected.

This problem is aggravated by the fact that investigators often go into the clinic or laboratory and collect data before clearly thinking out the specific question they wish to answer. As a result, after the data are collected and the investigators begin searching for a P value (often under the pressure of the deadline for submitting an

*J. Berkson, "Limitations of the Application of Fourfold Table Analysis to Hospital Data," *Biometrics,* **2:**47–53, 1946. For an additional (and less technical) discussion of Berkson's fallacy, see D. Mainland, "The Risk of Fallacious Conclusions from Autopsy Data on the Incidence of Diseases with Applications to Heart Disease," *Am. Heart J.,* **45:**644–654, 1953. For an example of how the differences between considering patients in a given clinic, all hospitalized patients, and all people in the community can alter the conclusions reached in an in-hospital study, see H. Muench's comments (*N. Engl. J. Med.,* **272:**1134, 1965) on H. Binder, A. Clement, W. Thayer, and H. Spiro, "Rarity of Hiatus Hernia in Achalasia," *N. Engl. J. Med.,* **272:**680–682, 1965.

abstract to a scientific meeting), they run into the fact that *P* values are associated with statistical *hypothesis tests* and that in order to test a hypothesis, you need a hypothesis to test. Surprisingly, very few investigators pause at the start of their work to carefully define a hypothesis; only 20 percent of the protocols approved by the committee on human research at one major health sciences center contained a clearly stated hypothesis.*

As discussed earlier in this chapter, the hypothesis (as embodied in the type of experiment) combined with the scale of measurement determines the statistical method to be used. Armed with a clearly stated hypothesis, it is relatively straightforward to design an experiment and determine the method of statistical analysis to be applied before one starts collecting the data. The simplest procedure is to make up the table that will contain the data before collecting it, assume that you have the numbers, and then determine the method of analysis. This exercise will ensure that after going to the trouble and expense of actually collecting the data, it will be possible to analyze it.

While this procedure may seem obvious, very few people follow it. As a result, problems often arise when the time comes to compute the prized *P* value, because the experimental design does not fit the hypothesis—which is finally verbalized when a feisty statistician demands it—or the design does not fit into the paradigm associated with one of the established statistical hypothesis tests. (This problem is especially acute when dealing with more complex experimental designs.) Faced with a desperate investigator and the desire to be helpful, the statistical consultant will often try to salvage things by proposing an analysis of a subset of the data, suggesting the use of less powerful methods, or suggesting that the investigator use his or her data to test a different hypothesis (i.e., ask a different question). While these steps may serve the short-term goal of getting an abstract or manuscript out on time, they do not encourage efficient clinical and scientific investigation. These frustrating problems could be easily avoided if investigators simply thought about how they were going to analyze their data at the *beginning* rather than the end of the process. Unfortunately, most do not.

*For a complete discussion of this problem and the role that committees on human research could play in solving it, should they choose to do so, see M. Giammona and S. Glantz, "Poor Statistical Design in Research on Humans: The Role of Committees on Human Research," *Clin. Res.*, **31**:571–577, 1983.

The result is the sorry state of affairs discussed throughout this book. As a result, you and other responsible individuals can rarely take what is published or presented at clinical and scientific meetings at face value.

When evaluating the strength of an argument for or against some treatment or scientific hypothesis, what should you look for? The investigator should clearly state*

- *The hypothesis being examined (preferably, as the specific null hypothesis to be analyzed statistically).*
- *The data used to test this hypothesis and the procedure used to collect them (including the randomization procedure).*
- *The population the samples represent.*
- *The statistical procedure used to evaluate the data and reach conclusions.*
- *The power of the study to detect a specified effect, particularly if the conclusion is "negative."*

As Chapter 1 discussed at length, one rarely encounters this ideal. In general, however, the closer a paper or oral presentation comes to it, the more aware the authors are of the statistical issues in what they are doing and the more confident you can be of their conclusions.

One should immediately be suspicious of a paper that says nothing about the procedures used to obtain "*P* values" or that includes meaningless statements like "standard statistical procedures were used."

Finally, the issues of ethics and scientific validity, especially as they concern human and animal subjects, are inextricably intertwined. Any experimentation that produces results that are misleading or incorrect as a result of avoidable methodologic errors—statistical or otherwise—is unethical. It needlessly puts subjects in jeopardy by not taking every precaution to protect them against unnecessary risk of injury, discomfort, and, in the case of humans, inconvenience. In addition, significant amounts of time and money can be wasted trying to reproduce or refute erroneous results. Alternatively, these results might be accepted without

*Indeed, some journals are moving to formalize the reporting of results from randomized controlled trials. For a description of one set of standards, see The Standards of Reporting Trials Group, "A Proposal for Structured Reporting of Randomized Controlled Trials," *JAMA* **272:**1326–1331, 1994.

further analysis and adversely affect not only the work of the scientific community, but also the treatment of patients in the future.

Of course, a well-designed, properly analyzed study does not automatically make an investigator's research innovative, profound, or even worth placing subjects at risk as part of the data collection process. However, even for important questions, it is clearly not ethical to place subjects at risk to collect data in a poorly designed study when this situation can be avoided easily by a little technical knowledge (such as that included in this book) and more thoughtful planning.

How can you help improve the situation?

Do not let people get away with sloppy statistical thinking any more than you would permit them to get away with sloppy clinical or scientific thinking. Write letters to the editor. Ask questions in class, rounds, and meetings. When someone answers that they do not know how or where P came from, ask them how they can be certain that their results mean what they say. The answer may well be that they cannot.

Most important, if you decide to contribute to the fund of scientific and clinical knowledge, take the time and care to do it right.

Appendix A

Computational Forms

TO INTERPOLATE BETWEEN TWO VALUES IN A STATISTICAL TABLE

If the value you need is not in the statistical table, it is possible to estimate the value by *linear interpolation.* For example, suppose you want the critical value of a test statistic, C, corresponding to ν degrees of freedom, and this value of degrees of freedom is not in the table. Find the values of degrees of freedom that are in the table that bracket ν, denoted a and b. Determine the fraction of the way between a and b that ν lies, $f = (\nu - a)/(b - a)$. Therefore, the desired critical value is $C = C_b + f(C_b - C_a)$, where C_a and C_b are the critical values that correspond to a and b degrees of freedom.

A similar approach can be used to interpolate between two P values at a given degrees of freedom. For example, suppose you want to estimate the P value that corresponds to $t = 2.620$ with 20 degrees of freedom. From Table 4–1 with 20 degrees of freedom $t_{.02} = 2.528$ and $t_{.01} = 2.845$. $f = (2.845 - 2.620)/(2.845 - 2.528) = 0.7098$, and $P = .01 + .07098$ $(.02 - .01) = .0171$.

VARIANCE

$$s^2 = \frac{\Sigma X^2 - (\Sigma X)^2/n}{n - 1}$$

ONE-WAY ANALYSIS OF VARIANCE

Given Sample Means and Standard Deviations

For treatment group t: n_t = size of sample, $\overline{X}_t$ = mean, s_t = standard deviation. There are a total of k treatment groups.

$$N = \Sigma n_t$$

$$\text{SS}_{\text{wit}} = \Sigma(n_t - 1)s_t^2$$

$$\nu_{\text{wit}} = \text{DF}_{\text{wit}} = N - k$$

$$s_{\text{wit}}^2 = \frac{\text{SS}_{\text{wit}}}{\text{DF}_{\text{wit}}}$$

$$\text{SS}_{\text{bet}} = \Sigma n_t \overline{X}_t^2 - \frac{(\Sigma n_t \overline{X}_t)^2}{N}$$

$$s_{\text{bet}}^2 = \frac{\text{SS}_{\text{bet}}}{\text{DF}_{\text{bet}}}$$

$$\nu_{\text{bet}} = \text{DF}_{\text{bet}} = k - 1$$

$$F = \frac{\text{SS}_{\text{bet}}/\text{DF}_{\text{bet}}}{\text{SS}_{\text{wit}}/\text{DF}_{\text{wit}}}$$

Given Raw Data

Subscript t refers to treatment group; subscript s refers to experimental subject.

$$C = (\Sigma_t \Sigma_s X_{ts})^2/N$$

$$\text{SS}_{\text{tot}} = \Sigma_t \Sigma_s X_{ts}^2 - C$$

$$\text{SS}_{\text{bet}} = \Sigma_t \frac{(\Sigma_s X_{ts})^2}{n_t} - C$$

$$\text{SS}_{\text{wit}} = \text{SS}_{\text{tot}} - \text{SS}_{\text{bet}}$$

Degrees of freedom and F are computed as above.

UNPAIRED *t* TEST

Given Sample Means and Standard Deviations

$$t = \frac{\bar{X}_1 - \bar{X}_2}{s_{\bar{X}_1 - \bar{X}_2}}$$

where

$$s_{\bar{X}_1 - \bar{X}_2} = \sqrt{\frac{n_1 + n_2}{n_1 n_2 (n_1 + n_2 - 2)} [(n_1 - 1)s_1^2 + (n_2 - 1)s_2^2]}$$

$$\nu = n_1 + n_2 - 2$$

Given Raw Data

Use

$$s_{\bar{X}_1 - \bar{X}_2} = \sqrt{\frac{n_1 + n_2}{n_1 n_2 (n_1 + n_2 - 2)} \left[\Sigma X_1^2 - \frac{(\Sigma X_1)^2}{n_1} + \Sigma X_2^2 - \frac{(\Sigma X_2)^2}{n_2}\right]}$$

in the equation for t above.

2 × 2 CONTINGENCY TABLES (INCLUDING YATES CORRECTION FOR CONTINUITY)

The contingency table is

$$\begin{matrix} A & B \\ C & D \end{matrix}$$

Chi Square

$$\chi^2 = \frac{N(|AD - BC| - N/2)^2}{(A + B)(C + D)(A + C)(B + D)}$$

where $N = A + B + C + D$

McNemar's Test

$$\chi^2 = \frac{(|B - C| - 1)^2}{B + C}$$

where B and C are the numbers of people who responded to only one of the treatments.

Fisher Exact Test

Interchange the rows and columns of the contingency table so that the smallest observed frequency is in position A. Compute the probabilities associated with the resulting table, and all more-extreme tables obtained by reducing A by 1 and recomputing the table to maintain the row and column totals until $A = 0$. Add all these probabilities to get the first tail of the test. If either the two-row sums or two-column sums are equal, double the resulting probability to obtain the two-tail P value. Otherwise, to obtain the second tail of the test, identify the smallest of elements B or C. Suppose that it is B. Reduce B by 1 and compute the probability of the associated table. Repeat this process until B has been reduced to 0. Identify those tables with probabilities equal to or less than the probability associated with the original observations. Add these probabilities to the first-tail probabilities to obtain the two-tail value of P. All the tables computed by varying B may not have probabilities below that of the original table, so many not all contribute to P.

Table A–1 lists values of $n!$ for use in computing the Fisher exact test. For larger values of n, use a computer or logarithms as $P = \text{antilog}\,[(\log 9! + \log 14! + \log 11! + \log 12!) - \log 23! - (\log 1! + \log 14! + \log 11! + \log 12!)]$, using tables of log factorials available in handbooks of mathematical tables.

LINEAR REGRESSION AND CORRELATION

$$SS_{tot} = \Sigma Y^2 - \frac{(\Sigma Y)^2}{n}$$

$$SS_{reg} = b\left(\Sigma XY - \frac{\Sigma X \Sigma Y}{n}\right)$$

Table A–1 Values of $n!$ for $n = 1$ to $n = 20$

n	$n!$
0	1
1	1
2	2
3	6
4	24
5	120
6	720
7	5040
8	40320
9	362880
10	3628800
11	39916800
12	479001600
13	6227020800
14	87178291200
15	1307674368000
16	20922789888000
17	355687428096000
18	6402373705728000
19	121645100408832000
20	2432902008176640000

$$s_{y \cdot x} = \sqrt{\frac{\text{SS}_{\text{tot}} - \text{SS}_{\text{reg}}}{n - 2}}$$

$$r = \sqrt{\frac{\text{SS}_{\text{reg}}}{\text{SS}_{\text{tot}}}} = \frac{\Sigma XY - n\overline{X}\,\overline{Y}}{\sqrt{(\Sigma X^2 - n\overline{X}^2)(\Sigma Y^2 - n\overline{Y}^2)}}$$

REPEATED-MEASURES ANALYSIS OF VARIANCE

There are k treatments and n experimental subjects.

$$A = \frac{(\Sigma_t \Sigma_s \Sigma_{ts})^2}{kn} \quad B = \Sigma_t \Sigma_s X_{ts}^2$$

$$C = \frac{\Sigma_t (\Sigma_s X_{ts})^2}{n} \quad D = \frac{\Sigma_s (\Sigma_t X_{ts})^2}{k}$$

$$\text{SS}_{\text{treat}} = C - A \qquad \text{SS}_{\text{res}} = A + B - C - D$$
$$\text{DF}_{\text{treat}} = k - 1 \qquad \text{DF}_{\text{res}} = (n - 1)(k - 1)$$
$$F = \frac{\text{SS}_{\text{treat}}/\text{DF}_{\text{treat}}}{\text{SS}_{\text{res}}/\text{DF}_{\text{res}}}$$

KRUSKAL-WALLIS TEST

$$H = \frac{12}{N(N + 1)} \Sigma\left(\frac{R_t^2}{n_t}\right) - 3(N + 1) \text{ where } N = \Sigma n_t$$

FRIEDMAN TEST

$$\chi_r^2 = \frac{12}{nk(k + 1)} \Sigma R_t^2 - 3n(k + 1)$$

where there are k treatments and n experimental subjects and R_t is the sum of ranks for treatment t.

Appendix B

Power Charts*

*These charts are adapted from E. S. Pearson and H. O. Hartley, "Charts for the Power Function for Analysis of Variance Tests, Derived from the Non-Central F Distribution," *Biometrika,* **38:**112–130, 1951.

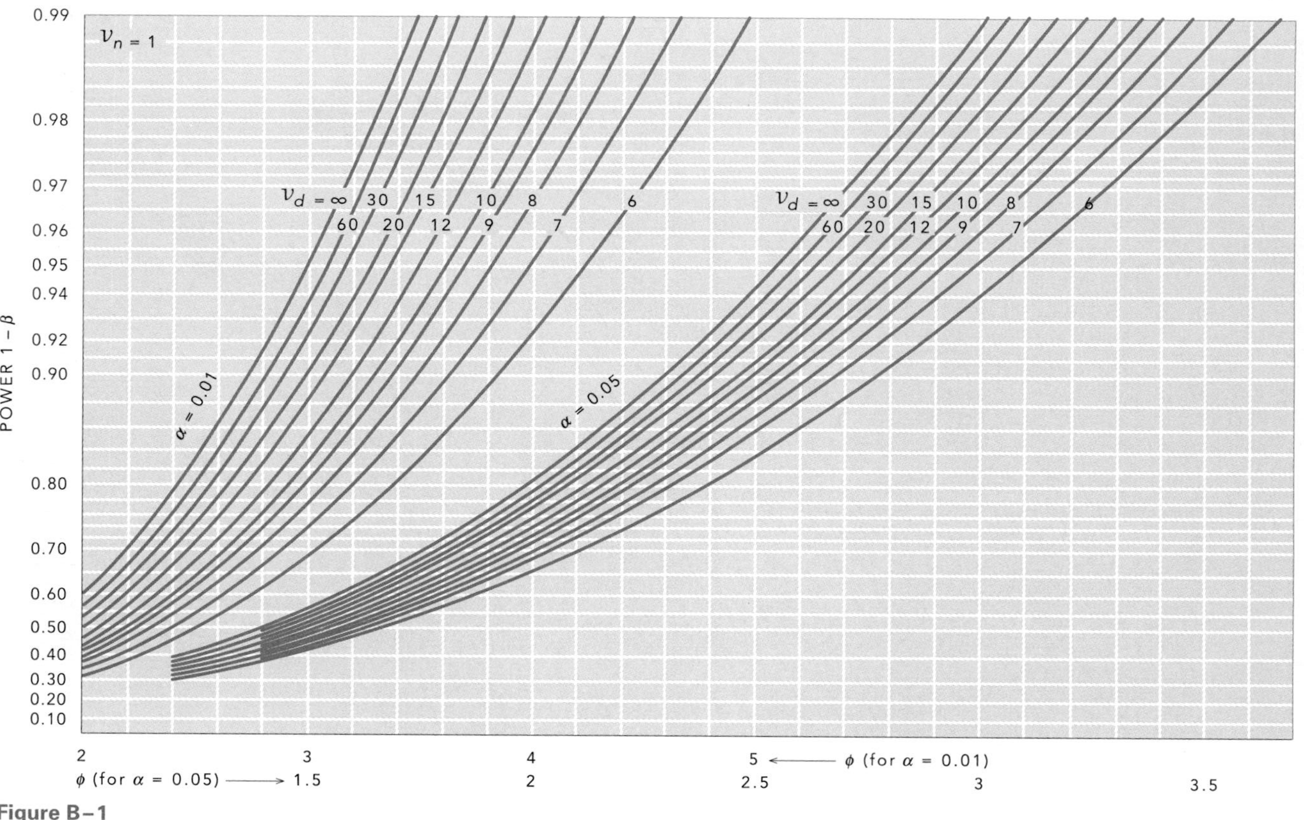

$\nu_n = 1$
$\nu_d = \infty$ 30 15 10 8 6
60 20 12 9 7
$\nu_d = \infty$ 30 15 10 8 6
60 20 12 9 7
$\alpha = 0.01$
$\alpha = 0.05$
POWER $1 - \beta$
0.99
0.98
0.97
0.96
0.95
0.94
0.92
0.90
0.80
0.70
0.60
0.50
0.40
0.30
0.20
0.10
2
3
4
5 ← ϕ (for α = 0.01)
ϕ (for α = 0.05) → 1.5
2
2.5
3
3.5

Figure B–1

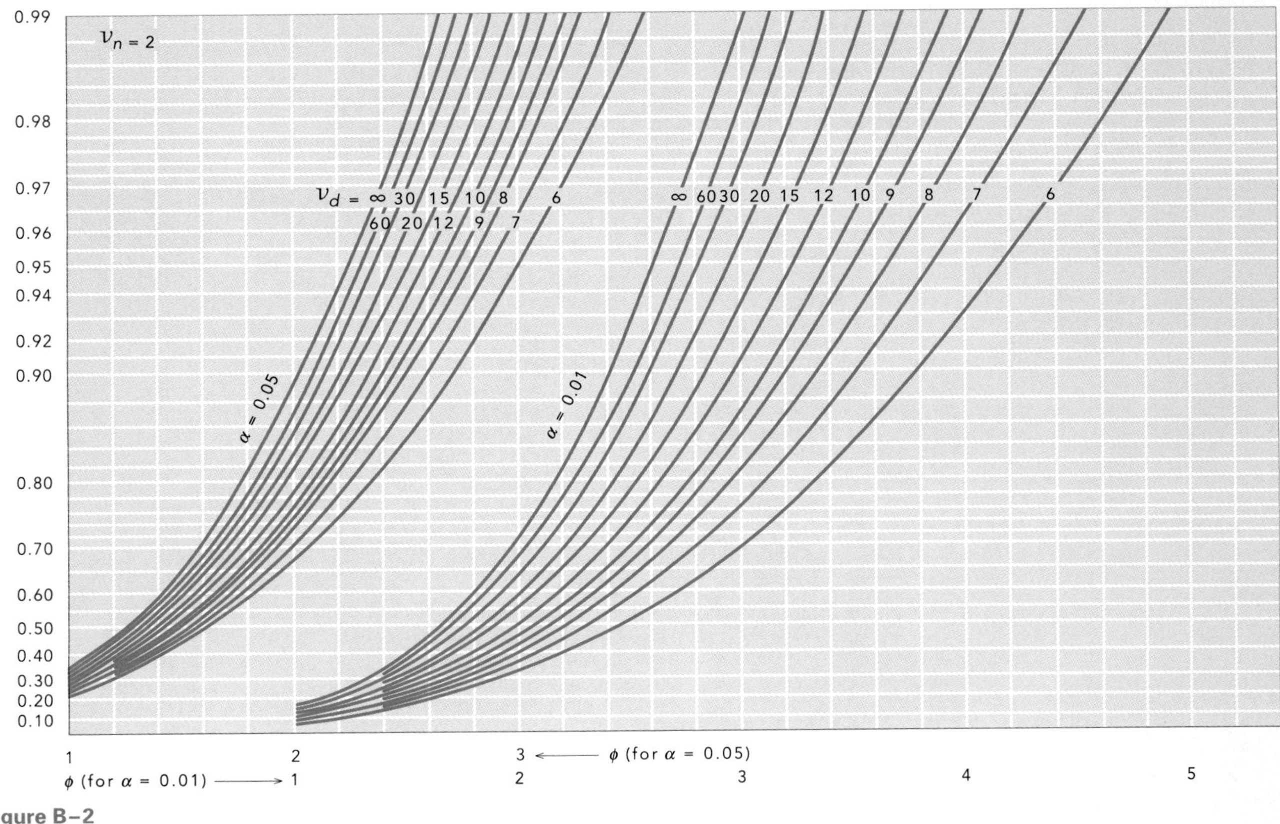

$\nu_n = 2$
POWER $1 - \beta$
0.99
0.98
0.97
0.96
0.95
0.94
0.92
0.90
0.80
0.70
0.60
0.50
0.40
0.30
0.20
0.10
$\nu_d = \infty$ 30 15 10 8 6
60 20 12 9 7
∞ 60 30 20 15 12 10 9 8 7 6
$\alpha = 0.05$
$\alpha = 0.01$
1 2 3 ← ϕ (for $\alpha = 0.05$)
ϕ (for $\alpha = 0.01$) → 1 2 3 4 5

Figure B–2

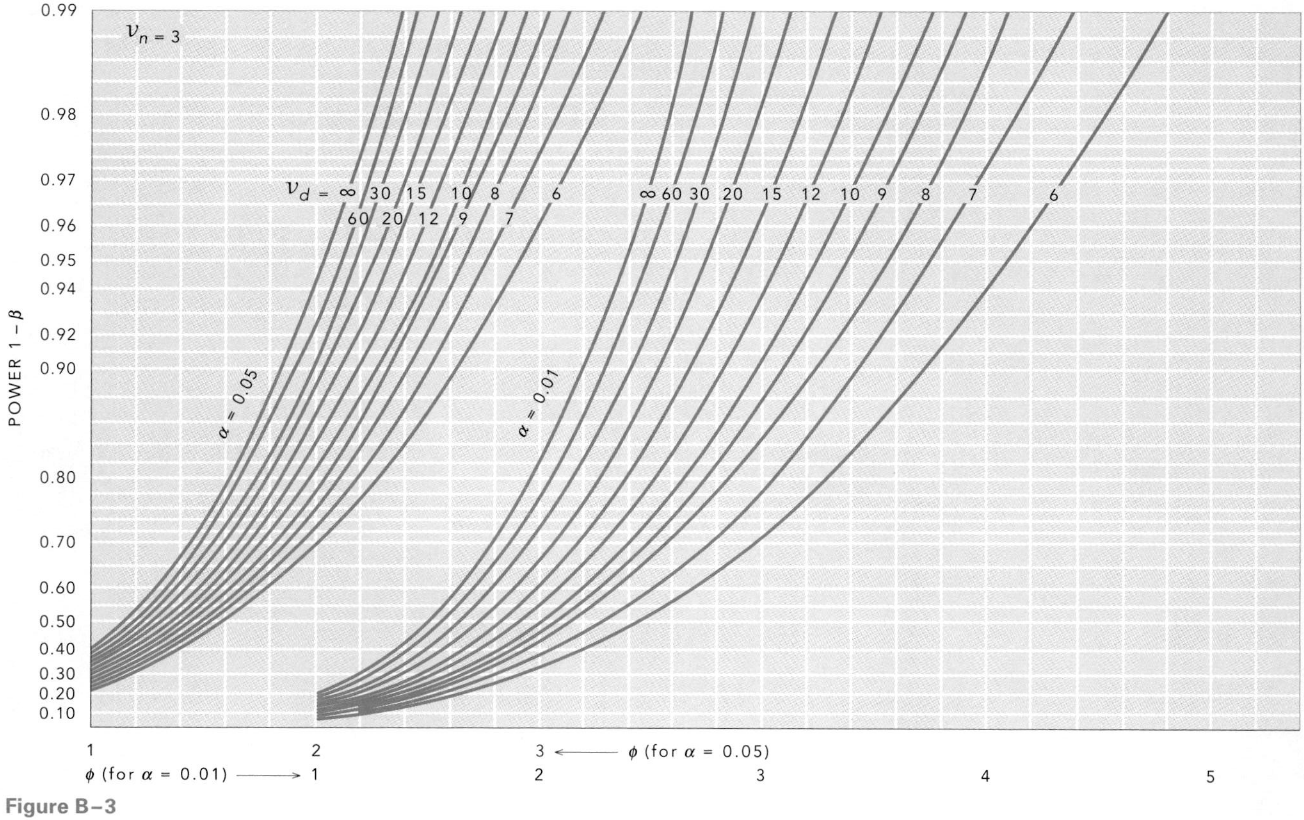

$\nu_n = 3$
$\nu_d = \infty$ 30 15 10 8 6
60 20 12 9 7
∞ 60 30 20 15 12 10 9 8 7 6
$\alpha = 0.05$
$\alpha = 0.01$
POWER $1 - \beta$
0.99
0.98
0.97
0.96
0.95
0.94
0.92
0.90
0.80
0.70
0.60
0.50
0.40
0.30
0.20
0.10
1 2 3 ⟵ ϕ (for α = 0.05)
ϕ (for α = 0.01) ⟶ 1 2 3 4 5

Figure B–3

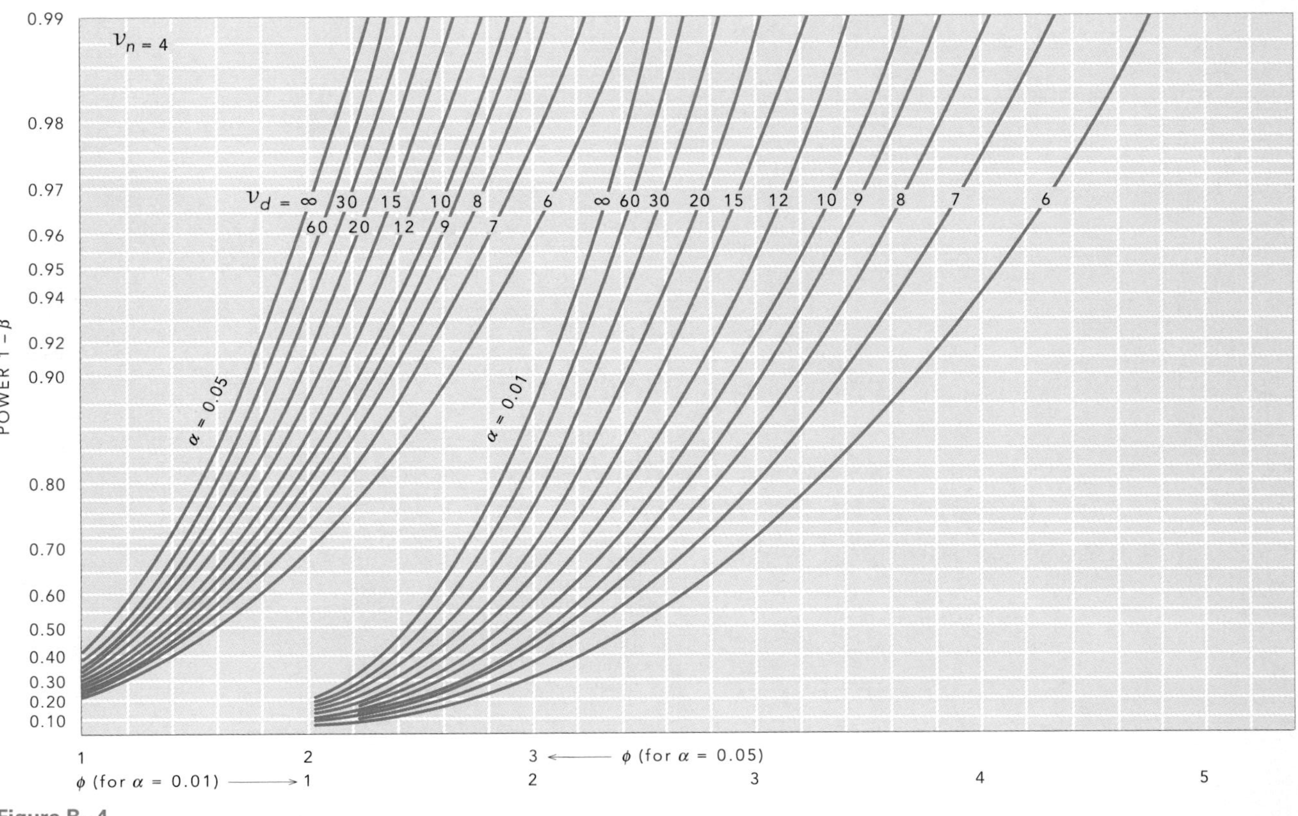

$\nu_n = 4$
$\nu_d = \infty$ 60 30 20 15 12 10 9 8 7 6
∞ 60 30 20 15 12 10 9 8 7 6
$\alpha = 0.05$
$\alpha = 0.01$
POWER 1 − β
0.99 0.98 0.97 0.96 0.95 0.94 0.92 0.90 0.80 0.70 0.60 0.50 0.40 0.30 0.20 0.10
1 2 3 ⟵ ϕ (for $\alpha = 0.05$)
ϕ (for $\alpha = 0.01$) ⟶ 1 2 3 4 5

Figure B–4

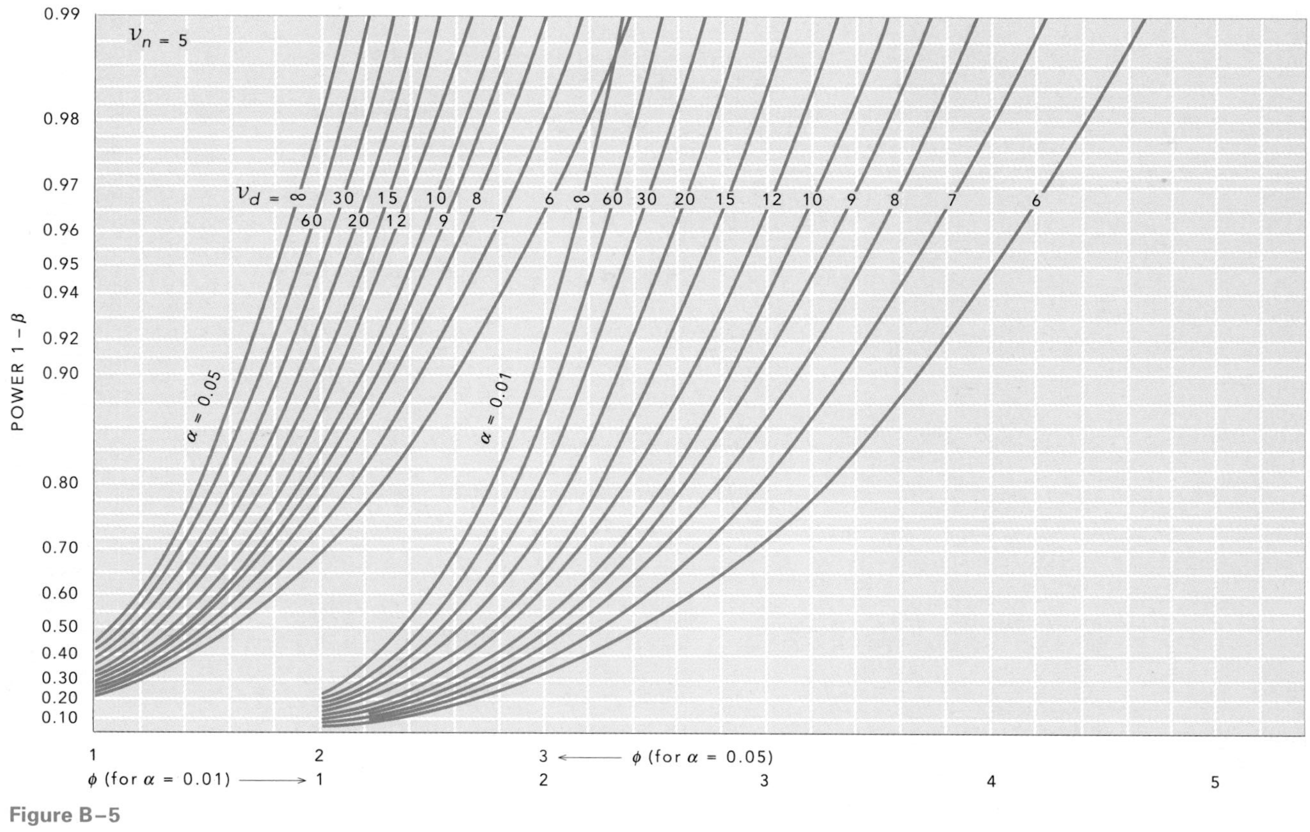

$\nu_n = 5$
$\nu_d = \infty$ 30 15 10 8 6 ∞ 60 30 20 15 12 10 9 8 7 6
60 20 12 9 7
$\alpha = 0.05$
$\alpha = 0.01$
POWER $1 - \beta$
0.99
0.98
0.97
0.96
0.95
0.94
0.92
0.90
0.80
0.70
0.60
0.50
0.40
0.30
0.20
0.10
1 2 3 ⟵ ϕ (for $\alpha = 0.05$)
ϕ (for $\alpha = 0.01$) ⟶ 1 2 3 4 5

Figure B–5

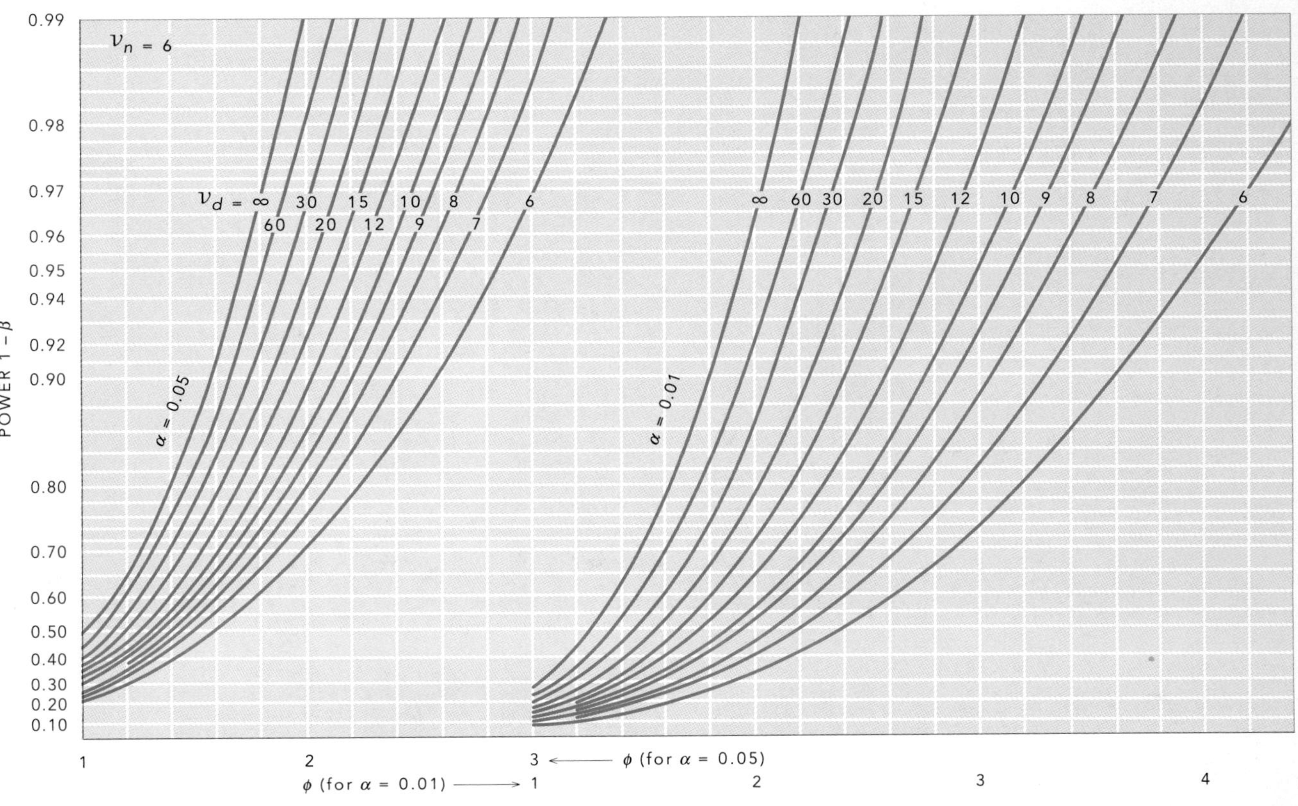
$\nu_n = 6$
$\nu_d = \infty$ 60 30 20 15 12 10 9 8 7 6
∞ 60 30 20 15 12 10 9 8 7 6
$\alpha = 0.05$
$\alpha = 0.01$
POWER $1 - \beta$
0.99
0.98
0.97
0.96
0.95
0.94
0.92
0.90
0.80
0.70
0.60
0.50
0.40
0.30
0.20
0.10
1 2 3
ϕ (for $\alpha = 0.01$) ⟶ 1
3 ⟵ ϕ (for $\alpha = 0.05$)
2 3 4

Figure B–6

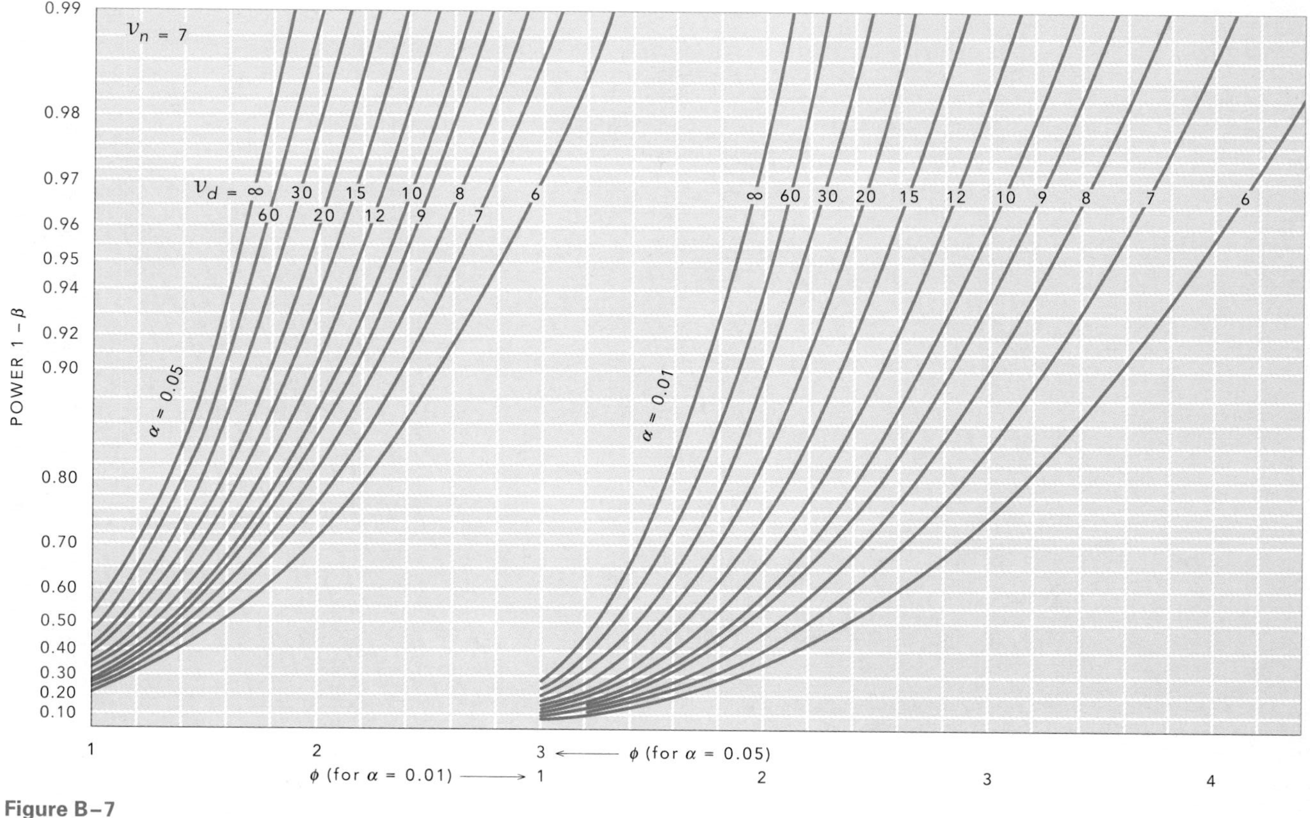

$\nu_n = 7$
$\nu_d = \infty$ 60 30 20 15 12 10 9 8 7 6
∞ 60 30 20 15 12 10 9 8 7 6
$\alpha = 0.05$
$\alpha = 0.01$
POWER $1 - \beta$
0.99
0.98
0.97
0.96
0.95
0.94
0.92
0.90
0.80
0.70
0.60
0.50
0.40
0.30
0.20
0.10
1 2 3
3 ⟵ ϕ (for $\alpha = 0.05$)
ϕ (for $\alpha = 0.01$) ⟶ 1 2 3 4

Figure B–7

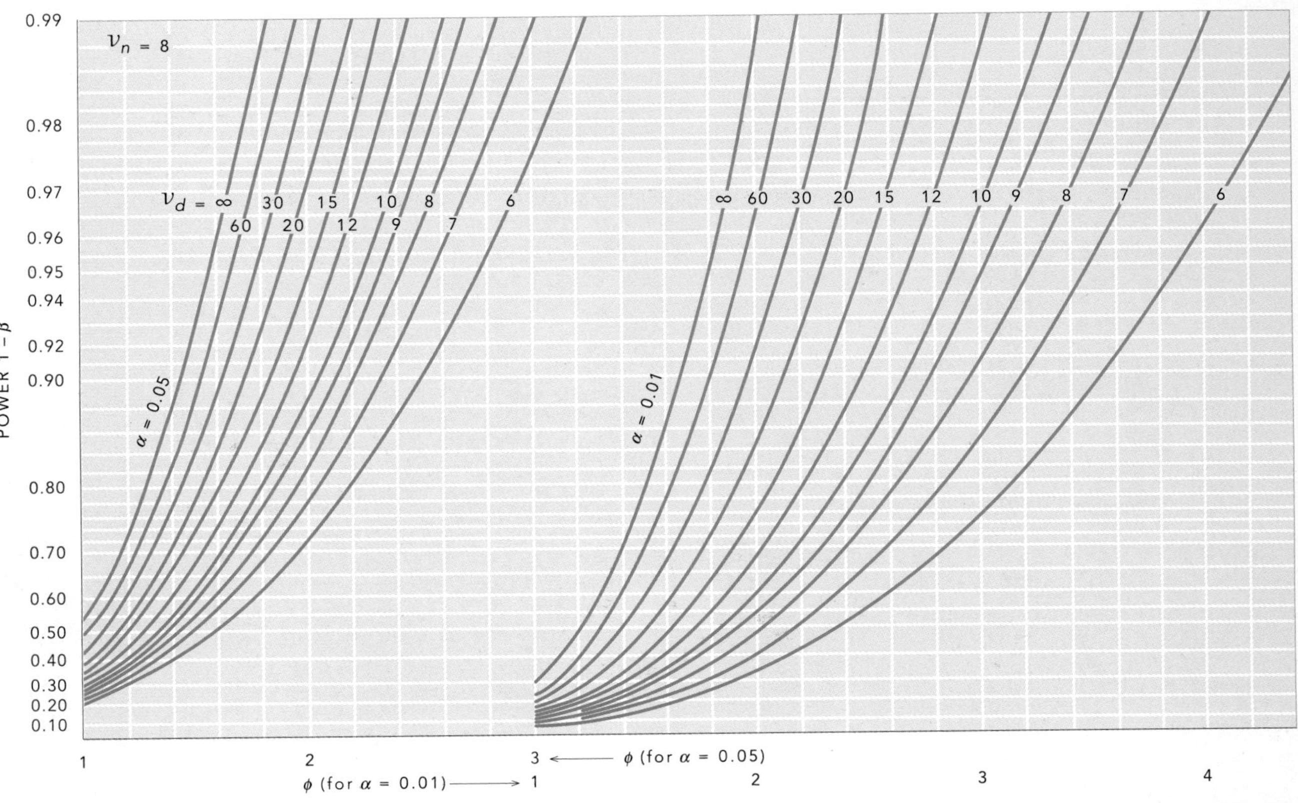

$\nu_n = 8$
$\nu_d = \infty$ 60 30 20 15 12 10 9 8 7 6
∞ 60 30 20 15 12 10 9 8 7 6
$\alpha = 0.05$
$\alpha = 0.01$
POWER $1 - \beta$
0.99
0.98
0.97
0.96
0.95
0.94
0.92
0.90
0.80
0.70
0.60
0.50
0.40
0.30
0.20
0.10
1
2
3 ← ϕ (for $\alpha = 0.05$)
ϕ (for $\alpha = 0.01$) → 1
2
3
4

Figure B–8

Appendix C

Answers to Exercises

2-1 Mean = 61,668, median = 13,956, standard deviation = 117,539, 25th percentile = 7861, 75th percentile = 70,133, mean − 0.67 standard deviations = 6623, mean + 0.67 standard deviations = 79,604. These data appear not to be drawn from a normally distributed population for several reasons. (1) The mean and median are very different. (2) All the observations are (and have to be, since you cannot have a negative viral load) greater than zero and the standard deviation is larger than the mean. If the population were normally distributed, it would have to include negative values of viral load, which is impossible. (3) The relationship between the percentiles and numbers of standards deviations about the mean are different from what you would expect if the data were drawn from a normally distributed population.

2-2 Mean = 4.30, median = 4.15, standard deviation = 0.67, 25th percentile = 3.93, 75th percentile = 4.79, mean − 0.67 standard deviations = 3.82, mean + 0.67 standard deviations = 4.90. These data appear to be drawn from a normally distributed population on the basis of the comparisons in the answer to Prob. 2-1.

2-3 Mean = 1709.3, median = 1750, standard deviation = 824.8, 25th percentile = 877.5, 75th percentile = 2350, mean − 0.67 standard deviations = 1156.7, mean + 0.67 standard deviations = 2261.9. These data appear to be drawn from a normally distributed population on the basis of the comparisons in the answer to Prob. 2-1.

2-4 There is 1 chance in 6 of getting each of the following values: 1, 2, 3, 4, 5, and 6. The mean of this population is 3.5.

2-5 The result is a sample drawn from the distribution of all means of samples of size 2 drawn from the population described in Prob. 2-4. Its mean is an estimate of the population mean, and its standard deviation is an estimate of the standard error of the mean of samples of size 2 drawn from the population in Prob. 2-4.

3-1 $F = 8.92$, $\nu_{\mathrm{n}} = 1$, $\nu_{\mathrm{d}} = 28$. These observations are not consistent with the null hypothesis that there is no difference in the average rate of ATP production in the two groups; we conclude that the rate of ATP production depends on insulin resistance ($P < .01$).

3-2 $F = 64.18$, $\nu_n = 4$, $\nu_d = 995$. Mean forced midexpiratory flow is not the same, on the average, in all of the experimental groups studied ($P < .01$).

3-3 $F = 35.25$, $\nu_n = 2$, $\nu_d = 207$. At least one group of men represents a different population from the others ($P < .01$).

3-4 $F = 8.02$, $\nu_n = 5$, $\nu_d = 36$. Different preconditioning treatments led to different mean infarct size ($P < .01$).

3-5 $F = 2.15$, $\nu_n = 1$, $\nu_d = 98$. This value of F is not large enough to reject the hypothesis that there is no difference in vertebral bone density between similarly aged men and women who have had vertebral bone fractures.

3-6 $F = 3.450$, $\nu_n = 3$, $\nu_d = 96$. Health professionals in at least one unit experience more burnout than those in the others ($P < .02$).

3-7 $F = 95.97$, $\nu_n = 3$, $\nu_d = 57$. At least one strain of mouse differs in response to estrogen ($P < .01$).

3-8 No. $F = 1.11$, $\nu_n = 4$, $\nu_d = 130$, which does not approach the critical value of F that defines the upper 5 percent of possible values under the null hypothesis of no difference among the groups, 2.37. Therefore, we cannot reject the null hypothesis that all these samples were drawn from the same population.

4-1 For mean arterial pressure $t = -1.969$, and for total peripheral resistance $t = -1.286$. There are 23 degrees of freedom in each case. With 23 degrees of freedom 2.069 defines the most extreme 5 percent of the possible values of the t distribution when the treatment has no effect. Thus, these data do not provide sufficient evidence to reject the hypothesis that different anesthetic agents did not produce differences in mean arterial pressure or total peripheral resistance.

4-2 Yes. $t = 3.14$, $\nu = 20$, $P < .01$. The blood pressure drops rather than increasing, however, so this change is not clinically desirable.

4-3 No. $t = 1.33$, $\nu = 20$, $P = .20$.

4-4 Prob. 3-1: $t = 3.967$, $\nu = 40$, $P < .01$; Prob. 3-5: $t = -1.467$, $\nu = 98$, $P < .01$. In both these cases, we can reject the null hypothesis of no difference between the groups. $t_2 = F$.

4-5 People who work in a smoky environment and light smokers form one subgroup; each of the other groups are distinct subgroups. Here are the results of the pairwise comparisons using a Holm t test (with $\nu = 995$) with 1 = Nonsmokers in smokefree environment, 2 = Worked in smoky environment, 3 = Light smokers, 4 = Moderate smokers, 5 = Heavy smokers:

Comparison	$P_{uncorrected}$	P_{crit}	$P < .05$
1 vs 5:	<.001	.005	Yes
1 vs 4:	<.001	.006	Yes
2 vs 5:	<.001	.006	Yes
1 vs 3:	<.001	.007	Yes
3 vs 5:	<.001	.008	Yes
1 vs 2:	<.001	.010	Yes
2 vs 4:	<.001	.013	Yes
3 vs 4:	<.001	.017	Yes
4 vs 5:	.018	.025	Yes
2 vs 3:	.212	.050	No

4-6 All the groups have worse lung function than the nonsmokers breathing clean air (the control group). Nonsmokers in smoky office; $q' = 6.249$, $p = 5$; light smokers: $q' = 7.499$, $p = 5$; moderate smokers: $q' = 12.220$, $p = 5$; heavy smokers: $q' = 14.558$, $p = 5$. All exceed the critical values of q' for $P < .01$ with $p = 5$ and 995 degrees of freedom: 3.00.

4-7 From Holm t tests with 207 degrees of freedom, the uncorrected P value for marathon runners versus inactive men is $< .001$, which is less than the .017 critical value; for joggers versus inactive men, it is $< .001$, which is compared to .025; and for marathon runners versus joggers, it is .010, which is compared to .050. Therefore, we conclude that all three groups are significantly different with a family error rate of less than $\alpha_T = 0.05$.

4-8 From Holm t tests with 207 degrees of freedom, the uncorrected P for the comparison of marathon runners to inactive men is $< .001$ compared to the critical P values of .025 and the uncorrected P value for comparison of joggers to inactive men is $< .001$ compared to a critical value of .05. Both groups are significantly different from the control group (inactive men). Therefore, the two nonsedentary groups are significantly different from the inactive men. No statement can be made about the possible difference between the joggers and runners because all comparisons are against the control group. Note that the values of uncorrected P computed from the data are the same as in Prob. 4-7. The critical value of P, however, is larger, reflecting the fact that there are fewer comparisons than in Prob. 4-7.

4-9 Because the problem asks which interventions have protective effects on the heart during a prolonged ischemic attack, we will look at all pairwise comparisons and not just comparisons to the control group. The two subgroups based on the Holm t-test are (1) control, 8-p- (sulfophenyl) theophylline, phenoxybenzamine, and polymyxin B and (2) ischemic preconditioning and phenylephrine. Use of the SNK test would also result in these subgroups. However, the subgroups become ambiguous if the Bonferroni t test is used. Polymyxin B and phenoxybenzamine can be grouped with both ischemic preconditioning and phenylephrine or control and 8-p- (sulfophenyl) theophylline. The reason for this ambiguity is the lower power of the Bonferroni t test compared to the other two multiple comparison procedures.

4-10 The results of the pair-wise comparisons are CD-1 vs. B6, $t = 19.031$; CD-1 vs. C17/JIs, $t = 15.770$; CD-1 vs. S15/JIs, $t = 11.825$; S15/JIs vs. B6, $t = 13.191$; S15/JIs vs. C17/JIs, $t = 7.619$; C17/JIs vs. B6, $t = 6.243$. Since there are 6 comparisons, these values of t should be compared with the critical value of t corresponding to $P = .05/6 = .0083$ with 57 degrees of freedom, 2.735, to keep the total chance of erroneously reporting a difference below 5 percent. Comparing the observed values of t with this critical value shows all the groups are significantly different from each other.

4-11 The results of the pairwise comparisons (in the order they should be done) are

SNK Comparisons

Comparison	Difference of means	p	q	$P < .05$
CD-1 vs. B6	142 − 38 = 104	4	22.837	Yes
CD-1 vs. S15/J1s	142 − 60 = 82	3	18.518	Yes
CD-1 vs. C17/J1s	142 − 82 = 60	2	13.370	Yes
S15/J1s vs. B6	82 − 38 = 44	3	10.147	Yes
S15/J1s vs. C17/J1s	82 − 60 = 22	2	5.255	Yes
C17/J1s vs. B6	60 − 38 = 22	2	5.167	Yes

Holm *t* test comparisons				
Comparison	Difference of means	P	P_{crit}	$P < .05$
CD-1 vs. B6	142 − 38 = 104	< .001	.008	Yes
CD-1 vs. S15/J1s	142 − 60 = 82	< .001	.010	Yes
CD-1 vs. C17/J1s	142 − 82 = 60	< .001	.013	Yes
S15/J1s vs. B6	82 − 38 = 44	< .001	.017	Yes
S15/J1s vs. C17/J1s	82 − 60 = 22	< .001	.025	Yes
C17/J1s vs. B6	60 − 38 = 22	< .001	.050	Yes

For $\alpha_T = .05$ and $\nu_d = 57$, the critical values of q (by interpolation in Table 4–3) are 3.745 for $p = 4$, 3.435 for $p = 3$, and 2.853 for $p = 2$. All comparisons are associated with values of q above the critical values. Therefore, there are four subgroups. Note that, in contrast to the results of the multiple comparisons using Bonferroni t tests, the SNK and Holm t test yield unambiguous definitions of the subgroups.

4-12 Use the SNK test for multiple comparisons because there are so many comparisons that the Bonferroni t test will be much too conservative. The results of these comparisons are

	Difference of means	q	p
G/M vs. G/S	65.2 − 43.9 = 21.3	5.362	6
G/M vs. SDU/M	65.2 − 46.4 = 18.8	4.733	5
G/M vs. ICU/S	65.2 − 49.9 = 15.3	3.852	4
G/M vs. ICU/M	65.2 − 51.2 = 14.0	3.525	3
G/M vs. SDU/S	65.2 − 57.3 = 7.9	1.989	2
SDU/S vs. G/S	57.3 − 43.9 = 13.4	3.374	5
SDU/S vs. SDU/M	57.3 − 46.4 = 10.9	2.744	4
SDU/S vs. ICU/S	57.3 − 49.9 = 7.4	1.863	3
SDU/S vs. ICU/M	57.3 − 51.2 = 6.1	1.536	2
ICU/M vs. G/S	51.2 − 43.9 = 7.3	1.838	4
ICU/M vs. SDU/M	51.2 − 46.4 = 4.8	1.208	3
ICU/M vs. ICU/S	51.2 − 49.9 = 1.3	0.327	2
ICU/S vs. G/S	49.9 − 43.9 = 6.0	1.511	3
ICU/S vs. SDU/M	49.9 − 46.4 = 3.5	0.881	2
SDU/M vs. G/S	46.4 − 43.9 = 2.5	0.629	2

For $\nu_d = 90$ and $\alpha_T = .05$, the critical values of q (by interpolation in Table 4-3) are 4.1 for $p = 6$, 3.9 for $p = 5$, 3.7 for $p = 4$, 3.4 for $p = 3$, and 2.8 for $p = 2$. Therefore, the first four comparisons in the preceding table are significant and none of the others are. Thus these results indicate that there are two groupings of units in terms of nursing burnout: One group consists of the general medical (G/M) and stepdown unit/surgical (SDU/S) units and the other group consists of both stepdown units (SDU/S and SDU/M), both intensive care units (ICU/S and ICU/M), and the general surgical unit (G/S). Note the ambiguity in the results with SDU/S appearing in both groups. This type of ambiguity arises sometimes in multiple-comparison testing, especially when there are many means (i.e., treatments) to be compared. One must simply use some judgment in interpreting the results.

4-13 **a** No, **b** No, **c** No, **d** Yes.

5-1 Yes. $\chi^2 = 1.247$, $\nu = 1$, $P = .264$; No.

5-2 Violent suicide: $\chi^2 = 1.380$, Yates corrected $\chi^2 = 0.870$, $\nu = 1$, $P > 0.25$; suicide under the influence of alcohol: $\chi^2 = 18.139$, Yates corrected $\chi^2 = 16.480$, $\nu = 1$, $P < .001$; BAC >= 150 mg/dL: $\chi^2 = 19.20$, Yates corrected $\chi^2 = 17.060$, $\nu = 1$, $P < .001$; suicide during weekend: $\chi^2 = 4.850$, Yates corrected $\chi^2 = 4.020$, $\nu = 1$, $P < .02$; parental divorce: $\chi^2 = 5.260$, Yates corrected $\chi^2 = 4.340$, $\nu = 1$, $P < .05$; parental violence: $\chi^2 = 9.870$, Yates corrected $\chi^2 = 8.320$, $\nu = 1$, $P < .01$; parental alcohol abuse: $\chi^2 = 4.810$, Yates corrected $\chi^2 = 3.890$, $\nu = 1$, $P < .05$; paternal alcohol abuse: $\chi^2 = 5.630$, Yates corrected $\chi^2 = 4.570$, $\nu = 1$, $P < .05$; parental suicidal behavior: $\chi^2 = 1.570$, Yates corrected $\chi^2 = 0.770$, $\nu = 1$, $P > .2$; institutional rearing: $\chi^2 = 4.000$, $P < .05$ Yates corrected $\chi^2 = 2.640$, $\nu = 1$, $P > .1$. The key factors seem to be suicide under the influence of alcohol, BAC >= 150 mg/dL, suicide during weekend, parental divorce, parental violence, parental alcohol abuse, and paternal alcohol abuse. Note that the significance of institutional rearing changed when the Yates correction was applied. Despite the high confidence we can have in reporting these differences, they probably are not stark enough to be of predictive value in any given adolescent.

5-3 There is a possibility that the fact that the families declined to be interviewed reflects a systematic difference between the 106 suicides that were included and the ones that we excluded. One way to investigate whether this situation leads to biases would be to compare what is known about the families that granted interviews and ones that did not (using variables such as age, socioeconomic status, gender of victim) to see if there were any systematic differences. If there were no differences, the lack of interviews is probably not a problem. If there are differences, the lack of interviews could bias the conclusions of the analysis.

5-4 For the three groups, $\chi^2 = 21.176$, $\nu = 2$, $P < .001$, so there is evidence that at least one group differs in the number of remissions. Subdividing the table to compare just nefazodone and psychotherapy yields:

	Remission	No remission
Nefazodone	36	131
Psychotherapy	41	132

$\chi^2 = 0.220$, Yates corrected $\chi^2 = 0.120$, $\nu = 1$, $P > .6$. There is not sufficient evidence to conclude that these two treatments produce different remission rates. Pool the results and compare them to the combination nefazodone and psychotherapy treatment.

	Remission	No remission
Nefazodone or psychotherapy alone	77	263
Nefazodone or psychotherapy combined	75	104

$\chi^2 = 20.990$, Yates corrected $\chi^2 = 20.070$, $\nu = 1$, $P < .001$ before the Bonferroni correction. Allowing for two comparisons, both P values should be doubled, to obtain .002 in both cases. Hence, the results remain significant even after accounting for multiple comparisons. (You would obtain similar results with using a Holm correction applied to the chi-square.) Thus, the combination of nefazodone and psychotherapy seems to work better than either treatment approach alone.

5-5 $\chi^2 = 74.93$, $\nu = 2$; $P < .001$. These data suggest that the rate at which people got sick was significantly associated with water consumption.

5-6 For honorary authors among all journals, the contingency table is:

Journal	No honorary authors	Articles with honorary authors
American Journal of Cardiology	115	22
American Journal of Medicine	87	26
American Journal of Obstetrics and Gynecology	111	14
Annals of Internal Medicine	78	26
Journal of the American Medical Association	150	44
New England Journal of Medicine	112	24

$\chi^2 = 11.026$, $\nu = 5$, $.10 < P < .05$, so we do not reject the null hypothesis that the rate of honorary authorship does not vary among journals. Since we did not reject the null hypothesis based on all the journals, there is no need to subdivide the table between small and large circulation journals. (This negative conclusion should be taken as tentative, since the critical value of χ^2 for $P = .05$ is 11.070, which the data just misses.) Overall, 156 of 809 articles (19 percent) included honorary authors.

For ghost authors among all journals, the contingency table is:

Journal	No Ghost Authors	Articles with Ghost Authors
American Journal of Cardiology	124	13
American Journal of Medicine	108	15
American Journal of Obstetrics and Gynecology	112	13
Annals of Internal Medicine	98	16
Journal of the American Medical Association	184	14
New England Journal of Medicine	114	22

$\chi^2 = 8.331$, $\nu = 5$, $.25 < P < .10$, so we do not reject the null hypothesis that the rate of ghost authorship does not vary among journals. Since we did not reject the null hypothesis based on all the journals, there is no need to subdivide the table between small and large circulation journals. Overall, 93 of 809 articles (11 percent) had ghost authors.

5-7 $\chi^2 = 4.880$, Yates corrected $\chi^2 = 4.450$, $\nu = 1$, $P < .05$; yes.

5-8 For people on therapy the expected number of patients in at least one cell is below 5, so the analysis should be done with the Fisher exact test, which yields $P = .151$. There is no significant difference in the responses for the two tests in people on therapy. The numbers of observations for people not receiving therapy are large enough to use the χ^2 test statistic; $\chi^2 = 2.732$ with 1 degree of freedom, $P = .098$, so we do not conclude that the responses to the two tests differ in people with ischemic heart disease who are not receiving therapy.

5-9 $\chi^2 = 5.185$, $\nu = 1$, $P < .025$; yes. $\chi^2 = 2.273$, $\nu = 1$, $.25 > P > .1$; the results do change because the "deleted" patients are not randomly distributed among the treatments. The study should be analyzed including the patients who were excluded from the original analysis because the outcome of the study is death or other complications and the excluded patients died.

5-10 $\chi^2 = 8.8124$, $\nu = 1$, $P < .005$. She would not reach the same conclusion if she observed the entire population because the sample would not be biased by differential admission rates.

5-11 OR = 1.40. $\chi^2 = 14.122$ with 1 degree of freedom; $P < .001$. Smoking significantly increases the odds of developing renal cell cancer.

5-12 OR = 0.74, $\chi^2 = 4.556$ with 1 degree of freedom; $P = .03$. Stopping smoking significantly reduces the risk of renal cell cancer.

5-13 RR = 0.61, $\chi^2 = 127.055$ with 1 degree of freedom; $P < .001$. Hormone replacement therapy is associated with a reduction in risk of death compared with nonusers.

5-14 RR = 1.00, $\chi^2 = .002$ with 1 degree of freedom; $P = .962$. Past use of hormone replacement therapy did not affect the risk of death compared to never users.

6-1 $\delta/\sigma = 1.1$ and $n = 9$; from Fig. 6-9, power = .63.

6-2 $\delta/\sigma = .55$ and power = .80; from Fig. 6-9, $n = 40$.

6-3 For mean arterial blood pressure: $\delta = .25 \times 76.8$ mm Hg = 19.2 mm Hg, $\sigma = 17.8$ mm Hg (based on pooled variance estimate), so $\delta/\sigma = 1.08$, $n = 9$ (the size of the smaller sample). From Fig. 6–9, power = .63. For total peripheral resistance, $\delta/\sigma = 553/1154 = .48$, $n = 9$. From Fig. 6–9, power = .13.

6-4 The power is 93 percent based on a difference in bone density of 14, which is 20 percent of 70.3.

6-5 Twenty people in each group, based on a difference of 21, which is 30 percent of 70.3.

6-6 Power = .80.

6-7 Power = .36 to detect a change of 5 mg/dL; power = .95 to detect a change of 10 mg/dL.

6-8 $N = 183$.

6-9 The desired pattern of the responses is

Antibiotic	Remission	No Remission	Total
Nefazodone	.098	.195	.293
Psychotherapy	.116	.232	.347
Both	.180	.180	.359
Total	.393	.607	1.000

$\phi = 2.1$, $\nu_n = (3 - 1)(2 - 1) = 2$, so from Fig. 6–10, power = .90.

6-10 $N \cong 140$.

7-1 95 percent confidence interval: 1233 to 2185 ng/g; 90 percent confidence interval: 1319 to 2100 ng/g.

7-2 95 percent confidence interval for the difference: .72 to 3.88 μ mol/g of muscle/min. Since this interval does not include 0, we reject the null hypothesis of no difference ($P < .05$).

7-3 95 percent confidence intervals: Anesthetic gel: 0 to .17; Placebo: .08 to .32; Difference −.28 to +.04. We cannot reject the null hypothesis of no difference in effect between the placebo and the anesthetic gel. This is the same conclusion we reached in Prob. 5-1.

7-4 Nonsmokers, clean environment: 3.03 to 3.31; nonsmokers, smoky environment: 2.58 to 2.86; light smokers: 2.49 to 2.77; moderate smokers: 2.15 to 2.43; heavy smokers: 1.98 to 2.26. Nonsmokers smoky environment, and light smokers overlap and can be considered one subgroup, as can moderate smokers and heavy smokers. Nonsmokers, clean environment, is a third subgroup.

7-5 1946: 17 to 31 percent; 1956: 22 to 36 percent; 1966: 43 to 59 percent; 1976: 48 to 64 percent.

7-6 95 percent confidence interval for 90 percent of the population: −517.67 to 3936.25 ng/g lipid; 95 percent confidence interval for 95 percent of the population: −930.07 to 4348.65 ng/g lipid. The negative numbers at the lower ends of the confidence intervals are possible members of the actual populations; these negative numbers reflect the conservative nature of this computation based on small sample sizes.

7-7 OR = 1.40. The 95 percent confidence interval is from 1.18 to 1.66, which does not include 1. Therefore, we conclude that smoking significantly increases the risk of renal cell cancer.

7-8 OR = 0.74. The 95 percent confidence interval is from .57 to .97, which does not include 1. Therefore, we conclude that stopping smoking significantly reduces the odds of developing renal cell cancer.

7-9 RR = 0.61. The 95 percent confidence interval is from .55 to .66, which does not include 1. Therefore, we conclude that hormone replacement therapy reduces the risk of death.

7-10 RR = 1.00. The 95 percent confidence interval is from .94 to 1.07, which includes 1. Therefore, we cannot conclude that past use of hormone replacement therapy affects the risk of death.

8-1 **a:** $a = 3.0$, $b = 1.3$, $r = .79$; **b:** $a = 5.1$, $b = 1.2$, $r = .94$; **c:** $a = 5.6$, $b = 1.2$, $r = .97$. Note that as the range of data increases, the correlation coefficient increases.

8-2 **a:** $a = 24.3$, $b = .36$, $r = .561$; **b:** $a = .5$, $b = 1.15$, $r = .599$. Part **a** illustrates the large effect one outlier point can have on the regression line. Part **b** illustrates that even though there are two different and distinct patterns in the data, this is not reflected when a single regression line is drawn through the data. This problem illustrates why it is important to look at the data before computing regression lines through it.

8-3 $a = 3.0$, $b = 0.5$, $r = .82$ for all four experiments, despite the fact that the patterns in the data differ from experiment to experiment. Only data from experiment 1 satisfies the assumption of linear regression analysis.

8-4 Yes. As maternal milk PCB levels increase, children's IQ at 11 years of age falls; the slope is $-.021$ (standard error .00754, so $t = -2.8$ with 12 degrees of freedom; $P < .05$). The Pearson product moment correlation, r, is $-.63$ (also $P < .05$). You could also have tested the hypothesis of no relationship with a Spearman rank-order correlation, which would yield $r_s = -.610$ ($P < .05$).

8-5 Use the Bland-Altman method to compare the two methods of estradiol measurement. The mean difference is -25 pg/mL and the standard deviation of the differences is 19 pg/mL. These results suggest that there is not particularly good agreement between the two methods, with the blood spot yielding lower results and a substantial amount of variability in the results of the two methods in comparison with the magnitude of the observations.

8-6 These regression results are computed after conducting the regressions of the Relaxation Force as the dependent variable against $\log_{10}$ (arginine level) as the independent variable:

	Slope	Intercept	$s_{y \cdot x}$	P
Acetylcholine	−7.85	−50.5	13.80	.024
A23187	−10.4	−57.5	15.10	.010
Common estimate	−9.06	−54.1	14.16	.001

To do the overall test of coincidence, we compute

$$s^2_{y \cdot x_p} = \frac{(11 - 2)13.80^2 + (13 - 2)15.10^2}{11 + 13 - 4} = 211.40$$

and

$$s^2_{y \cdot x_{imp}} = \frac{(11 + 13 - 2)14.16^2 - (11 + 13 - 4)211.40}{2} = 91.56$$

so that $F = 91.56/211.40 = 4.33$ with $\nu_n = 2$ and $\nu_d = 20$, which does not even approach the critical value of 3.49 required to reject the null hypothesis of no difference with $P < .05$. Therefore, we cannot reject the null hypothesis that there is no difference between the two relationships; given the very small value of F, we can be reasonably confident in concluding that the two different stimuli have similar effects on force levels (arterial relaxation).

8-7 There is a significant relationship. $r_s = .912$, n = 20, $P < .001$.

8-8 Yes. $r_s = 0.899$; $P < .001$. Higher clinical scores are associated with larger amounts of plaque.

8-9 $r_s = .472$, n = 25, $P = .018$. There is a significant relationship between these two different ways of measuring the extent of cancer, but the correlation is weak enough that they cannot be used interchangeably for clinical purposes.

8-10 Power = .999.

8-11 $n = 20$, so this study could have been done with a smaller sample size than was actually used.

8-12 To answer the question, we fit linear regressions to the two groups of men, then do an overall test of coincidence. For controls $I = -1.77R + 2.59$, $r = 0.800$, $s_{\text{slope}} = 0.369$, $s_{\text{intercept}} = 0.336$, $s_{I \times R} = 0.125$, $n = 15$. For relatives: $I = -0.18\ R + 0.932$, $r = 0.075$, $s_{\text{slope}} = 0.651$, $s_{\text{intercept}} = 0.932$, $s_{I \times R} = 0.219$, $n = 15$. For common regression: $I = -1.09\ R + 1.88$, $r = 0.432$, $s_{\text{slope}} = 0.441$, $s_{\text{intercept}} = 0.405$, $s_{I \times R} = 0.211$, $n = 30$. Overall test of coincidence: $F = 6.657$ with $\nu_n = 2$ and $\nu_d = 26$; $P < .01$; the relationships are different. Test for difference in slopes: $t = -2.137$, $\nu = 26$, $P < .05$. Test for difference in intercepts: $t = 2.396$, $\nu = 26$, $P < .05$. Therefore, the slopes and intercepts of the two lines are significantly different. The relationship between physical fitness and insulin index is different in these two groups of men.

9-1 Yes. The paired t test yields $t = 4.69$ with $\nu = 9$, so $P < .002$.

9-2 There is a significant difference. $t = 6.160$ with $\nu = 7$, $P < .001$.

9-3 $\delta = 9$ msec (half the 18 msec difference observed in Prob. 9-2) and $\sigma = 8.3$ msec, the standard deviation of the differences before and after breathing secondhand smoke so the noncentrality parameter $\phi = 9/8.3 = 1.1$. From the power chart in Fig. 6-9, the power is .75.

9-4 $F = 37.94$, $\nu_n = 1$, $\nu_d = 7$, $P < .01$. $F = t^2$.

9-5 $F = 0.519$, $\nu_n = 2$, $\nu_d = 6$. This value falls far short of 5.14, the critical value that defines the greatest 5 percent of possible values of F in such experiments. Thus, we do not have sufficient evidence to conclude that there are differences in C reactive protein over time ($P > .50$).

9-6 There are significant differences between the different experimental conditions ($F = 50.77$, $\nu_n = 3$, $\nu_d = 33$). Multiple comparisons using the residual mean square and Holm t test show that testosterone levels are greater before capture than at any time after. In addition, testosterone levels after 48 hours of capture are decreased compared to time of capture and 12 hours post-capture, which do not differ.

9-7 Repeated measures analysis of variance yields $F = 4.56$ with $\nu_n = 2$ and $\nu_d = 12$, so $P < .05$ and the food intake appears different among the different groups. Multiple comparisons (using either Bonferroni t tests or the SNK test) reveal that food intakes at pressures of 10 and 20 mm Hg are both significantly different from intake at a pressure of 0 mm Hg, but they are not different from each other. The subjects were not told the true goal or design of the study in order to avoid biasing their responses.

9-8 $\delta = 100$ mL, $\sigma = \sqrt{MS_{res}} = \sqrt{5483} = 74$ mL. $\phi = 1.45$. Power = .50 or a 50 percent chance of finding the target effect with the study as designed.

9-9 By McNemar's test: $\chi^2 = 4.225$, $\nu = 1$, $P < .05$. No; indomethacin is significantly better than placebo.

9-10 When the data are presented in this format, they are analyzed as a 2×2 contingency table. $\chi^2 = 2.402$, $\nu = 1$, $P < .10$, so there is no significant association between drug and improvement of shunting. This test, in contrast to the analysis in Prob. 9-8, failed to detect an effect because it ignores the paired nature of the data, and so is less powerful.

10-1 For mean annual lab charges: $W = -72$, $n = 12$ (there is one zero in the charges), $P < .02$. For drug charges: $W = 28$, $n = 13$, $P > .048$. Therefore, the audit seemed to reduce the amount of money spent on laboratory tests but not drugs. There was not a significant relationship between money spent on laboratory tests and money spent on drugs ($r_s = .201$, $P > .5$).

10-2 $z_T = 2.003$, $P < .05$; there is a significant difference in the level of adhesions between the two groups. (Adjusting for ties, $z_T = 2.121$, $P < .05$.)

10-3 A Kruskal-Wallis test yields $H = 15.161$ with $\nu = 3$, $P = .002$. There is a significant difference among the treatments. Using a Student-Newman-Keuls test reveals that there are three different subgroups: (1) Baseline, (2) Information, and (3) Pocket Cards plus Weekly Lectures and Pocket Cards only.

10-4 Problem 9-5: Endotoxin and salbutamol did not affect CRP levels ($\chi_r^2 = 1.5$, $k = 3$, $n = 4$, $P > .05$). Problem 9-6: Capture produced significant differences in testosterone levels ($\chi^2 = 27.3$, $\nu = 3$, $P < .001$). Using the SNK test with $\alpha_T = .05$, there are two subgroups: The testosterone levels before capture are highest; the levels at the other three times are not significantly different from each other.

10-5 $T = 195.0$, $n_S = 15$, $n_B = 15$; $z_T = 1.519$ and $.1 > P > .05$. They do not appear to have different cholesterol levels.

10-6 The Mann-Whitney rank-sum test yields $z_T = 3.864$ ($P < .001$), so problem gambling substance abusers exhibit riskier sexual behavior than non-problem gambling substance abusers.

10-7 $H = 17.633$ with 3 degrees of freedom; $P < .01$, so there is strong evidence that weight satisfaction is different among these four groups of students. The pair-wise comparison with Dunn's test, shows that 5th grade boys, 5th grade girls, and 8th grade boys are one subgroup, and 8th grade girls are the other subgroup.

10-8 Yes, G is a legitimate test statistic. The sampling distribution of G when $n = 4$:

G	Possible ways to get value	Probability
0	1	1/16
1	4	4/16
2	6	6/16
3	4	4/16
4	1	1/16

When $n = 6$:

G	Possible ways to get value	Probability
0	1	1/64
1	6	6/64
2	15	15/64
3	20	20/64
4	15	15/64
5	6	6/64
6	1	1/64

G cannot be used to conclude that the treatment in the problem had an effect with $P < .05$ because the two most extreme possible values (i.e., the two tails of the sampling distribution of G), 1 and 4, can occur $1/16 + 1/16 = 1/8 = 0.125 = 12.5$ percent of the time, which exceeds 5 percent. G can be used for $n = 6$, where the extreme values, 1 and 6, occur $1/64 + 1/64 = 2/64 = .033$ percent of the time, so the (two-tail) critical values (closest to 5 percent) are 1 and 6.

11-1 Here is the survival curve in tabular form.

			95% Confidence interval	
Month	Cumulative survival, $\hat{S}(t)$	Standard error	Lower	Upper
1	0.971	0.0291	0.919	1.000
2	0.946	0.0406	0.866	1.000
3	0.858	0.0611	0.738	0.978
4	0.828	0.0657	0.699	0.957
5	0.799	0.0697	0.662	0.936
6	0.769	0.0732	0.626	0.912
7	0.739	0.0761	0.590	0.888
8	0.680	0.0807	0.522	0.838
9	0.651	0.0824	0.490	0.813
12	0.586	0.0861	0.417	0.755
13	0.521	0.0879	0.349	0.693
15	0.488	0.0883	0.315	0.661
16	0.455	0.0882	0.282	0.628
20	0.358	0.0854	0.191	0.525
21	0.260	0.0785	0.106	0.414
28	0.233	0.0756	0.085	0.381
34	0.186	0.0716	0.046	0.326
56	0.124	0.0695	0.000	0.260
62	0.062	0.0559	0.000	0.172
84	0.000	0.0000	0.000	0.000

The median survival time is 14 months.

11-2 The survival curves for the two groups are:

High IADL score		Low IADL score	
Month	Survival, $\hat{S}_{Hi}(t)$	Month	Survival, $\hat{S}_{Lo}(t)$
14	0.988	6	0.967
20	0.963	12	0.934
24	0.925	18	0.867
28	0.913	24	0.85
30	0.887	28	0.782
38	0.861	32	0.714
48	0.834	36	0.643
		42	0.584
		47	0.522
		48	0.48

Use the log-rank test to compare the two survival curves. The sum of the differences between expected and observed number of survivals at each time is −13.243; the standard error of the differences is 3.090, so $z = -4.285$ (or −4.124 with the Yates correction). We conclude that there are significant differences in survival between these two groups of people, $P < .001$.

11-3 (a) The survival curves and 95% confidence intervals are:

Diagnosed 1975–1979					Diagnosed 1980–1984				
Month	Surival	SE	Low 95% CI	High 95% CI	Month	Survival	SE	Low 95% CI	High 95% CI
2	0.940	0.034	0.873	1.000	2	0.920	0.038	0.846	0.994
4	0.860	0.049	0.764	0.956	4	0.900	0.042	0.763	0.928
6	0.800	0.057	0.688	0.912	6	0.840	0.052	0.738	0.942
8	0.720	0.063	0.597	0.843	8	0.640	0.068	0.507	0.773
12	0.679	0.066	0.550	0.808	12	0.560	0.070	0.423	0.697
14	0.617	0.069	0.482	0.752	14	0.500	0.071	0.361	0.639
18	0.575	0.071	0.436	0.714	22	0.457	0.071	0.318	0.596
24	0.552	0.071	0.413	0.691	24	0.435	0.071	0.296	0.574
30	0.508	0.072	0.367	0.649	30	0.391	0.070	0.254	0.528
36	0.486	0.072	0.345	0.627	36	0.326	0.068	0.193	0.459
54	0.462	0.073	0.322	0.604	48	0.283	0.065	0.156	0.410
56	0.438	0.073	0.299	0.581	56	0.236	0.062	0.114	0.358
60	0.413	0.073	0.276	0.558	60	0.212	0.060	0.094	0.330

(b) The median survival time for the children diagnosed in 1974 to 1979 is 36 months and those diagnosed in 1980 to 1984 is 14 months. (c) The log rank test yields $z = 1.777$ (1.648 with Yates correction). This value of z does not exceed the critical value of z for $\alpha = 0.05$, 1.960, so we cannot conclude that there is a significant difference between children diagnosed in 1974 to 1979 and 1980 to 1984. (d) The power to detect the specified difference is 0.62. (e) If steady state death rate in second group is 0.20, there need to be 104 deaths and a total of 149 subjects in the study; if the steady state death rate is 0.15, there need to be 65 deaths and 89 subjects.

Index

The *n* after a page number indicates footnote.